CONTEMPORARY PROFESSIONAL NURSING

CONTEMPORARY PROFESSIONAL NURSING

Joseph T. Catalano, RN, PhD, CCRN
Professor of Nursing
East Central University
Ada, Oklahoma

 F. A. DAVIS COMPANY • Philadelphia

F. A. Davis Company
1915 Arch Street
Philadelphia, PA 19103

Printed in the United States of America

Last digit indicates print number: 10 9 8 7 6 5 4 3 2

Nursing Developmental Editor: Melanie Freely
Production Editor: Rose Gabbay
Cover Designer: Steven R. Morrone
Cover Art: untitled photo collage by Judy Engle

As new scientific information becomes available through basic and clinical research, recommended treatments and drug therapies undergo changes. The author and publisher have done everything possible to make this book accurate, up to date, and in accord with accepted standards at the time of publication. The author, editors, and publisher are not responsible for errors or omissions or for consequences from application of the book, and make no warranty, expressed or implied, in regard to the contents of the book. Any practice described in this book should be applied by the reader in accordance with professional standards of care used in regard to the unique circumstances that may apply in each situation. The reader is advised always to check product information (package inserts) for changes and new information regarding dose and contraindications before administering any drug. Caution is especially urged when using new or infrequently ordered drugs.

Library of Congress Cataloging-in-Publication Data
Catalano, Joseph T.
    Contemporary professional nursing / Joseph T. Catalano.
      p.   cm.
    Includes bibliographical references and index.
    ISBN 0-8036-0091-7
    1. Nursing—Vocational guidance—United States.   2. Nursing—Practice—United States.   3. Nursing—Social aspects—United States.   4. Nursing—Philosophy.
5. Nursing—History. I. Title.
    [DNLM: 1. NURSING.   WY 16 C357c 1996]
RT82.C33 1996
610.73—dc20
DNLM/DLC
for Library of Congress   95-46673
                                                      CIP

To all those dedicated students with high stress levels who are the hope and future of our profession.

PREFACE

As the world prepares to begin a new century, many exciting changes are occurring in the health care system. The profession of nursing, as a vital part of that health care system, is also experiencing many changes. Change brings with it new challenges, and those preparing to work in a changing profession are faced with increasing demands to learn more, do more, and be more. Students entering nursing schools today come from diverse cultural, personal, and educational backgrounds. Yet, they are required to master a tremendous amount of information and learn a wide variety of skills so that they can successfully pass the licensure examination and become competent registered nurses. Most of the courses taken in nursing school focus mainly on the practice aspect of the profession and less on the theoretical.

Contemporary Professional Nursing focuses primarily on the theoretical elements that help comprise the totality called professional nursing. The purpose of this book is to present an overview and synthesis of the important issues and trends that are basic to the development of professional nursing and affect nursing both today and into the future. Courses that cover this material are sometimes taught at the beginning of the student's educational process as an "Introduction to Nursing" course, or toward the end of the process as an "Issues and Trend" course. This text would be appropriate and useful for either type of course.

This text is organized into 14 chapters. Chapter 1 introduces the student to the concept of profession, empowerment, accountability, and professionalism. Chapter 2 presents fundamental background information about theories and models in nursing, why they are important to a profession, and how they can be used in client care. In Chapter 3, the concept of critical thinking is introduced, and ways in which critical thinking can be used in nursing are discussed. The nursing process is also presented in this chapter as a client health care problem-solving approach. Chapter 4 discusses the history and development of nursing education, the current types of nursing education found in the United States in light of the American Nurses Association's Position Paper on Education for Nursing, advanced nursing education, and its implications for the future of the profession. In Chapter 5, the reader is initiated into the language and concepts of professional ethics as it applies to health care and nursing. Chapter 6 builds directly on Chapter 5, and allows the students to apply ethical principles to some of the more common bioethical issues found in today's health care system, such as abortion, genetic research, fetal tissue experimentation, organ transplantation, use of scarce resources, assisted suicide, and AIDS. The goal of the Chapter 7 is to help students through the transition process from student to registered nurse by increasing students' awareness of the realities in the workplace. Several methods of lessening role transition shock are presented as well as the topic of burnout. Chapter 8 discusses the purpose of licensure and certification, current roles, membership requirements, and services offered by the major nursing organizations. The goal of Chapter 9 is to acquaint the student with the purpose and format of the NCLEX examination, and present several study strategies as well as selected test-taking strategies. Chapter 10 defines key terms used in describing health care delivery, discusses the prime members of the health care team, and presents the main factors that influence current health care delivery practices, including payment systems for health care. In Chapter 11, the student is introduced to the political process in general, and its effect on health care in particular. A model for political activism for professional nurses is presented. Chapter 12 discusses collective bargaining and its relationship to professional nursing. This chapter also presents the concept of governance, the roles of nurses in governance, and several different models for governance. The goal of Chapter 13 is to introduce the student to the legal world, its terminology, and how law relates to health care and nursing practice. Standards of care and the nurse practice act are presented as the legal standards to which nurses are held. In Chapter 14, the student is acquainted with several of the important issues that affect health care today, including care delivery models, the use of computers in health care, nursing research, the legal and ethical obligations in dealing with the chemically impaired nurse, and how nurses can improve their image. The chapter concludes with a discussion of the future of nursing and how nurses can prepare for it and participate in it.

Rather than presenting the history of health care and nursing in one long chapter, the reader will find 13 short sections throughout the book called "Historical Perspectives." These present many of the important historical developments that had a major impact on health care. The reader will also notice the presentation of current issues in the "A Closer Look" and "Issues in Practice" boxes throughout the book. These interesting, and current, issues help the reader relate the chapter content to the real world of professional nursing. Finally, each chapter concludes with "Critical Thinking Exercises." These exercises will allow students to use their higher-level thinking skills in resolving complex questions.

The profession of nursing is standing on the threshold of the future. We can either move forward and attain the full professional status we deserve and have worked so hard and so long for, or retreat into the safety of the past, with its outdated modes of thinking and acting. During 14 years of teaching nursing students, I have observed that students who graduate with a clear understanding of what it means to be a professional, and a willingness to meet the requirements and demands of that status, have developed into the leaders that will guide the profession into the next century. It is hoped that this book can play a part in preparing these future leaders.

Joseph T. Catalano

ACKNOWLEDGMENTS

I would like to express my thanks to all of my students and colleagues who have shaped my thoughts and ideas about the nursing profession over the years. I would particularly like to acknowledge Peggy Hart, PhD, RN, a co-professor for many years, for her insights, dedication, and support. Finally, this text would never have been completed without the direction, encouragement, and support of Melanie Freely.

CONTRIBUTORS

Tonia Aiken, RN, BSN, JD
President and CEO,
Aiken Development Group
New Orleans, Louisiana

Anne Davis, RNC, PhD
Associate Professor
East Central University
Ada, Oklahoma

Mary Evans, RN, JD
316 N. Tejon
Colorado Springs, Colorado

Deborah L. Finfgeld, RN, PhD
Associate Professor of Nursing
Illinois Wesleyan University
Bloomington, Illinois

Kathleen Winter, RN, PhD
Associate Professor
Duquesne University
Pittsburgh, Pennsylvania

CONSULTANTS

Judith A. Allender, RNC, EdD
Associate Professor
California State University at Fresno
Fresno, California

Troy W. Bradshaw, RNC, MS
Assistant Professor
Angelo State University
San Angelo, Texas

Mary Louise Brown, RN, PhD
Dean Academic Affairs
St. Joseph College of Nursing
Joliet, Illinois

Elizabeth Deitz, RN, CS, EdD
Professor, Nurse Practioner
San Jose State University
San Jose, California

Dr. Barbara Kellum, RN, MS
Instructor
Orange County Community College
Middletown, New York

Grace Laubach, RN, MA
Associate Professor
Milton Hershey Medical Center
Hershey, Pennsylvania

Hope Moon, RN, MSN
A.D.N. Faculty
Lorain County Community College
Elyria, Ohio

Mary L. Richards, RN, PhD
Associate Professor
Arizona State University
Tempe, Arizona

Mabel Smith, RN, PhD, JD
Coordinator and Associate Professor
University of Southern Mississippi
Long Beach, Mississippi

Golden Tradewell, RN, MSN
Assistant Professor
McNeese University
Lake Charles, Louisiana

CONTENTS

1

THE DEVELOPMENT OF NURSING AS A PROFESSION

Learning Objectives

After completing this chapter, the reader will be able to:

1 Define the terms **position, job, occupation,** and **profession.**
2 Compare the three approaches to defining a profession.
3 Name the key elements in the "Trait Approach" to defining a profession.
4 Analyze those traits defining a profession that nursing has attained.
5 Evaluate why nursing has failed to attain some of the traits that define a profession.
6 Correlate the concept of power with its important characteristics.
7 Analyze the seven sources of power.
8 Discuss four ways that nurses can increase their power.

Since the time of Florence Nightingale, each generation of nurses, in its own way, has fostered the movement to professionalize the image of nurses and nursing. The struggle to change the status of nurses from that of female domestic servants to that of high-level health care providers basing their protocols on scientific principles has been a primary goal of nursing's leaders for many years. Yet some people, both inside and outside of nursing, question if the search for and attainment of professional status is worth the effort and price that must ultimately be paid.

At some levels in nursing, the question of professionalism takes on immense significance. Yet to the practicing nurse who is trying to figure out how to give six bed baths, pass the 0900 medications to 24 clients, supervise two aides, a licensed practical nurse (LPN), and a nursing student, the issue may not seem very significant at all.

Indeed, when nurses were first developing as an entity separate from that of physicians, there was no thought about their being part of a profession. But over the years, as the scope of practice has expanded and the responsibilities have increased, nurses have increasingly begun to view what they do as professional activities.

This chapter presents some of the current thinking concerning professions, and where nursing stands in relationship to this thinking.

APPROACHES TO DEFINING A PROFESSION

Terminology and the definition of terms, as with most complex and controversial issues, play an important part in any discussion of nursing as a profession. In common usage, terms such as position, job, occupation, professional, profession, and professionalism are often used interchangeably and incorrectly. The following definitions will clarify what is meant by these terms within this text.

- Position—group of tasks assigned to one individual.
- Job—a group of positions that are similar in nature and level of skill that can be carried out by one or more individuals.
- Occupation—a group of jobs that are similar in type of work, and that are usually found throughout an industry or work environment.
- Profession—a type of occupation that meets certain criteria (discussed later in this chapter) that raise it to a level above that of an occupation.
- Professional—a person who belongs to and practices a profession. (The term **professional** is probably the most misused of all these terms when describing people who are clearly involved in jobs or occupations, such as a "professional truck driver," "professional football player," or even a "professional thief.")
- Professionalism—the demonstration of high-level personal, ethical, and skill characteristics of a member of a profession.

Expert social scientists have been attempting to develop a "foolproof" approach to determining what constitutes a profession for nearly 100 years, but with only minimal success. Three common models are the process approach, the power approach, and the most widely accepted trait approach.

The Process Approach

The process approach views all occupations as points of development into a profession along a continuum ranging from position to profession.

Continuum of Professional Development:
Position———————————————→Profession

Using this approach, the question becomes not whether nursing and truck driving are professions, but where they are located along the continuum. Occupational fields, such as medicine, law, and the ministry, are widely accepted by the public as being closest to the professional end of the continuum (Moloney, 1986). Other occupations may be less clearly defined.

The major difficulty with this approach is that it lacks criteria on which to base judgments. Final determination of the status of an occupation or profession depends almost completely on public perception of the activities of that occupation. Nursing has always had a rather poor public image when it comes to being viewed as a profession.

The Power Approach

The power approach uses just two criteria to define a profession: (1) how much independence of practice does this occupation have and (2) how much power does this occupation control? The concept of power is discussed later in this chapter, but in this context it refers to political power. Political power goes hand in hand with income levels and monetary resources. Therefore, an important contributing characteristic to determine if an occupation qualifies as a profession according to this approach is the amount of money the person in that occupation earns (Smith, 1994).

Using this determinant, occupations such as medicine, law, and politics would clearly be considered professions. The members of these occupations earn high incomes, practice their skills with a great deal of independence, and exercise significant power over individuals, the public, and the political community, both individually and in organized groups. The ministry, except for a few individuals such as television evangelists, would probably not be considered a profession because of its relatively low income levels. Nursing, of course, with its relatively poor salaries, low membership in organizations, and perceived lack of political power, would clearly not meet the power criteria for a profession.

The question that comes to mind is whether power, independence of practice, and high incomes are the only elements that determine professional status. Although those three factors confer status in our culture, other elements can be considered as significant in how a profession is viewed. For example, for many, the clergy have a great deal of power when they act as counselors, speakers of the truth, and community leaders.

The Trait Approach

Of the many researchers and theorists who have attempted to identify the traits that define a profession, three are most widely accepted as the leaders in the field. They are Flexner (1915), Bixler (1959), and Pavalko (1971). The following list is a synthesis of the common characteristics these three social scientists have determined to be important:

- Activities involve functioning at a high intellectual level.
- Activities involve high levels of individual responsibility and accountability.
- Activities are based on a specialized body of knowledge.

- Activities can be and are learned in institutions of higher education.
- Activities serve the public and are generally altruistic.
- Motivation of the individual is public service over financial gain.
- Activities conducted involve a relatively high degree of autonomy and independence of practice.
- A well-organized and strong organization represents the members of the profession and controls the quality of practice.
- A code of ethics guides the members of the profession in their practice.
- Members have a strong professional identity and are committed to their professional development.
- Members have demonstrated competency in the profession and have a legally recognized license to practice it.

NURSING AS A PROFESSION

How does nursing compare as a profession when measured against these widely accepted traits for a profession? Looking at the criteria individually, nursing meets most of them.

WHEN NURSING MEETS THE CRITERIA OF A PROFESSION

Activities Involve Functioning at a High Intellectual Level

In the early stages of the development of the practice of nursing, this statement was not true. Most of the tasks of early nurses are generally considered, by today's standards, as menial and routine. As health care has advanced and made great strides in technology, pharmacology, and all branches of the physical sciences, however, a high level of intellectual functioning is required for even relatively simple nursing tasks, like taking a client's temperature or blood pressure using automated equipment. Nurses use assessment skills and knowledge, use the ability to reason, and make routine judgments based on clients' conditions daily. Without a doubt, professional nurses must and do function at a high intellectual level.

Activities Involve a High Level of Individual Responsibility and Accountability

Not too long ago, nurses were rarely, if ever, named as defendants in malpractice suits. The public, in general, did not view nurses as having enough knowledge to be held accountable for errors that were made in client care. That is not the case in today's health care system. Nurses are often the primary, and frequently the only, defendants named when errors that result in injury to the client are made. Nurses must be accountable and demonstrate a high level of individual responsibility for the care and services they provide.

The concept of accountability has legal, ethical, and professional implications that include accepting responsibility for actions taken in providing client care as well as accepting responsibility for the consequences of actions that are not performed. No longer can a nurse say "the physician told me to do it" as a method of avoiding responsibility for his or her actions.

Activities Are Based on a Specialized Body of Knowledge

Nursing has been and always will be an eclectic science that draws a large portion of its knowledge from many other areas of science. In the early history of nursing, most of the skills practiced by so-called nurses were based either on traditional ways of doing things or on the intuitive knowledge of the individual nurse. As nursing has developed into an identifiable, separate discipline, a specialized body of knowledge called "nursing science" was compiled through the research efforts of nurses who hold advanced educational degrees. Although this body of specialized nursing knowledge is relatively small at present, it does form a theoretical basis for the practice of nursing today. As more and more nurses obtain advanced degrees, conduct research, and develop philosophies and theories about nursing, this body of knowledge will increase in scope.

Activities Serve the Public and Are Generally Altruistic

Almost all major nursing theorists, when defining nursing, include a statement that refers to a goal of helping clients to adapt to illness and to achieve their highest level of functioning. The public (variously referred to as patients, clients, man, individuals, or human beings) is the focal point of all nursing models and nursing practice. The public service function of nursing has always been recognized and acknowledged by society. This acknowledgment has been manifested by society's willingness to continue to educate nurses in public, tax-supported institutions as well as in private schools.

In addition, nursing has universally been viewed as being an altruistic profession. From its earliest days, when dedicated nurses provided care for victims of deadly plagues, with little regard for their own welfare, to today, when nurses are found in remote, and often hostile, areas of the planet, providing care for the sick and dying, the perception is that nurses are selfless individuals who place the lives and well-being of their clients above their personal physical safety.

Motivation of the Individual Is Public Service Over Personal Gain

Very few individuals enter nursing in order to become rich and famous. It is likely that those who do so for these reasons quickly become disappointed. Although the pay scale has increased tremendously over the last decade, nursing is, at best, a middle-income occupation. Recent surveys among students entering nursing programs continue to indicate that the primary reason for wishing to become a nurse is to "help others" or "make a difference" in someone's life, and "job security." Rarely do these beginning students include "to make a lot of money" as their motivation (Bunting, 1990).

A Well-Organized and Strong Professional Organization Represents the Members of the Profession, and Controls the Quality of Professional Practice. Nursing has never been at a loss for nursing organizations. The National League for Nursing (NLN) and the American Nurses Association (ANA) are the two major national organizations that represent nursing in today's health care system. The NLN is primarily responsible for regulating the quality of the educational programs that prepare nurses for the practice of nursing, whereas the ANA is more concerned with the quality of nursing practice in the day-to-day health care setting. These organizations are discussed in more detail in Chapter 6.

Both of these organizations are well organized, but neither can be considered *powerful* when compared with other professional organizations, such as the American Medical Association (AMA) or the American Bar Association (ABA). A reason for their lack of strength is that less than 15% of all nurses in this country are members of any professional organization at the national level (Smith, 1994). Many nurses do belong to specialty organizations that represent a specific area of practice, but these lack sufficient political clout to produce changes in health care laws and policies at the national governmental level.

A Code of Ethics Guides the Members of the Profession Within Their Professional Practice

Nursing has several codes of ethics that are used in guiding practice. The ANA Code for Nurses, the most widely used in the United States, was first published in 1971, and last updated in 1985. This code of ethics is recognized by other professions as a standard with which others are compared. The nurses' code of ethics and its implications are discussed in greater detail in Chapter 8.

Members Have Demonstrated Competency in the Profession and Hold a License. Members of the profession have demonstrated competency in practice and have a legally recognized license to practice the profession. Nurses must pass a national licensure examination to demonstrate that they are qualified to practice nursing. Only after passing this examination are nurses allowed to practice. Interim permits granted several years before the advent of the computerized examination are used today in only a few locations. The granting of a nursing license is a legal activity conducted by the individual state under the regulations contained in that state's nurse practice act.

WHEN NURSING FALLS SHORT OF MEETING THE CRITERIA OF A PROFESSION

Activities Are Learned in Institutions of Higher Education

Before Florence Nightingale, educating nurses through independent nursing programs in publicly supported educational institutions was considered unnecessary, if not outright dangerous. As nursing has developed, particularly in the United States, the recognition of the intellectual nature of the practice, as well as the vast amount of material nurses must know, has led to a belief by some nursing leaders that college education for nurses is now a necessity. Many attempts since 1950, however, to require all nurses to be educated in institutions of higher education, have been resisted and ultimately rejected by the more numerous diploma and associate degree programs.

Nursing is the only major discipline that does not require its members to hold at least a baccalaureate degree in order to obtain licensure. Although the number of diploma programs in nursing has decreased tremendously over the past decade, enrollment in associate degree programs continues to remain large and large numbers of graduates are produced. At issue is whether the baccalaureate degree should be the minimum requirement for entry-level nurses.

Activities Conducted Involve a Relatively High Degree of Autonomy and Independence of Practice

Historically, the handmaiden or servant relationship of nurse to physician was widely accepted. It was based on several factors, including social norms: women became nurses, men became physicians, women were subservient to men, the nature of the work involved (nurses cleaned, physicians cured), and the relative levels of education of the two groups (the average nursing program, 1 year; physician education, 6 to 8 years). Unfortunately, despite efforts to expand nursing practice into more independent areas through updated nurse practice legislation, nursing retains its subservient image.

In reality, nursing is both an independent and interdependent discipline. Nurses in all health care settings must work closely with physicians, hospital administrators, pharmacists, and other groups in the provision of care. In some instances, nurses in advanced practice roles, such as nurse practitioners, can and do establish their own independent practices. Actually, most state practice acts allow nurses more independence in their practice than they realize. Until nurses recognize their right to practice independently, are recognized by other disciplines as independent practitioners, and actually do begin to practice nursing independently, however, nursing will probably not be acknowledged as a true profession.

Members Have a Strong Professional Identity and Are Committed to the Profession and to Professional Development

This statement refers to the issue of job versus career. A **job** is a group of tasks that are organized so that one individual can carry them out. There is relatively little commitment to a job, and many individuals move from one job to another with little regard to the long-term outcomes of what they are doing. A **career,** on the other hand, is usually viewed as a person's major lifework that progresses and develops as the person ages. Career and **profession** have many of the same characteristics including a formal education, full-time employment, requirement for lifelong learning, and a dedication to what is being done. Although an increasing number of nurses view nursing as their life's work, many still treat it more as a job.

The problem becomes circular. The reason that nurses lack a strong professional identity and consider nursing a life-long career is because nursing does not have full status as a profession. But until nurses are fully committed to the profession of nursing, identify with it as a profession, and are dedicated to its future development, it probably will not achieve professional status.

FUTURE TRENDS IN THE NURSING PROFESSION

Clearly, it would be difficult to make an airtight case for nursing as a profession. Yet nursing does meet many of the criteria proposed for profession. Although it would probably be most accurate to call nursing a developing or aspiring profession, for the purposes of this book nursing will be referred to as a profession. Only when nurses begin to think of nursing as a profession and themselves as professional will the shift become a reality. The movement of any discipline from the status of occupation to one of profession is a dynamic, and ongoing, process with many considerations.

Perhaps the current oversupply of nurses will force nursing leaders to reconsider the educational requirements. The current nursing education system is producing about 40,000 graduates from diploma and associate degree programs every year (American Nurses Association, 1992). Is this level of education going to prepare nurses to meet the challenges of a rapidly changing and demanding health care system into the next century?

As the national employment picture changes, and financial resources become stressed, perhaps more nurses will begin to look on what they do as a lifelong commitment. Professional commitment is a complicated issue, but little doubt exists that nurses will not have an increased independence of practice until they begin to demonstrate that they are professionals committed to the field of nursing.

EMPOWERMENT IN NURSING

One of the concerns that has plagued nurses and nursing almost from its development as a separate health care specialty is the relatively large amount of personal responsibility shouldered by nurses. This is combined with a relatively small amount of control over their practice. Even in the more enlightened atmosphere of today's society with its concerns about equal opportunity, equitable pay, and collegial relationships, many nurses still seem uncomfortable with the concepts of power and control in their practice. Their discomfort may stem from the belief that nursing is a helping and caring profession whose goals are separate from issues of power. Historically, nurses have never had much power, and past attempts at gaining power and control over their practice have been met with much resistance from groups who benefit from keeping nurses powerless. Nevertheless, all nurses use power in their daily practice, even if they do not realize it. Until nurses understand the sources of their power, how to increase it, and how to use it in providing client care, they will be relegated to a subservient position in the health care system.

THE NATURE OF POWER

The term **power** has many meanings. From the standpoint of nursing, power is probably best defined as the ability or capacity to exert influence over another person or group of persons. In other words, power is the ability to get other people to do things even when they do not want to do them. Although power in itself is neither good nor bad, it can be used to produce either good or bad results.

Power is always a two-way street. By its very definition, when power is exerted by one person, another person is affected, that is, the use of power by one person requires that another person give up some of his or her power. Always in a state of change, individuals are either increasing their power or losing some, but rarely does the balance of power remain static. Empowerment refers to the increased amount of power that an individual, or group, is either given or gains.

ORIGINS OF POWER

If power is such an important part of nursing and the practice of nurses, where does it come from? Although there are many sources, some of them would be inappropriate or unacceptable for those in a helping and caring profession. The following list, compiled from several authors (Fitzpatrick, 1983; Kalish & Kalish, 1982; Smith, 1994), includes some of the more accessible and acceptable sources of power that nurses should consider using in their practice. These sources are:

- Referent
- Expert

- Reward
- Coercive
- Legitimate
- Expert
- Collective

Referent Power

The referent source of power depends on establishing and maintaining a close personal relationship with someone. In any close personal relationship, one individual, because of the relationship, often will do something he or she would really rather not do. This ability to be able to change the actions of another is an exercise of power. Nurses often obtain power from this source when they establish and maintain good therapeutic relationships with their clients. Clients take medications, tolerate uncomfortable treatments, and participate in demanding activities that they would clearly prefer to avoid *because* the nurse has a good relationship with them. Likewise, nurses who have good collegial relationships with other nurses, departments, and physicians are often able to obtain what they want from these individuals or groups, in providing care to clients.

Expert Power

The expert source of power derives from the amount of knowledge, skill, or expertise that an individual or group of individuals has. This power source is exercised by the individual or group when knowledge, skills, or expertise is either used or withheld in order to influence the behavior of others. Nurses should have at least a minimal amount of this type of power because of their education and experience. It follows logically that increasing the level of nurse's education, will, or should, increase this expert power. As nurses attain and remain in positions of power longer, the increased experience will also aid with the use of expert power. Nurses in advanced practice roles are good examples of the use of expert power. Their additional education and experience provide them with the ability to practice skills at a higher level than nurses prepared at the basic education level.

Nurses access this expert source of power when they use their knowledge to teach, counsel, or motivate clients to follow a plan of care. Nurses can also use this source of power when dealing with physicians. By demonstrating their knowledge of the client's condition, recent laboratory tests, and other elements that are vital in the client's recovery, nurses increase the amount of respect they are given by physicians.

Power of Rewards

The reward source of power depends on the ability of one person to grant another some type of reward for specific behaviors or changes in behavior. The rewards themselves can take on many different forms, including personal favors, promotions, money, expanded privileges, and eradication of punishments. Nurses, in their day-to-day provision of care, can use this source of power to influence client behavior. For example, a nurse can give a client extra praise for completing the prescribed range-of-motion exercises. There are many aspects of the daily care of clients over which nurses have a substantial amount of reward power. This reward source of power also is the underlying principle in the process of behavior modification.

Coercive Power

The coercive source of power is the flip-side of the reward source. The ability to punish, withhold rewards, or threaten punishment are key elements underlying the coercive source of power. Although nurses do have access to this source of power, it is probably one which they use minimally, if at all. Not only does use of the coercive source of power destroy therapeutic and personal relationships, it can also be considered unethical and even illegal in certain situations. Threatening clients that they will get a shot if they do not take their oral medications may motivate them to take those medications, but it is generally not considered to be a good example of therapeutic communication technique.

Legitimate Power

The legitimate source of power depends on a legislative or legal act that gives the individual or organization a right to make decisions they might not otherwise have the authority to make. Most obviously, political figures and legislators have this source of power. But this power can also be disseminated and delegated to others though legislative acts. In nursing, the state board of nursing has access to the legitimate source of power because of its establishment under the nurse practice act of that state. Similarly, nurses have access to the legitimate source of power when they are licensed by the state under the provisions in the nurse practice act, or when they are appointed to positions within a health care agency. Nursing decisions made about client care can only come from individuals who have a legitimate source of power to make those decisions, that is, licensed nurses.

Collective Power

The collective source of power is often employed in a broader context than individual client care and is the underlying source for many other sources of power. When a large group of individuals who have similar beliefs, desires, or needs becomes organized, a collective source of power exists. For individuals who belong to professions, the professional organization is the focal point for this source of power. The main goal of any organization is to influence those policies that affect the members of the organization. This influence is usually in the form of political activities carried out by politicians and lobbyists.

Professional organizations that can deliver large numbers of votes have a powerful means of influencing politicians. The use of the collective source of power has elements of reward, coercive, expert, and even referent sources in it. Each source may come into play at one time or another.

HOW TO INCREASE POWER IN NURSING

Despite some feelings of powerlessness, nurses really do have access to some important, and rather substantial, sources of power. What can nurses, either as individuals or as a group, do in order to increase their power?

Professional Unity

Probably the first, and certainly the most important, way nurses can gain power in all areas is through professional unity. The most powerful groups are those that are best organized and most united. The power that a professional organization has is directly related to the size of its membership. There are approximately 3,000,000 nurses in the United States (Kalish, 1992). It is not difficult to imagine the power that the ANA could have to influence legislators and legislation if all of those nurses were members of the organization rather than the 250,000 who actually do belong. This point, that nurses need to belong to their nursing national organization, cannot be emphasized too much.

Political Activities

A second way nurses can gain power is by becoming involved in political activities. Although this produces discomfort in many, nurses must realize that they are influenced by politics and political decisions in every phase of their daily nursing activities.

The simple truth is that if nurses do not become involved in politics and participate in important legislation that influences their practice, someone other than nurses will be making those decisions for them. Nurses need to become involved in political activities from local to national levels. The average legislator knows little about such issues as client's rights, national health insurance, quality of nursing care, third-party reimbursement for nurses, and expanded practice roles for nurses. Yet, they make decisions about these issues almost daily. It would seem logical that more informed and better decisions could be made if nurses took an active part in the legislative process.

Accountability and Professionalism

A third means of increasing power is by demonstrating the characteristics of accountability and professionalism. Nursing has made great strides in these two areas in recent years. Nurses, through professional organizations, have been working hard to establish standards for quality client care. More importantly, nurses are now concerned with demonstrating competence and delivering high-quality client care through processes such as peer review and evaluation. By accepting responsibility for the care they provide, and by setting the standards to guide that care, nurses are taking the power to govern nursing away from nonnursing groups.

Networking

Finally, nurses can gain power through establishing a nurse support network. It is common knowledge that the "old boy" system remains alive and well in many segments of our seemingly enlightened 20th-century society. The "old boy" system, found in most large organizations ranging from universities to businesses and governmental agencies, provides individuals, usually men, with the encouragement, support, and nurturing that allows them to move up quickly through the ranks in the organization to achieve high administrative positions. Nursing and nursing organizations have never really had this type of system for the advancement of nurses. Part of this system of doing business involves never criticizing another "old boy" in public, even though there may be major differences of opinion in private. Presenting a united front is extremely important in maintaining power within this system.

Part of the difficulty in establishing a nurse support network stems from the fact that nurses really have not been in high-level positions for very long. The framework for a support system for nurses is now in place, however, and with some commitment to the concept and activity, it can grow into a well-developed network to allow the brightest, best, and most ambitious in the profession to achieve high level positions.

SUMMARY

Proposed changes in the health care system will have a major impact on how, where, and even who practices nursing. Unless nurses become involved in decisions about where health care is going, band together as a profession, and exert some of the tremendous potential power that they have access to, politicians, physicians, hospital administrators, and insurance companies will ultimately be shaping their future.

Nursing has taken great strides forward in achieving professional status in the health care system. Currently, many nurses accept the premise that nursing is a profession and therefore are not much concerned about furthering the process. Even as nursing has reached a heightened level of maturity and evolved

CHALLENGES OF AN AGING NATION

The complexity of issues in today's health care system challenges the professional nurse to look beyond the narrow confines of the individual client to a more comprehensive perspective of each situation. The following case study demonstrates some of the elements that need to be evaluated in the care of an elderly client.

CASE STUDY

Clara, 108 years old, is admitted through the hospital emergency room (ER) for nonspecific complaints of chest pain and dizziness. This is the third time she has come to the hospital with this complaint in the last month, and although previous examinations and tests showed no acute disease process, the ER physician felt that because of her age and long history of coronary artery disease, she should be monitored and evaluated more closely. She has no private insurance, but is covered under Medicare, parts A and B, with supplemental coverage from a small insurance company in her state.

Despite her age, Clara is mentally alert and competent, lives by herself in a small apartment, and manages basic daily care, including shopping and cleaning, with only minimal assistance from friends. She has no living family members except for a few aging cousins in a distant state. She is taking several medications at home, including diltiazem (Cardizem) for her heart problems, ranitidine (Zantac) for a hiatal hernia, and papaverine (Pavabid) to increase her general circulation.

After a complete physical examination, including several tests and an electrocardiogram (ECG), she is scheduled for a cardiac catheterization. A significant block is seen in one of the major coronary arteries, and it is decided to perform angioplasty on the artery. She is admitted to the intensive care unit (ICU) after the procedure, where she also receives 2 units of blood for anemia. She recovers without incident and is discharged 5 days after her admission. The total cost for her hospitalization, including tests and angioplasty, is in excess of $15,000.

Clara is not a typical client for her age group. Many medical experts would categorize the treatment given her as *overtreatment* because of the current emphasis on quality of life, death with dignity, and the futility of treating the hopelessly ill. Yet, as the population of this country continues to age, it is more likely that Clara will become the norm rather than the exception. Many issues—ethical, financial, and others—surround this case.

In an era of cost containment and reform, financial concerns are always near the top. Almost everyone admits that the Medicare reimbursement system is, at best, arbitrary and inconsistent, and at worst, disorganized and wasteful. Because of the concern about paying for expensive complicated procedures, such as angioplasty, which may not necessarily improve the quality of life, and for which less expensive alternatives may exist, the system seems to force physicians to select modes of care that the elderly often consider substandard. In general, angioplasty on a 108-year-old person would be classified as excessive; yet given this client's mental state and quick return to a normal life, it would appear to have been the correct course of action.

Related to the cost issue is the ethical issue of distributive justice. The terms currently used to define this problem are the **rationing of health care** and **limiting access to health care.** The elderly, through the various entitlement programs, consume a large proportion of the national budget. This cost is borne largely by young and middle aged workers through their taxes. Is it fair that the young be required to carry the burden for the care of the old?

The problems posed by an ever-aging population will only worsen as the next century approaches. Decisions will have to be made about where best to spend the limited resources for health care. Basic questions, such as is it better to spend 65¢ to immunize a 4-year-old child or to spend $10,000 to perform an angioplasty on a 108-year-old woman, will challenge health care providers of the future. It seems that blanket policies, such as are used now, will be inadequate to deal with these complex issues. Development of geriatric consultation teams at all facilities will make it possible to evaluate on an individual basis the case of each client 65 years or older who is admitted to the facility. Decisions could then be made about which type of care would be most appropriate, including the client's input, as well as what can be done to improve the quality of that individual's life. This will allow clients like Clara to live their lives to the fullest and to end their days with dignity and respect.

Modified from Curtin, LH: How much is enough? Nursing Management 25:30–31, 1994.

into a field of study with an identifiable body of knowledge, however, the questions and problems that have plagued it in the past persist. In addition, advances in technology, management, and society in general have raised new questions about the nature and role of nursing in the health care system. Only by understanding and exploring the issues of professionalism will nurses be prepared to practice effectively in the present and meet the complex challenges of the future.

ISSUES IN PRACTICE
Misplaced Loyalty

Tisha S., a senior nursing student, was acting as the team leader during her final clinical experience. Jamie D., a close friend of Tisha's, was one of three junior nursing students in Tisha's team that day. Because of some personal problems, Jamie had been late and unprepared for several clinical experiences. She was informed by her instructor that she might fail unless she showed marked improvement during clinical training.

Clarie B., a 64-year-old patient with diabetes and possible renal failure, was one of Jamie's clients. Mrs. B. was having a 24-hour urine test to help determine her renal function. After the test was completed later that afternoon, she was to be discharged and treated through the renal clinic. Jamie understood the principles of the 24-hour urine test and realized that all the urine for the full 24 hours needed to be saved. But she became busy caring for another client, and accidently threw away the last specimen before the test was to end. She took the specimen container to the laboratory anyway.

At the end of the shift, when Jamie was giving her report to Tisha, she confided that she had thrown away the last urine specimen but begged Tisha not to tell the instructor. This mistake would mean that the test would have to be started over again, and Mrs. B. would have to spend an extra day in the hospital. Out of friendship, Tisha agreed not to tell the instructor, rationalizing that they had gotten almost all the urine and she was going to be treated for renal failure anyway. When the instructor asked Tisha for her final report for the day, she specifically asked if there had been any problems with the 24-hour urine test. What would be the consequences of telling the truth? Of not telling the truth?

CRITICAL THINKING EXERCISES

1   Distinguish between an occupation and a profession.
2   Is nursing a profession? Defend your position.
3   Discuss four ways nursing can improve its professional status.
4   Name the three sources of power to which nurses have the most access. Discuss how nurses can best use these sources of power to improve nursing, nursing care, and the health care system in general.

BIBLIOGRAPHY

American Nurses Association: Nursing's Agenda for Health Care Reform. Kansas City, 1992.
Bernard, LA and Walsha, M: Leadership, the Key to the Professionalization of Nursing. John Wiley and Sons, New York, 1981.

Brink, PJ: The difference between a job and a career. West J Nurs Res 10:5–6, 1988.
Bunting, S and Campbell, J: Feminism and nursing: Historical perspectives. Adv Nurs Sci 12:11–24, 1990.
Fitzpatrick, ML. Prologue to Professionalism. Robert J. Brady, Bowie, MD, 1983.
Hudek, K: Nursing, Making it a career. Can Nurse 86:18–19, 1990.
Kaler, SR, Levy, DA and Schall, M: Stereotypes of professional roles. Image, Nurs Scholarship 21:85–89, 1989.
Kalish, BJ and Kalish, PA: The Politics of Nursing. JB Lippincott, Philadelphia, 1982.
McCloskey, M: Many issues influence profession. Amer Nurse 22:7, 1992.
Moloney, MM: Professionalization of Nursing. JB Lippincott, Philadelphia, 1986.
Smith, GR: Power and health care reform. J Nurs Educ 33:194–197, 1994.
Webster, ML: Professional style: An update. Nurs Life 5:63, 1985.

HISTORICAL PERSPECTIVES

Why the Study of History Is Important to Professional Nurses

Many of the issues found in the health care system today, in general, and in the profession of nursing, in particular, have their roots in the historical process that has developed over centuries. Knowledge of these historical roots can help in understanding the profession and may even point toward solutions.

One of the difficulties in studying history is that much of the information seems to be unrelated. History is often presented as a series of isolated facts. One effective way of connecting information that may at first seem unrelated is to find common themes or historical threads that are present to some degree at all times and in all places. The history of health care and nursing has three elements to be aware of. They are:

1   The group or society's beliefs regarding the causes of illness
2   The value placed on individual life
3   The role of women in that society

In addition, war and its consequences has had a major effect on the direction of health care.

Health Care Without Nurses

From the viewpoint of modern health care, it is difficult to envision a health care system without nurses. Yet, nursing as it is practiced today is a relatively recent historic development. The major concern of most early civilizations was the survival of the human species. The most fundamental needs of survival were nourishment, shelter, and procreation. Illness and injury threatened survival at a very basic level, and so was also one of the major concerns of early civilizations. Early human history is marked by a trial-and-error process for meeting the basic needs for survival at all levels. Much of primitive health care grew out of this process.

Development of the Modern Nurse (1350–1600)— Influences of the Renaissance

Although the seeds of modern nursing had been planted during the medieval period with the development of religious nursing orders, not until the Renaissance did nursing assume a form recognizable to us. Its development was marked by rapid growth offset by setbacks. Major political changes caused by the chaos following the Reformation had the most effect on health care in that period.

The Renaissance was a time of intellectual reawakening for much of Europe. Starting in Italy in the 14th century, the curtains of ignorance and superstition of the medieval period were slowly rolled back across all of Western Europe as new discoveries, inventions, and philosophies were developed. Names associated with this period include Galileo, Copernicus, Descartes, and Newton. Crude forms of such inventions as the microscope, thermometer, pendulum clock, and telescope can be traced to this period that eventually led to discovery of other new knowledge. Within this renewed interest in learning lay the philosophical, political, and religious seeds of a discontent that were to come to full bloom some 100 years later.

Initially, the health care establishment that had developed during the Middle Ages had great difficulty in applying the new learning to the actual care of patients. Most health care in the early Renaissance was still being provided in hospitals maintained by religious orders. With some 500 years of tradition and development, these hospitals viewed the primary goal of care as the salvation of the sick individual's soul, with the restoration of health and cure of illness seen as only a secondary goal. Use of more modern methods of diagnosis and treatment of disease were often viewed as disrespectful, improper, or even the work of the devil.

THEORIES AND MODELS OF NURSING

Learning Objectives

After completing this chapter, the reader will be able to:

1 Explain why theories and models are important to the profession of nursing.
2 Analyze the four key concepts found in nursing theories and models.
3 Interrelate systems theory as an important element in understanding nursing theories or models.
4 Evaluate how the four parts of all systems interact.
5 Synthesize three nursing theories, identifying how the different nursing theorists define the key concepts in their theories.

WHY THEORIES AND MODELS ARE IMPORTANT TO NURSING

For many nurses, and for most nursing students, the terms **theory** and **model** evoke images of thick textbooks filled with abstract, obscure words and convoluted sentences. The visceral response is often "Why is this important, I want to take care of real people!" The simple answer is: "Understanding and using nursing theories or models will help you to be a better nurse and provide better care to real people."

Although the terms **theory** and **model** are not exactly synonymous, in nursing practice they are often used interchangeably. Strictly speaking, a theory refers to a speculative statement concerning some element of reality that has not been proven. For example, the theory of relativity has never been proven, although the results have often been observed. The nursing profession tends to use the term theory when attempting to explain apparent relationships between observed behaviors and their effect on a patient's health. In this nursing context, the goal of a theory is to describe and explain a particular nursing action in order to predict its effect on a patient outcome, such as improved health or recovery from illness. For example, turning unresponsive clients from side to side every 2 hours should help prevent skin breakdown and improve respiratory function.

A model, on the other hand, is a hypothetical representation of something that exists in reality. The purpose of a model is to attempt to explain a complex reality in a systematic and organized manner. For example, a hospital organizational chart is a model that attempts to demonstrate the interrelationships of the various levels of the hospital's administration.

Although a model tends to be more concrete than a theory, their common element is that they help explain and direct nursing actions. This ability, using a systematic and structured approach, is one of the key elements that raises nursing from a task-oriented job to the level of a real profession. With the use of a conceptual model, nurses can provide intelligent and thoughtful answers to the question: "What do nurses do?" (Nightingale/Harrison, 1966).

Consider this scenario: Mr. X had surgery for intestinal cancer 4 days ago. He has a colostomy and needs to learn how to take care of it at home because he is going to be discharged in 2 days. When the nurses attempt to teach him colostomy care, he looks away, makes sarcastic personal comments about the nurses, and generally displays a belligerent and hostile attitude.

Without an understanding of the underlying dynamics involved, the nurses' very human response to this client's behavior might be to become sarcastic and scold the client about his behavior, or to simply keep the amount of contact with him to a minimum (Aguilera, 1990). This type of response will not improve Mr. X's health status at all.

If the nurses knew, however, and understood the dynamics of the grief theory, they would realize that Mr. X was probably in the anger stage of the grief process. This understanding would direct the nurses to allow, or even to encourage, Mr. X to express his anger without condemnation, and to help him deal with his feelings in a constructive manner. Once Mr. X gets past the anger stage, he can move on to taking a more active part in his care, and thereby improve his health status. The goals of the nurses would then be achieved.

KEY CONCEPTS COMMON TO NURSING MODELS

Although nursing models vary in terminology and approach to health care, there are four concepts that are common to almost all of them. These concepts are patient or client (individual, or collective), health, nursing, and environment. Each nursing model has its own specific definition of these terms, but the underlying definitions of the concepts are similar.

Client

The concept of client (or patient) is central to all nursing models because it is the client who is the primary recipient of nursing care. Although the term **client** is usually used to refer to a single individual, it can also refer to small groups or to a large collective of individuals (for community health nurses, the community is the client).

The concept of client has changed over the years as the knowledge and understanding of human nature developed and increased. A client is more than simply a person who comes to a health care facility with an illness to be cured. Clients are now seen as complex entities affected by a variety of interrelating factors, such as the mind and body, the individual and the environment, and the person and the person's family. When nurses talk about clients, the term **biopsychosocial** is often used to express the complex relationship between the body, mind, and environment.

A client, in many of the nursing models, does not have to have an illness in order to be the central element of the model (this explains the current preference of using the term **client** over the term **patient**). This is also one of the clearest distinctions between medical models and nursing models. Medical models are almost exclusively devoted to curing diseases and to restoring health. Nursing models are concerned with disease cure and health restoration, but they also focus on prevention of disease and maintenance of health. A healthy person is just as important to many nursing models as the person with a disease.

Health

Health is the second common concept found in nursing models. Like the concept of client, the concept of health has undergone much development and change over the years as knowledge has increased. Originally thought of as an absence of disease, today's more realistic view often sees health as a continuum ranging from a completely healthy state where there is no disease, to a completely unhealthy state, which ends in death. At any given time in their lives, everyone is located somewhere along the health continuum and may move closer to one side or the other depending on circumstances and health status (Mitchell & Grippano, 1993).

Health is difficult to define because it varies so much from individual to individual. For example, a 22-year-old bodybuilder who has no chronic diseases perceives health differently than an 85-year-old who has diabetes, congestive heart failure, and problems seeing. The perception of health also varies from culture to culture, and at different historical periods within the same culture. In some past cultures, a sign of health was pure white skin, whereas in the American culture, a dark bronze suntan has been more desirable as a sign of health, until recently.

Environment

The concept of **environment** is also an element in most current nursing models. Nursing models often broaden the concept of environment from the simple physical environment to elements such as living conditions, public sanitation, and air and water quality. Also included are factors such as interpersonal relationships and social interactions.

Some internal environmental factors that affect health include the personal psychologic processes, religious beliefs, sexual orientation, personality, and emotional responses. It has long been known that individuals who are highly self-motivated and internally goal directed (i.e., type A personality) tend to develop ulcers and have myocardial infarctions at a higher rate than the general population. Medical models, which are primarily illness oriented, although acknowledging this factor, may not consider it treatable. Nursing models that consider personality as one of the environmental factors that affect health are more likely to attempt to modify the individual's behavior (internal environment) to decrease the risk of disease.

Like the other key concepts found in nursing models, the concept of environment is used so that it is consistent within a particular model's overall context. Nursing models try to show how various aspects of environment interrelate and how they affect the client's health status. In addition, nursing models treat environment as an active element in the overall health care system and assert that positive alterations in the environment will improve the client's health status.

Nursing

The culminating concept in all the various nursing models is **nursing** itself. After consideration of what it means to be a client, what it means to be healthy, and how the environment influences the client's health status either positively or negatively, the concept of nursing delineates the function and role nurses have in their relationship with clients. Historically, the profession of nursing has been interested in providing basic physical care (i.e., hygiene, activity, nourishment), psychologic support, and relief of discomfort for clients. But modern nursing, although still including these basic elements of client care, has expanded into areas of health care only imagined a generation ago.

In the modern nurse-client relationship, the client is no longer the passive recipient of nursing care. The relationship has been expanded to include clients as key partners in curing and in the health maintenance process. In conjunction with the nurse, clients set goals for care and recovery, take an active part in achieving those goals, and help in evaluating whether or not those actions have achieved the goals (McCann-Flynn & Heffron, 1984).

Because of the broadened understanding of environment, several nursing models include manipulation of environmental elements affecting health as an important part of the nurse's role. The environment may be directly altered by the nurse with little or no input from the client, or the client may be taught by the nurse to alter the environment in ways that will contribute to curing disease, increasing comfort, or improving the client's health status (Riehl-Sisca, 1989).

When attempting to analyze and understand any nursing model, it is important to look for these four key concepts, client, health, environment, and nursing. These concepts should be clearly defined, closely interrelated, and mutually supportive. Depending on the particular nursing model, one element may be emphasized more than another. The resulting role and function of the nurse depend on which element is given greater emphasis.

GENERAL SYSTEMS THEORY

A widely accepted method for conceptualizing and understanding the world and what is in it is derived from a systems viewpoint. Generally understood as an organized unit with a set of components that interact and affect each other, a system acts as a whole because of the interdependence of its parts (Putt, 1978). As a result, when part of the system malfunctions or fails, it interrupts the function of the whole system rather than affecting merely one part. Humans, plants, cars, governments, the health care system, the profession of nursing, and almost anything that exists can be viewed as a system. The terminology and principles of systems theory pervade American society.

Although general systems theory in its pure form is rarely, if ever, used as a nursing model, its process and much of its terminology underlie many nursing models. Elements of general systems theory in one form or another have found their way into many textbooks and much of the professional literature. General systems theory often acts as the unacknowledged framework for many educational programs. Understanding the mechanisms and terminology of general systems theory is helpful in providing an orientation to understanding nursing models.

General systems theory, sometimes referred to simply as systems theory, is an outgrowth of an innate intellectual process. The human mind has difficulty comprehending large, complex entities as a single unit. As a result, the mind automatically divides that entity into smaller, more manageable fragments, and then examines each fragment separately. This is similar to the process of deductive reasoning in which a single complex thought or theory is broken down into smaller, interrelated pieces. All scientific disciplines, from physics to biology, and social sciences, such as sociology and psychology, use this method of analysis.

But systems theory takes the process a step further. After analyzing or breaking down the entity, systems theory attempts to put it back together by showing how the parts work individually and together within the *system*. This interrelationship of the parts makes the system function as a unit. And often, particularly where the system involves biologic or sociologic entities, the system that results is greater than the sum of its parts.

Although the early roots of general systems theory can be traced as far back as the 1930s, Ludwig von Bertalanffy is usually credited with the formal development and publication of general systems theory around 1950 (Stevens, 1984). His major achievement was to standardize the definitions of the terms used in system theory, and make the concept useful to a wide range of disciplines. Systems theory is so widely applicable because it reflects the reality that underlies the basic human thought processes.

WHAT IS A SYSTEM?

Very simply, a **system** is defined as a set of interacting parts. The parts that compose a system may be similar or they may vary a great deal from each other, but they all have the common function of making the system work well to achieve its overall purpose. A school is a good example of how the dynamics and interrelatedness of a system works. A school as a system is composed of a large number of units including buildings, administrators, teachers, students, and a variety of other individuals, such as counselors, financial aid personnel, bookkeepers, and maintenance persons. Each of these individuals has a unique job but also contributes to the overall goal of the school, which is to provide an education for the students, and also to further the development of knowledge through research.

All systems are composed of four key parts. These parts are the system itself (that is, whether open or closed), input and output, throughput, and a feedback loop.

Open and Closed Systems

A system is categorized as either being open or closed. In reality, very few systems are completely open or completely closed. Rather, they usually are a combination of both open and closed systems.

Open systems are those in which relatively free movement of information, matter, and energy into and out of the system exists. In a completely open system there would be no restrictions on what moves in and out of the system, thus making its boundaries difficult to identify. Most systems have some control on the movement of information, energy, and matter around them. This control is maintained through the semipermeable nature of their boundaries, which allows some things in and keeps some things out, as well as allowing some out while keeping others in. This control on input and output leads to the dynamic equilibrium found in most well-functioning systems.

Theoretically, a closed system prevents any movement into and out of the system. In this case the system would be totally static and unchanging. Probably no absolutely closed systems exist in the real world, although there are systems that may tend to be closed to outside elements. A stone, for example, considered as a system, seems to be very nearly a perfectly closed system. It does not take anything in or put anything out. It does not change very much over long periods. In reality, though, it is affected by a number of elements in nature. It absorbs moisture when it is damp, freezes when cold, and becomes hot in the summer. Over long periods, these factors may cause the stone to crack, break down, and eventually turn into topsoil.

Systems that nurses deal with frequently are relatively open. Primarily, the client can be categorized as a highly open system that requires certain input elements and has output elements also. Other systems that nurses commonly work with, such as hospital administrators and physicians, are generally considered to be open systems, although their degree of openness may vary widely.

Input and Output

The processes by which a system interacts with elements in its environment are called input and output. **Input** is defined as any type of information, energy, or material that enters the system from the environment through its boundaries. Conversely, **output** is defined as any information, energy, or material that leaves the system and enters the environment through the system's boundaries. Open systems require relatively large amounts of input and output.

Throughput

A third term, sometimes used in relationship to the system's dynamic exchange with the environment, is **throughput.** Throughput is a process that allows the input to be changed so that it is useful to the system. For example, most automobiles run on some form of liquid fossil fuel (input) such as gasoline or diesel. Going to the gas station and pouring liquid fuel on the roof of the car probably will not produce the effects desired when most people buy fuel for their cars. But if the fuel is put into the gas tank, it can be transformed by the carburetor or fuel injection system into a fine mist, which when mixed with air and ignited by a spark plug burns rapidly to produce the force necessary to propel the car. Without this internal process (throughput) found in the car, liquid fuel is not a useful form of energy.

Feedback Loop

The fourth key element of a system is the **feedback loop.** The feedback loop allows the system to monitor its internal functioning so that it can either restrict or increase its input and its output. The feedback loop also provides for the system to monitor and regulate its own internal process so that it is maintained at the highest level of functioning.

Two basic types of feedback exist. Positive feedback leads to change within the system, with the goal of improving the system. Students in the classroom, for example, receive feedback from the teacher in a number of ways; it may be in the form of direct verbal statements such as "good work on this assignment," or feedback by examination and homework grades.

Feedback is considered positive if it produces a change in students' behavior, such as motivating them to study more, spend more time on assignments, or prepare for class in a more thorough manner. Negative feedback maintains stability; that is, it does not produce change. Negative feedback is not necessarily bad for a system. Rather, when a system has reached its peak level of functioning, negative feedback helps it maintain that level. For example, an athlete who has reached his or her peak level of performance through long hours of practice knows what type of practice is required to stay at that level of ability. Negative feedback in the form of optimal times in the case of runners, or number of pounds lifted in the case of weight lifters, indicates that no changes in practice patterns are required.

The feedback loop is an important element in systems theory. It makes the process circular, and links the various elements of the system together. Without a feedback loop, it is virtually impossible for the system to have any meaningful control over its input and output.

Other Terms Used in Systems Theory

Other terms used in speaking of systems theory carry over into nursing models in some degree.

The **hierarchy** of systems is an important concept. It is evident that there are some very large systems, some very small systems, and many intermediate-sized ones. Although these terms are somewhat relative to the overall system they are a part of, they do have distinct definitions.

The term **subsystem** is defined as one of the smaller, or less complex, systems that make up the total system. The study of human anatomy and physiology is a classic example of how the subsystem concept is used. Physiologic systems such as the nervous, cardiovascular, and endocrine systems are all subsystems of the total system we call the human being.

The smallest subsystems are called microsystems. The microsystem is the most basic, and least complex, element of the larger system. In human anatomy or physiology, the cell is usually considered a microsystem. Yet, the cell itself is composed of even smaller elements, such as cell membranes, nucleus, and mito-chondria, which in turn could also be considered microsystems in themselves.

Equifinality is a term that is used in systems theory to describe the progressive complexity of interactions found in most systems. There is an innate tendency for systems to become more complex as they grow. Their increasing complexity is a result of the system's attempt to reach a final goal, regardless of the means. When the first self-rule government was established for the new United States of America, it was much less complex than it is now. Its primary goals were to keep internal order, to allow people to have a say in what happened to them, and to protect the country from invaders. Over the years as the country grew in population and developed as a nation, the goals remained the same, but the government, to carry out these goals, necessarily became more complex. Today, the government of the United States is an extremely complex macrosystem, with literally millions of subsystems in the form of agencies, bureaus, and programs.

Another term used in systems theory is **entropy**, the tendency systems have to become disorganized and nonfunctional over time. As systems grow, an internal differentiation takes place within its subsystems. If input, particularly in the form of energy, does not keep pace with the growth and differentiation within the system, the increasing number of subsystems have fewer and fewer resources with which to carry out their functions. Unless the process is stopped or reversed, at some point the system stops functioning or may actually destroy itself. For the human body, the ultimate example of entropy is death and the subsequent deterioration of the body into its basic chemical elements.

The opposite of entropy is the process termed **negentropy** (negative entropy). Negentropy allows a system to control its input and output and maintain its internal equilibrium, thereby retaining a high degree of organization and functioning. Because negentropy goes against the natural, internal forces of the system, the system requires a very strong feedback loop and effective internal controls to make negentropy successful. Again, using the human body as an example of a system, negentropy is demonstrated in the complex subsystems that help keep that body healthy. The gastrointestinal system is designed to provide the nutrients that build, rebuild, and maintain the body. The endocrine system, regulated by the neurologic system, produces hormones that maintain the internal metabolic and electrolyte balances needed for normal functioning. The circulatory system distributes nutrients and hormones to the proper tissues at the proper time. The whole process requires a large amount of energy; a failure in any part of it affects all the other parts.

In systems theory, the term **nonsummativity** is defined as the degree of interdependence among the system's subsystems or parts. The higher the nonsummativity, the greater is the amount of interdependence of the system's parts. In a system with low nonsummativity, the parts of the system have a low degree of interdependence.

Some subsystems may be more important to generalized functioning than others. If a person suffers a severe head injury, major disruption of almost all the other subsystems usually occurs, whereas a skin laceration has less effect on other subsystems. All parts of a system need some degree of nonsummativity to remain even minimally functional (Putt, 1978).

MAJOR NURSING THEORIES AND MODELS

At last count, at least 15 published nursing models (or theories) have been used to direct nursing education and nursing care (Fawcett, 1989). The six nursing models discussed here (Table 2–1) have been selected because they are the most widely accepted and are good examples of how the concepts of client, health, environment, and nursing are used to explain and guide nursing actions. Discussion of these theories is not intended to be exhaustive, but rather to provide an overview of the theorists' main concepts. It is important to understand the terms used in the theories *as defined by their authors* and to see the interrelationship be-

TABLE 2–1. Comparison of Selected Nursing Models

Nursing Theory	Client	Health	Environment	Nursing
Roy Adaptation Model	Man—as a dynamic system with input and output	A continuum—the ability to adapt successfully to illness	Both internal and external stimuli that affect behaviors	Multistep process that helps the client adapt and reach the highest level of functioning
Orem Self-Care Model	Humans—biologic, psychologic social beings with the ability for self-care	Ability to live life to the fullest through self-care	The medium through which the client moves	Helping the client achieve health through assistance in self-care activities
King Model of Goal Attainment	Person—exchanges energy and information with the environment to meet needs	Dynamic process to achieve the highest level of functioning	Personal, interpersonal, and social systems and the external physical world	Dynamic process to identify and meet the health care needs of the person
Watson Model of Human Caring	Individual—has needs, grows, and develops to reach a state of inner harmony	Dynamic state of growth and development leading to full potential as a human being	Those factors the client must overcome to achieve health	Science of caring that helps clients reach their greatest potential
Johnson Behavioral System Model	Person—a behavioral system that is an organized and integrated whole composed of seven subsystems	A balanced and steady state within the behavioral system of the client	All those internal and external elements that affect client behavior	Activities that manipulate the environment and help clients achieve the balanced state of health
Neuman Health Care Systems Model	An open system that constantly interacts with internal and external environment	Relatively stable internal functioning of the individual in a high state of wellness (stability)	Internal and external stressors that produce change in the client	Identifies boundary disruption and helps clients in activities to restore stability

tween the elements in each theory as well as the similarities and differences among the various different models.

The Roy Adaptation Model

As developed by Sister Callista Roy, the Roy Adaptation Model of Nursing is very closely related to systems theory (Roy, 1991). The main goal of this model is to have the client reach his or her highest level of functioning through adaptation.

Client

The central element in the Roy Model is **man** (a generic term referring to human beings in general, or the client in particular). Man is viewed as a dynamic entity with both input and output. As derived from the context of the four modes in the Roy Model, the client is defined as a biopsychosocial being who is affected by a variety of stimuli and displays behaviors to help adapt to the stimuli. Because the client is constantly being affected by stimuli, adaptation is a continual process (Roy & Andrews, 1991).

Input are called stimuli, and include internal stimuli that arise from within the client's environment, as well as stimuli coming from external environmental factors such as physical surroundings, family, and society. The output in the Roy Model is the behavior that the client demonstrates as a result of stimuli that are affecting him or her

Output, or behavior, is a very important element in the Roy Model because it is the primary source of information about the client that the nurse is able to obtain through assessment techniques. In the Roy Model, the output (behavior) is always modified by the client's internal attempts to adapt to the input, or stimuli. Roy has identified four internal adaptational activities that clients use, and has termed these the four **adaptational modes.** These modes are the **physiologic mode** (using internal physiologic process), the **self-concept mode** (developed throughout life by experience), the **role function mode** (dependent upon the client's relative place in society), and the **interdependence mode** (indicating how the client relates to others).

Health

In the Roy Model, the concept of health is defined as the location of the client along a continuum between perfect health and complete illness. Health, in the Roy Model, is rarely an absolute. Rather, a person's ability to adapt to stimuli, such as injury, disease, or even psychologic stress, determines the level of that person's health status. For example, a client who was in an automobile accident, had a broken neck, and was paralyzed but who eventually went back to college, obtained a law degree, and became a practicing lawyer would, in the Roy Model, be considered to have a high degree of health because of the ability to adapt to the stimuli imposed.

Environment

The Roy Model's definition of environment is synonymous with the concept of stimuli. The environment consists of all those factors that influence the client's behavior, either internally or externally. The Roy Model categorizes these environmental elements, or stimuli, into three groups: (1) focal, (2) contextual, and (3) residual.

Focal stimuli are environmental factors that most directly affect the client's behavior, and require most of his or her attention. **Contextual stimuli** form the general physical, social, and psychologic environment from which the client emerges. **Residual stimuli** are factors in the client's past, such as personality characteristics, past experiences, religious beliefs, and social norms that have an indirect affect on the client's health status. Residual stimuli are often very difficult to identify because they may remain hidden in the person's past memory, or may be an integral part of the client's personality.

Nursing

In the Roy Model, nursing becomes a multistep process to aid and support the client in the attempt to adapt to stimuli in one or more of the four adaptive modes. To determine what type of help is required to promote adaptation, the nurse must first assess the client. The primary assessments the nurse makes are of the client's behavior (output). Basically, the nurse should try to determine if the client's behavior is adaptive or maladaptive in each of the four adaptational modes previously defined. Some first-level assessments of the pneumonia client might include a temperature of 104°F, a cough productive of thick green sputum, chest pain on inspiration, weakness, and signs of weakness or physical debility, such as the inability to bring in wood for the fireplace or to visit friends.

A second-level assessment should also be made to determine what type of stimuli (input) are affecting the client's health care status. In the case of the pneumonia client, this might include a culture and sensitivity of the sputum to identify the invasive bacteria, assessment of the client's clothes to determine if they were adequate for the weather outside, and an investigation to find out if any neighbors could help the client upon discharge.

After performing the assessment, the nurse analyzes the data and arranges them in such a way so as to be able to make a statement about the client's adaptive or maladaptive behaviors, that is, identifies the problem. In current terminology, this identification of the problem is called a **nursing diagnosis.** After the problem has been identified, goals for optimal adaption are established. Ideally, these goals should be a collaborative effort between nurse and client. Determining the actions that need to be taken to achieve the goals is the next step in the process. The focus should be on manipulation of the stimuli to promote optimal adaptation. Finally, an evaluation is made of the whole process to see if the goals have been met. If not, then the nurse must determine *why*, not *how*, the activities should be modified to achieve the goals (Stevens, 1984).

Orem Self-Care Model

Dorthea E. Orem's model of nursing is based on the belief that health care is each individual's own responsibility. The model is aimed at helping clients direct and carry out activities that either help maintain their health, or improve it (Orem, 1991).

Client

As with most other nursing models, the central element of the Orem Model is the client who is a biologic, psychologic, and social being with the capacity for self-care. **Self-care** is defined as the practice of activities that individuals initiate and perform on their own behalf to maintain life, health, and well-being. Self-care is a requirement for both maintenance of life and optimal functioning.

Health

In the self-care model, **health** is defined as the person's ability to live fully within a particular physical, biologic, and social environment, achieving a higher level of functioning that distinguishes the person from lower life forms. Quality of life is an extremely important element in this model of nursing. A person who is healthy is living life to the fullest and has the capacity to maintain that life through self-care. An unhealthy person is an individual who has a self-care deficit. This deficit is indicated by the inability to carry out one or more of the key health care activities. These activities have been categorized into six groups:

1   Air, water, and food
2   Excretion of waste
3   Activity and rest
4   Solitude and social interactions
5   Hazards to life and well-being
6   Being normal mentally under universal self-care

This group of unhealthy individuals also includes adults with diseases and injuries, young and dependent children, the elderly, and the disabled.

Universal Self-Care

In the Orem model, self-care is a two-part concept. The first type of self-care is called universal self-care and includes those elements commonly found in everyday life that support and encourage normal human growth, development, and functioning. Individuals who are healthy, according to the Orem Model, carry out the activities listed in order to maintain a state of health. To some degree, all these elements are necessary activities in maintaining health through self-care (Leininger, 1992).

The second type of self-care comes into play when the individual is unable to conduct one or more of the six self-care activities. This second type of self-care is called **health-deviation self-care.** Health-deviation self-care includes those activities carried out by individuals who have diseases, injuries, physiologic or psychologic stress, or other health care concerns. Activities such as seeking health care at an emergency room or clinic, entering a drug rehabilitation unit, joining a health club or weight control program, or going to a physician's office fall into this category.

Environment

Environment, in the self-care model, is the medium through which clients move as they conduct their daily activities. Although less emphasized in this model, the environment is generally viewed as a negative factor on a person's health status because many environmental factors detract from the ability to provide self-care. Environment includes social interactions with others, situations that must be resolved, and those physical elements that affect health.

Nursing

The primary goal of nursing in the Orem Model is to help the client conduct self-care activities in such a way as to reach the highest level of human functioning. Because there is a range of levels of self-care ability, three distinct levels, or systems, of nursing care are delineated, based on the individual's ability to undertake self-care activities. As clients become less able to care for themselves, their nursing care needs increase.

An individual who is able to carry out few or no self-care activities falls into the wholly compensated nursing care category in which the nurse must provide for most or all of the client's self-care needs. Examples of clients who require this level of care include comatose and ventilator-dependent clients in an intensive care unit, clients in surgery and the immediate recovery period, women in the labor and delivery phases of child birth, or clients with emotional and psychologic problems so severe as to render them unable to conduct normal activities of daily living.

Clients in the partially compensatory category of nursing care can meet some to most of their own self-care needs, but still have certain self-care deficits that require nursing intervention. The nurse's role becomes one of identifying these needs and carrying out activities to meet them until the client reaches a state of health and is able to meet the needs personally. Examples of this level of nursing care include the post-operative client who can feed himself and do basic activities of daily living (ADLs) but is unable to care for his catheter and dressings, or a client with newly diagnosed diabetes who has not yet learned the technique of self-administered insulin injections.

Clients who are able to meet all of their basic self-care needs require very little or no nursing interventions. These clients are recipients of the supportive-developmental category of nursing care, in which the nurse's main functions become teaching the client how to maintain or improve health, offering guidance in self-care activities, and providing emotional support and encouragement. Also, the nurse may adjust the environment to support the client's growth and development toward self-care, or may identify community resources to help in the self-care process. Conducting prenatal classes, arranging for discharge planning, providing child screening programs through a community health agency, and organizing aerobic exercise classes for post-coronary clients are all nursing actions that belong in the supportive-developmental category of care.

Nursing care is carried out through a three-step process in the Orem Model. Step 1 determines whether nursing care is needed. This step includes basic assessment of the client and identification of self-care problems and needs. Step 2 determines the appropriate nursing care system category and plans nursing care according to that category. Step 3 provides the indicated nursing care or actions to meet the client's self-care needs.

Five Methods. In the Orem Model, step 3, the provision of nursing care (implementation phase) is carried out by helping the client through one or a combination of five nursing methods (Fawcett, 1989). These five methods are:

1   Acting for or doing for another
2   Guiding another
3   Supporting another (physically or psychologically)
4   Providing an environment that promotes personal development
5   Teaching another

King Model of Goal Attainment

The current widely accepted practice of establishing health care goals for clients, and directing client care to meet these goals, has its origins in the nursing model developed by Imogene M. King. It is also called the King Intervention Model (King, 1991).

The King Model also noted that nursing must function in all three systems levels found in the environment: personal, interactional, and social. Nursing's primary function is at the personal systems level, where care of the individual is the main focus. But nurses can effectively provide care at the interactional systems level, where they deal with small- to moderate-size groups in activities such as group therapy and in health promotion classes. Finally, nurses can provide care at the social systems level through activities such as community health. In addition, the role of nursing at the social systems level can be expanded to include involvement in policy decisions that have an effect on the health care system as a whole.

Client

As in other nursing models, the focal point of care in the King Model is the person or client. The client is viewed as an open system that exchanges energy and information with the environment, a personal system with physical, emotional, and intellectual needs that change and grow during the course of life. Because these needs cannot be met completely by the client alone, interpersonal systems are developed through interactions with others depending on the client's perceptions of reality, communications with others, and transactions to reduce stress and tension in the environment.

Environment

Environment is an important concept in the King Model and encompasses a number of interrelated elements. The interpersonal systems or groups are central to King's conception of environment. They are formed at various levels according to internal goals established by the client.

Personal System. At the most basic level are the personal systems, where an interchange takes place between two individuals who share similar goals. An example of such a personal system is a client-nurse relationship.

Interpersonal System. At the intermediate level are the interpersonal systems that involve relatively small groups of individuals who share like goals, for example, a formal weight-loss program in which the members have the common goal of losing weight. Human interactions, communications, role delineation, and stress reduction are essential factors at this level.

Social System. At the highest level are social systems that include the large, relatively homogeneous elements of society. The health care system, government, and society in general are some important social systems. These social systems have as their common goals organization, authority, power, status, and decision. Although the client may not be in direct interaction with the social systems, these systems are important because the personal and interpersonal systems necessarily function within larger social systems. Evoking the principle of nonsummativity, whenever one part of an open system is changed, all the other parts of the system feel the effect. For example, a decision made at the governmental level to reduce Medicare payments may affect when and how often a client can use health care services such as doctor's office visits, group therapy, or emergency room care.

The King Model also includes the external physical environment that affects a person's health and well-being. As the person moves through the world, the physical setting interacts with the personal system to either improve or degrade the client's health care status.

Health

Viewed as a dynamic process that involves a range of human life experiences, health exists in people when they can achieve their highest level of functioning.

Health is the primary goal of the client in the King Model. It is achieved by continually adjusting to environmental stressors, maximizing the use of available resources and setting and achieving goals for one's role in life. Anything that disrupts or interferes with people's ability to function normally in their chosen roles is considered to be a state of illness.

Nursing

The King Model views nursing as a dynamic process and a type of personal system based on interactions between nurse and client. During these interactions, the nurse and the client jointly evaluate and identify the health care need(s), set goals for fulfillment of the needs, and consider actions to take in achieving the goals. Nursing is a multifaceted process that includes a range of activities such as the promotion and maintenance of health through education, the restoration of health through care of the sick and injured, and preparation for death through care of the dying (Stevens, 1984).

The process of nursing in the King Model includes five key elements considered central to all human interactions:

1 Action
2 Reaction
3 Interaction
4 Transaction
5 Feedback

Watson Model of Human Caring

Although the concept of caring has always been an important, if somewhat obscure, element in the practice of nursing, the Watson Model of Human Caring defines caring in a detailed and systematic manner. In the development of her model, Jean Watson used a philosophic approach rather than the systems theory approach seen in many other nursing models. Her main concern in the development of this model is to balance the impersonal aspects of nursing care that are found in the technologic and scientific aspects of practice with the personal and interpersonal elements of care that grow from a humanistic belief in life (Watson, 1985).

Client

The concept of client or person, in the Watson Model, is not well developed as separate from the concept of nursing. The individuality of the client is a key concern. The Watson Model views the client as someone who has needs, who grows and develops throughout life, and who eventually reaches a state of internal harmony. The client is also seen as a gestalt, or whole, who has value because of inherent goodness and capacity to develop. This gestalt, or holistic, view of the human being is a recurring theme in the Watson Model; it emphasizes that the total person is more important to nursing care than the individual injury or disease process that produced the need for care.

Environment

Environment in the Watson Model is a concept that is also closely intertwined with the concept of nursing. Viewed primarily as a negative element in the health care process, environment consists of those factors that the client must overcome to achieve a state of health. The environment can be both external—physical and social elements—and internal—psychologic reactions that affect health.

Health

To be healthy in the Watson Model, the individual must be in a dynamic state of growth and development that leads to reaching full potential as a human being. As with other nursing models, health is viewed as a continuum along which a person at any point may tend more toward health or more toward illness. Illness, in the Watson Model, is the client's inability to integrate life experiences and the failure to achieve full potential or inner harmony. In this model, the state of illness is not necessarily synonymous with the disease process. If the person reacts to the disease process in such a way as to find meaning, then that response is considered to be healthy. A failure to find meaning in the disease experience leads to a state of illness.

Nursing

Watson makes a clear distinction between the science of nursing and the practice of curing (medicine) (Fawcett, 1989). She defined nursing as the science of caring in which the primary goal is to assist the client reach the greatest level of personal potential. The practice of curing involves the conduct of activities that have the goal of treatment and elimination of disease.

The process of nursing in the Watson Model is based on the systematic use of the scientific problem-solving method for decision making. In order to understand and best perceive nursing as a science of caring, the nurse should hold certain beliefs and be able to initiate certain caring activities.

Values. Basic to the beliefs necessary for the successful practice of nursing in the Watson Model is the formation of a humanistic-altruistic system of values based on the tenet that all people are inherently valuable because they are human. In addition, the nurse should have a strong sense of faith and hope in human beings and their condition because of the human potential for development.

Caring. A number of activities are important when practicing nursing according to Watson's caring way. These include establishing a relationship of help and trust between the nurse and the client; encouraging the client to express both positive and negative feelings with acceptance; manipulating the environment to make it more supportive, protective, or corrective for the client with any type of disease process; and assisting in whatever way deemed appropriate to meet the basic human needs of the client.

Johnson Behavioral System Model

By integrating systems theory with behavioral theory, Dorothy E. Johnson has developed a model of nursing that views client behavior as the key to preventing illness, and also to restoring health when illness occurs. Johnson holds that human behavior is really a type of system in itself that is influenced by input factors from the environment and has output that in its turn affects the environment (Fawcett, 1989).

Client

Drawing directly on the terminology of systems theory, the Johnson Model describes the person, or client, as a behavioral system that is an organized and integrated whole. The whole is greater than the sum of its parts because of the integration and functioning of its subsystems. In the Johnson Model, the client as a behavioral system is composed of seven distinct behavioral subsystems. In turn, each of these seven behavioral subsystems contains four structural elements that guide and shape the subsystem.

Security. The first behavioral subsystem is the attachment or affiliate subsystem, which has security as its driving force. The type of activity that this subsystem undertakes is, for the most part, inclusion in social functions, and the behavior that is observed from this subsystem is social interactions.

Dependency. The second behavior subsystem is the dependency subsystem and has as its initiating force the goal of assisting or helping others. The primary type of activity involved is nurturing and promoting self-image, and the observable behaviors resulting from this activity include approval, attention, and physical assistance of the person.

Taking In. The third behavioral subsystem is named the ingestive and has as its driving force the meeting of the body's basic physiologic needs of food and nutrient intake. Correspondingly, its primary activity is seeking and eating food, which manifests itself in the external behavior of eating.

Evaluative. The fourth behavioral subsystem is the eliminative; its goal is removal of waste products from the system. Its primary activity is means of elimination, which is observed as the behavior of expelling waste products.

Sexual. The fifth behavioral subsystem is the sexual, found in the Johnson Model's description of the person. The sexual subsystem has gratification and procreation of the species as its goals. It involves the complex activities of identifying gender roles, sexual development, and actual biologic sexual activity. It manifests itself in courting and mating behaviors.

Self-Protection. The sixth behavioral subsystem is called the aggressive and has as its driving force the goal of self-preservation. All the actions that individuals undertake to protect themselves from harm, either internal or external, derive from this subsystem, and are shown in actions toward others and the environment in general.

Achievement. The seventh, and final, behavioral subsystem is identified as achievement. Achievement has as its driving force the broad goal of exploration and manipulation of the environment. Gaining mastery and control over the environment is the primary activity of this subsystem; it can be demonstrated externally when the individual shows that learning has occurred and higher-level accomplishments are being produced (Schaefer, 1991).

As with all open systems, the behavioral system that makes up the person seeks to maintain a dynamic balance by regulating input and output. This regulation process takes the form of adapting to the environment and responding to others. However, the Johnson Model sees human behavior as being goal directed, which leads the person to constant growth and development beyond the maintenance of a mere steady state.

Health

A state of health exists, according to the Johnson Model, when balance and steady state exist within the behavioral systems of the client. Under normal circumstances, the human system has enough inherent flexibility to maintain this balance without external intervention. At times, however, the system's balance may be disturbed to such a degree by physical disease, injury, or emotional crisis as to require external assistance. This *out-of-balance* state is the state of illness.

Environment

In the Johnson Model the environment is defined as all of those internal and external elements that have an affect on the behavioral system. These environmental elements include obvious external factors, such as air temperature and relative humidity; sociologic factors, such as family, neighborhood, and society in general; and the internal environment, such as bodily processes, psychologic states, religious beliefs, and political orientation. All seven behavioral subsystems of the client are involved with his or her relationship to the environment through the regulation of input and output. The client is continually interacting with the environment in the attempt to remain healthy by maintaining an internal dynamic balance.

Nursing

In the Johnson Model, nursing is an activity that helps the individual achieve and maintain an optimal level of behavior (state of health) through the manipulation and regulation of the environment (Stevens, 1984). Nursing has functions in both health and illness. Nursing interventions to either maintain or regain health involve four activities in the regulation of the environment. These four nursing activities include restricting harmful environmental factors, defending the client from negative environmental influences, inhibiting adverse elements from occurring, and facilitating positive internal environmental factors in the recovery process.

As a professional, the nurse in the Johnson Model provides direct services to the client. By interacting with, and sometimes intervening in, the multiple subsystems that are found in the client's environment, the nurse acts as an external regulatory force. The goal of nursing is to promote the highest level of functioning and development in the client at all times. Nursing actions include helping the client to act in a socially acceptable manner, monitoring and aiding with biologic processes necessary for maintenance of a dynamic balance, demonstrating support for medical care and treatment during illness, and taking actions to prevent illness from recurring. In this model, nursing makes its own unique contribution to the health and well-being of individuals and provides a service that is complementary to that provided by other health care professionals.

Neuman Health Care Systems Model

As envisioned by Betty Neuman, the Health Care Systems Model focuses on the individual and his or her environment and is applicable to a variety of health care disciplines apart from nursing. Drawing from systems theory, the Neuman Model also includes elements from stress theory with an overall holistic view of humanity and health care (Neuman, 1989).

Client

In this model, the client is viewed as an open system that interacts constantly with internal and external environments through the system's boundaries. The client-system's boundaries are called lines of defense and resistance in the Neuman Model, and may be represented graphically as a series of concentric circles that surround the basic core of the individual. The goal of these boundaries is to keep the basic core system stable by controlling system input and output.

Neuman classifies these defensive boundaries according to their various functions. The internal lines of resistance are the boundaries that are closest to the basic core and thus protect the basic internal structure of the system. The normal lines of defense are outside the internal lines of resistance; they protect the system from common, everyday, environmental stressors. The flexible line of defense surrounds the normal line of defense and protects it from extreme environmental stressors. The general goal of all of these protective boundaries is to maintain the internal stability of the client.

Health

Health, then, in the Neuman Model is defined as the relatively stable internal functioning of the client. Optimal health exists when the client is maintained in a high state of wellness or stability. As in other nursing models, health is not considered an absolute state, but rather a continuum that reflects the client's internal stability while moving from wellness to illness and back. It takes a considerable amount of physical and psychologic energy to maintain the stability of the person who is in good health.

The opposite of a healthy state, illness exists when the client's core structure becomes unstable through the effects of environmental factors that overwhelm and defeat the lines of defense and resistance. These environmental factors, whether internal or external, are called **stressors** in this model.

Environment

The environment is composed of internal or external forces or stressors that produce change or response in the client. Stressors may be helpful or harmful, strong or weak.

Stressors are also classified according to their relationship to the basic core of the client-system. Stressors that are completely outside the basic core are termed **extrapersonal stressors** and are either physical in nature, such as atmospheric temperature, or sociologic, such as living in either a rural or urban setting. **Interpersonal stressors** arise from interactions with other human beings. Marital relationships, career expectations, or friendships are included in this group of interpersonal stressors. Those stressors that occur within the client are called **intrapersonal** and include involuntary physiologic responses, psychologic reactions, and internal thought processes.

Nursing

The nurse's role, in the Neuman Model, is to identify at what level or in which boundary a disruption in the client's internal stability has taken place, and then to aid the client in activities that strengthen or restore the integrity of that particular boundary. The Neuman Model expands the concept of client from the individual to include families, small groups, the community, or even society in general.

Nursing's main concern in this model is either to identify stressors that will disrupt a defensive boundary in the future (prevention), or to identify a stressor that has already disrupted a defensive boundary, thereby producing present instability (illness) (Neuman, 1989). The Neuman Model is based on the nursing process, and identifies three levels of intervention: primary, secondary, and tertiary.

Intervention. Primary intervention has as its main goal the prevention of possible symptoms that could be caused by environmental stressors. Teaching clients about stress management, giving immunizations, or encouraging aerobic exercises to prevent heart disease are examples of primary interventions. Secondary interventions are aimed at treating symptoms that have already been produced by stressors. Many of the actions that nurses perform in the hospital or clinic, (e.g., giving pain medications, or teaching a client with cardiac disease about the benefits of a low-sodium diet) fall into this secondary intervention category. Actions carried out at the tertiary intervention level seek to restore the client's system to an optimal state of balance by adapting to negative environmental stressors. Teaching a client how to care for a colostomy at home after discharge from the hospital is an example of nursing activities at the tertiary level.

 ## CRITICAL THINKING EXERCISES

CASE STUDY

Mrs. McCann, 88 years old, has been a resident of St. Martin's Village, a lifetime care community, since her husband died 8 years ago. Her health status is fair. She has adult-onset diabetes controlled by oral medication and a scar from a tumor behind her left ear that was removed surgically. The wound from this tumor removal has never healed completely, and it has continuously oozed a serous fluid requiring a dressing.

At St. Martin's Village, Mrs. McCann has her own apartment, which she maintains with minimal assistance, receives one hot meal per day in a common dining room, and has access to a full range of services such as a beauty shop, recreational facilities, and a chapel. She is generally happy in this setting. She has no immediate family nearby, and the cost of the facility was covered by a large, one-time gift from her now deceased husband.

Recently, she has become much weaker and has had difficulty walking, attending activities including meals, and changing the dressing on her ear. The Village's nurse is sent to evaluate this client.

1 Select two nursing models and apply the principles of the model to this case study. Make sure to include the concepts of client, health, environment, and nursing.

2 Apply the principles of systems theory to a county health department as a system, including input, output, feedback, entropy, and nonsummativity, among others.

3 Select three nursing theories and analyze how systems theory influences the development of each theory.

A Closer Look

SIMPLE APPROACHES TO PATIENT-CENTERED CARE

The implementation of nursing models to actual patient care seems to be a difficult if not impossible task to many nurses. Yet, several inexpensive and rather simple changes can help make nursing care much more patient centered.

At the Robert Wood Johnson University Hospital in New Brunswick, NJ, the ICU nurses recognized that the families of trauma victims brought very little personal care items with them in their rush to get to the hospital. The staff set as its goal the reduction of stress and easing the transition of these families into the hospital atmosphere. The nurses in the unit also wanted to let these family members know that they cared about their needs and comfort, and that they were an important and welcomed part of the healing process.

With a small grant of $500.00, the nurses now have available for trauma patients' families packets containing such items as a pen and pad of paper, toothbrush, tissue, lotion and small change for the phone or vending machines. In addition, the ICU now has two beepers that families can borrow if they are waiting to hear from physicians, or are outside the ICU waiting area during surgical procedures. Family members can now go for a walk or go to the cafeteria and not worry about missing the physician.

In an attempt to personalize the very impersonal and often threatening atmosphere of the ICU, the nurses have posted a board outside the Unit with the names and pictures of the nurses. Business cards with the number of the Unit are also distributed so that family members can more easily reach the Unit to ask questions about their loved ones.

The initial response has been very positive. Family members appreciate being given these comfort items when their loved ones are hospitalized in the ICU.

Modified from Gray, B: Patient driven system. Crit Care Nurs 15:94, 1995.

SUMMARY

As nursing takes its rightful place among the other helping professions, nursing theory will take on added importance. Nursing theory and models are the systematic conceptualizations of nursing practice and how it fits into the health care system. Nursing theories help describe, explain, predict, and control nursing activities to achieve the goals of patient care. By understanding and using nursing theory, nurses will be better able to incorporate theoretic information into their practice to provide new ways of approaching nursing care and improving nursing practice.

The development of nursing theory and models indicates a maturing of the

A Closer Look

REMEMBER GRADUATION DAY?—WHAT HAPPENED TO THE DREAM?

Graduation day is a big event in most individuals' lives. Graduation day from a school of nursing often leaves an indelible imprint on the graduating nurse's brain. The keynote speaker congratulates the shiny new nurses on their achievements in nursing school and for their choice of such a noble profession.

By 1 year after graduation, many of these same new graduates would have difficulty visualizing themselves in a noble profession. Because of the hours, the stress, and the seeming lack of rewards, nurses quickly fall into the view that nursing is a job rather than a profession. It becomes essential to reexamine periodically why they chose this profession in the first place.

There is no greater calling than to help those in need. Care of the patients and their families should always be foremost in the nurse's mind and heart. If the nurse does not do it, who else will care, clean a draining wound, and speak softly to a grieving family? Who else will convert the unspoken movements and gestures of a patient into a nursing diagnosis and care plan? Who else will look past the myriad of tubes, wires, and machines to acknowledge a frightened, helpless patient?

Only nurses have the education, the strength, and the ability to deliver high-quality care to every patient who seeks help. If the patient is viewed as the hub in the wheel of health care, and the members of the health care team as spokes focused on the care of the patient, then the importance of the profession of nursing becomes evident. All members of the health care team, as the spokes of the wheel, touch, support, and guide the patient along his or her path to recovery.

Many of the things that nurses do as part of their daily tasks take on a great deal of significance to the patients under their care. Simple tasks such as introducing themselves as the primary care provider, calling the patient by name, touching the patient with a reassuring hand, and explaining what will happen to the patient and what can be expected next are small, but vital elements in patient care. Through these types of actions, nurses lessen the fear and hasten the recovery of those under their care.

Modified from Lasscar, DA: What ever happened to nursing? Am Nurse 27(1):4, 1995.

profession. As the knowledge associated with the profession increases, becomes unique, more complex, and better organized, the general body of nursing science knowledge also increases. Only when nursing has this well-developed body of specialized knowledge will it be fully recognized as a separate scientific discipline and a true profession.

A Closer Look

WHAT DO NURSES REALLY DO?

At first glance, it would seem that everybody knows that nurses take care of clients. But what constitutes care? A recent study conducted by the faculty of the University of Iowa called the Nursing Interventions Classification (NIC) or simply the Iowa Project, has identified some 336 tasks or interventions that nurses are responsible for in their care of patients. Not all nurses carry out all 336 of these tasks all the time, but during an average career, a nurse would likely be involved in the majority of these tasks (see Closer Look Tables 1 and 2).

This project is an excellent example of how a nursing theory led to a research project which developed information that can be used by nurses in their day-to-day practice. Based on the belief that nursing interventions are specific actions that a nurse can perform to bring about the resolution of a potential or actual health care problem, the NIC attempted to identify and classify nursing interventions. It also attempted to rank those interventions according to the number of times a nurse was likely to perform one during a working day. The goal of this project is to develop by 1997 a nursing information system that can be incorporated into the current information systems of all clinical facilities. By using the NIC system, hospital administrators, physicians, nurses, and even the public should be better able to recognize and evaluate the multiple interventions that nurses are responsible for in their daily work.

It is a generally acknowledged fact that nurses, as the largest single group of health care providers, are essential to the welfare and care of most clients. Yet, in an age of health care reform, nurses are finding it increasingly difficult to delineate the specific contributions they make to health care. And if nurses themselves are unable to define the care they provide, how are the reformers, politicians, and even the public going to be able to identify the unique contribution made by nursing?

Unfortunately, many of the contributions that nurses make to health care are currently invisible because there is no method of classification for them in computerized database systems now in use. Commonly used nursing interventions such as active listening, emotional support, touch, skin surveillance, or even family support cannot to be measured and quantified by most current information systems.

The large number of different interventions used daily by nurses demonstrates the complex and demanding nature of the profession. The breadth and depth of knowledge and skills demanded of nurses on a daily basis is much greater than is found in many other health care professions.

One study found that nurses working in general medical/surgical units, during a 6-month period, were likely to care for 500 clients with over 600 individual diagnoses (many clients have multiple diagnoses). These researchers also found that the physical demands of the work were actually less difficult and tiring than dealing with the emotional and technical demands of handling the huge amounts of information generated by the care given.

Modified from Bulechek, G.M., et al.: Nursing interventions used in nursing practice. Am J Nurs 94(10):59–61, 1994.

CLOSER LOOK TABLE 1. Interventions Frequently Used By Individual Nurses

Intervention	% who use	Intervention	% who use
Several times a day		Family support	26
Active listening	80	Teaching: procedure	26
Medication administration	65	Presence	26
Emotional support	64	Mutual goal setting	25
Infection control	62	*Weekly*	
Medication administration: parenteral	60	Diarrhea management	27
Medication administration: oral	59	Urinary catheterization	27
Touch	57	Referral	26
Positioning	57	Blood products administration	26
Analgesic administration	55	Fever treatment	25
Intravenous (IV) therapy	53	*Monthly*	
Skin surveillance	53	Postmortem care	34
Presence	53	Dying care	33
Pressure management	51	Culture brokerage	33
Daily		Seizure management	30
Hope instillation	32	Guilt work facilitation	30
Family involvement	31	Ostomy care	28
Decision-making support	30	Urinary retention care	26
Sleep enhancement	28	Spiritual support	25
Family mobilization	27	Seizure precautions	25
Teaching: disease process	27	Amputation care	25
Foot care	27	Wound irrigation	25

CLOSER LOOK TABLE 2. **Interventions with Highest Use Rates**

Intervention	% who use	Intervention	% who use
Survey of organizations (n = 28)		Medication administration: topical	90
Active listening*	100	Medication management	90
Referral	100	Teaching: procedure/treatment*	90
Limit setting	97	Anxiety reduction	90
Communication enhancement	97	Calming technique	90
Emotional support*	97	Simple relaxation therapy	90
Support system enhancement	97	Infection protection	90
Discharge planning	97	Vital signs monitoring*	90
Health system guidance	97	Intravenous (IV) insertion	90
Patient rights protection	97	IV therapy	90
Teaching: disease process*	97	*Survey of individuals (n = 277)*	
Health screening	97	Emotional support	98
Risk identification	97	Presence	98
Coping enhancement	93	Active listening	97
Counseling*	93	Decision-making support	94
Decision-making support	93	Hope instillation	92
Hope instillation	93	Family involvement	92
Touch	93	Coping enhancement	91
Family involvement	93	Teaching: disease process	91
Medication administration: parenteral	93	Anxiety reduction	91
Teaching: prescribed medication	93	Communication enhancement	91
Teaching: individual*	93	Teaching: prescribed medication	90
Environmental management	93	Touch	90
Environmental management: safety	93	Infection control	90
Infection control*	93	Counseling	88
Specimen management	93	Environmental management: safety	87
Self-responsibility facilitation	90	Teaching: individual	87
Humor	90	Vital signs monitoring	87
Values clarification	90	Humor	86
Caregiver support*	90	Infection protection	86
Admission care	90	Environmental management: comfort	85
Analgesic administration*	90	Pain management	85
Medication administration	90	Security enhancement	85
Medication administration: oral	90	Discharge planning	85

*These interventions, along with Pain management, Airway management, and Nutrition management, were reported most often among all reporting organizations. Taken together, they represent core interventions across nursing specialities.

BIBLIOGRAPHY

Aguilera, DC: Crisis Intervention: Theory and Methodology. CV Mosby, St. Louis, 1990.
Fawcett, J: Analysis and Evaluation of Conceptual Models of Nursing. FA Davis, Philadelphia, 1989.
King, IM: King's theory of goal attainment. Nurs Sci 5:19–25, 1992.
Leininger, MM (ed.): Cultural Care Diversity and Universality: A Theory of Nursing. National League for Nursing, New York, 1992.
McCann-Flynn, JB and Heffron, PB: Nursing: From Concept to Practice. Robert J. Brady, Bowie, MD, 1984.
Mitchell, PR, Grippando, GM. Nursing Perspectives and Issues. Delmar, Albany, NY, 1993.
Neuman, B: The Neuman Systems Model. Appleton & Lange, Norwalk, Conn., 1989.
Nightingale, F: Notes On Nursing: What It Is and What It Is Not. Harrison, London, 1859 (JB Lippincott, reprinted Philadelphia, 1966).
Orem, DE: Nursing: Concepts of Practice. Mosby-Year Book, St. Louis, 1991.
Putt, A: General Systems Theory Applied to Nursing. Little Brown, Boston, 1978.
Riehl-Sisca, JP: Conceptual Models for Nursing Practice. Appleton-Lange, Norwalk, CT, 1989.
Roy, C and Andrews, HA: The Roy Adaptation Model: The Definitive Statement. Appleton-Lange, Norwalk, CT, 1991.
Schaefer, KM and Pond, JB: Levine's Conservation Model: A Framework for Nursing Practice. FA Davis, Philadelphia, 1991.
Stevens, BJ: Nursing Theory: Analysis, Application, Evaluation, Little, Brown, Boston, 1984.
Watson, J: Nursing: Human Science and Human Care—A Theory of Nursing. Appleton Century Crofts, Norwalk, CT, 1985.

HISTORICAL PERSPECTIVES

Influences of the Reformation (1517)

The origins of the Reformation are usually attributed to Martin Luther (1483–1546), in Germany. Although widespread discontent with certain religious and political structures of the Roman Catholic Church had been stewing for many years, Martin Luther, a Catholic monk, brought the issue to a head.

Health care in the Catholic nation-states, including Italy, France, and Spain, generally remained unchanged from that of care established during the Middle Ages. The religious hospitals run by monks and nuns still provided a consistent, if somewhat primitive, form of health care. During this period, the number of male nursing orders gradually decreased, so that by 1500 almost all the health care providers were nuns. New technologies were generally shunned, and nursing education continued under an apprenticeship form. There was little education for physicians beyond the knowledge gathered in the libraries and hospitals of monasteries.

Major changes in health care occurred, however, in the nation-states that broke away from the Catholic Church, such as England, Germany, and the Netherlands. The large monastery and convent hospitals had been rich and powerful centers of the Catholic faith. They were now seen as a security threat to the new Protestant leadership. The property the monasteries rested on was confiscated, and the monks and nuns of the nursing orders were expelled from these countries.

With no other health care structures in place to assume their functions, health care in these countries soon degenerated to a point worse than that given in the early Middle Ages. Under Protestant political and religious leadership, the status of women was gradually reduced from one of importance in the care of the sick and homeless to a level of subordination and dependence. Women were forbidden to work outside the home, and it was believed that their primary role was the care of the home, the bearing of children, and fulfillment of their husbands' needs.

Eventually, crude hospitals were established in larger metropolitan areas to provide care for those who could not be attended at home. Because women of the upper classes were forbidden to work outside the home, these hospitals were often staffed by those members of society who belonged to the lower socioeconomic groups. These groups included prostitutes, alcoholics, opium addicts, and convicted prisoners. Working in these rudimentary hospitals was hard, with long hours and poor pay. Often the nurses supplemented their meager earnings with property and money taken from the patients. The hospitals were often filthy, filled with fouled linens and human excrement. The care provided was substandard, and nursing in these countries was viewed as the lowest and most menial form of work that a woman could undertake. Male caregivers were not to be found in these hospitals, and the male nurse all but disappeared during this period.

Out of the health care chaos of this period developed secular nursing orders of nuns who gradually took over the care duties in these hospitals. The most famous of these orders, the Sisters of Charity, was established in 1600. Although the care and services provided by these orders was minimal, the general sanitation and ethical standards of the hospitals improved greatly. Also seen in hospitals run by these nursing orders was the development of a nursing hierarchy. The primary nurses were called sisters, and those designated to help the sisters provide care were called helpers and watchers. Although often no clear distinction in duties among these groups was made, the overall benefit of competent, skilled nursing care was beginning to be recognized.

Other positive developments in health care that occurred during this period included the writing of the first nursing textbooks and the organization and widespread use of midwives in the delivery of babies. William Harvey (1578–1657), called the father of modern medicine, was born in England, where he made major contributions to medical practice. A more modern understanding of the microbial origin of many diseases developed. Joseph Lister began to understand how disease was spread, and developed aseptic practices that are still used today. In France, Louis Pasteur discovered that bacterial organisms could be killed by heat, and the process of pasteurization was born. Although medical education was developing, it was still under an apprenticeship system, and involved the use of many home remedies. There were no standards for care for either nurses or physicians, and many abuses existed. Although hospitals were gaining importance, the majority of health care was still given in the home.

CRITICAL THINKING AND THE NURSING PROCESS

Learning Objectives

After completing this chapter, the reader will be able to:

1 Discuss the theoretical origins of the nursing process.
2 Use the steps of the nursing process in planning client care.
3 Analyze the use of the nursing process in a client-care situation.
4 Differentiate between a medical diagnosis and a nursing diagnosis.
5 Evaluate the three parts of a nursing diagnosis.
6 Identify four practices to be avoided in formulating a nursing diagnosis.
7 Formulate a properly written nursing diagnosis.

As the social, technologic, educational, and political environments of health care have changed, so has the practice of nurses. Historically, the practice of nursing has always involved multiple roles. Nurses have traditionally been concerned with client comfort, hygiene, environment, health, activity, diet, and family interactions. With the development of specialization in health care, other groups (e.g., dietitians, physical therapists, social workers) provide many of the care elements formerly provided by nurses. As a result, the nurse's role is equally divided between being provider of care and coordinator of care. The nurse now, theoretically, has more time to provide the type of care that is unique to nursing and to enhance client care by involving the ancillary care services.

One way in which nurses can accomplish this double-edged task in client care is through use of the nursing care plan and nursing diagnosis. Through the nursing process, nurses can apply the theory and models developed by nursing leaders to actual client care. By viewing the client through the framework of the nursing process, the nurse can meet the unique needs of each client. In addition, the nursing process is useful in defining the scope of nursing practice and developing standards for nursing care.

CRITICAL THINKING

One of the most important responsibilities that nurses have is to make correct and safe decisions in a variety of client care situations. The decisions made by nurses affect the health status, recovery time, and even the life or death of a client. For example, the critical care nurse must decide when to give certain medications, based on changes in the client's condition. The emergency room nurse must decide which client is treated first, based on the extent of injuries. The hospital staff nurse must decide what PRN (as needed) medication to give for which set of symptoms. The community health nurse must decide when to call the physician about a change in a client's condition.

The process by which these decisions are made involves the use of critical thinking. Critical thinking is based on reason and reflection, knowledge, and instinct derived from experience (Tappen, 1995). It reflects both an attitude about and an approach to solving problems. Critical thinking helps nurses make decisions about problems for which no simple solutions exist. Often nurses have to make these decisions with less than complete information.

An important element in critical thinking is creativity. Nurses who think creatively explore new ideas and alternate ways of solving client-care problems. Creative thinkers are able to bring together bits of knowledge or information that initially may seem unrelated, and to reformulate them into a plan that solves the problem.

Process

Although different approaches exist to develop critical thinking skills, certain steps are common to every process. Some individuals seem to have an innate ability to work through these steps, whereas others have difficulty with the process. As with most skills, practice and repetition increase efficiency.

Step 1: Identify the Problem

The adage "it's hard to know if you have arrived if you don't know where you are going" applies particularly well to critical thinking. If the underlying problem has not been identified, it is impossible to develop a plan to solve it. One way to identify the underlying problem is to try to restate the issue as a pro-and-con statement. For example, sexually transmitted disease (STD) in teenagers is a growing problem in our society. But what is the underlying problem? Is it a lack of education about STDs? Is there a lack of morals in our society? Or does it result from the atmosphere of permissiveness and egocentrism that is pervasive in the popular media? It may be a combination of all these factors.

Step 2: Identify the Underlying Beliefs

Everybody, including nurses, has an opinion and a belief about all issues. Some of these beliefs are personal, some cultural, some are stated overtly whereas others remain deeply rooted but hidden in the unconscious. In any case, these beliefs influence how situations are perceived and what decisions are made.

In order to make solid decisions based on critical thinking, nurses must examine their own beliefs and value systems. Value clarification is an important element in critical thinking. At some point in the nurse's career, preferably in the early stages, the nurse should make a list of all the things he or she considers valuable. This list might include such factors as family, education, job, honesty, good health, respect, and leisure time. After as complete a list as possible has been composed, the items should be ranked according to priority. It should also be recognized that this list is not static, that items will be added, deleted, or will change in priority with time.

Nurses also need to learn and evaluate the value systems of those they are working with. Even though they may not agree with those values, it is important to recognize them and work with them when attempting to affect health. For example, in teaching a group of high school students about STDs, it would be essential to know the students' attitudes toward sex and health. In all likelihood, these attitudes would differ from those of the nurse. An education program organized around only the nurse's beliefs and value system would be doomed to failure. Presenting the information from a student's viewpoint will help nurses better understand and perhaps be more willing to accept the student's worldview.

Step 3: Find Support for the Beliefs

All people have reasons why they believe certain things, rather than others. These reasons can be based on opinions or fact, and may be accurate or inaccurate. If the nurse tries to support a belief, but discovers a lot of inconsistencies, contradictions, stereotypes and biases, then there may be major weaknesses in that belief system. For example, a nurse working with teenagers may hold the stereotyped belief that all teenagers are rebellious, uncooperative, and promiscuous. In reality, there are large numbers of teenagers who work well with others, are highly productive, and have high moral standards.

There are a variety of places where support for various beliefs can be obtained. Written reports, surveys, and published articles are valuable sources of information. Additional data may also be obtained from others informally, such as during discussions with individuals who work in a particular field, or feedback from the clients who are receiving the care. No matter what the source, information needs to be evaluated critically for accuracy, consistency, cause and effect, and inherent biases.

The information is accurate if it conforms with facts. Is the nurse correct in thinking all teenagers rebellious, uncooperative, and promiscuous? Reviewing the literature and analyzing studies about teenage beliefs and activities will probably lead the nurse to conclude that this is an inaccurate stereotype.

The information is consistent with reality when there are several sources that support the same conclusions. Articles that summarize similar research and evaluate the findings are highly useful in assessing consistency of beliefs.

Often factors are considered causes when in reality they are merely associated effects. For example, lack of morals in the family setting might be considered a cause for the increase in teenage pregnancies, when in reality both the lack of morals in the family and teenage pregnancies are caused by the wider attitude of society toward promiscuous behavior. It is important when attempting to use critical thinking in solving a problem to identify the real cause, and then to direct the interventions toward resolving that issue.

Biases are unjustified personal opinions or prejudices. Biases and stereotypes, however, are sometimes taken as fact. Just because a belief existed for a long time does not make it true. In order to use effective critical thinking, the nurse must identify and eliminate these biases and stereotypes.

Step 4: Identify Where the Value Systems Conflict

A nurse using critical thinking will often be able to identify more than one solution for a particular problem. If this is the case, then the nurse must take a look at the solutions proposed to see if one or more of them conflict with a personal value system. For example, possible solutions to the teenage pregnancy problem include providing condoms for all high school students, performing tubal ligations on sexually active girls, or establishing strict night-time curfews. Although all of these solutions may be effective, the nurse would have to evaluate the accuracy, cause-and-effect relationship, and value positions of each of these courses of action. A nurse who is a critical thinker will consider each one of these before implementing a course of action.

Critical Thinking in Decision Making

Although critical thinking is used in all aspects of decision making, it is particularly important in the nursing process. As a way of looking at the world, critical thinking allows the nurse to consider new ideas, and then to evaluate those ideas in light of accepted information and personal value systems. Critical thinking makes the nursing process an orderly and effective solving tool for client problems.

THE NURSING PROCESS

The seeds of the concept now called the nursing process were first planted by the early nurse theorists in the late 1940s and early 1950s. As nursing has moved toward a profession with a unique knowledge base and a distinct theoretical orientation, the nursing process has developed into one of the essential frameworks underlying the profession (Avant, 1990).

Actually, the nursing process is not unique or original to nursing. Like other aspects of nursing, it was adapted from other areas of the sciences. The biologic and physical sciences have long used one of two systematic approaches in dealing with problems and questions. These approaches are termed the **scientific method** and the **problem-solving method.**

Although these processes may appear strictly theoretic, most individuals use a form of the problem-solving method every day to deal with all kinds of problems. For example, a nurse is on the way to work at the hospital by car when there is a strange thumping noise from the rear of the car. The nurse stops, gets out, and sees that there is a large nail sticking out of the rear tire, accompanied by a loud hissing sound as the air leaks out from around the nail (gathering information through observation). The nurse concludes that the tire is flat (analyzing the information and identifying the problem), and then decides that it will be necessary to take the spare tire and jack out of the trunk, jack the car up and change the tire (planning a course of action). After opening the trunk, the nurse actually does proceed in the changing of the tire (carrying out the plan). As the nurse lets the car down off of the jack, it is obvious that the spare tire is also flat, never having been repaired after the last time it was used (evaluation).

The steps of the nursing process are really identical to the steps in the problem-solving method except that they use different terminology, and are oriented toward the care of clients. When this systematic process is used in client care, it helps identify client behaviors indicating health care needs, define the specific health care need, develop a plan to meet that need, carry out the plan, and then evaluate its effectiveness. Using the nursing process in the provision of nursing care has the advantage of combining the various complex aspects of client care, including the psychologic, social, physical, and spiritual, in a coherent and organized way with the client as the central focus.

Many of the activities that nurses perform to care for clients are borrowed from or shared with other health care disciplines such as medicine, respiratory therapy, physical therapy, and pharmacology. Using the nursing process helps identify those activities that are unique to nursing and for which nurses are held accountable. After these activities are identified as elements of nursing practice, then standards of performance can be established (Moritz, 1991). Public accountability for specific actions is one of the first steps in making the transformation from nursing as a job to nursing as a profession.

The nursing process is not difficult to use. Beginning nursing students are instructed in its use starting with the most basic nursing courses. Because of its flexibility, even the most advanced nursing theorist can use the nursing process in the development of theoretic models, research, or advanced nursing practice. Of course, factors such as the knowledge and skill level of the nurse, as well as the health care setting of the nursing practice, affect how the nursing process is used.

Steps in the Nursing Process

Assessment

Assessment is the gathering of all types of information or data that relate to a client. There are many ways of making an assessment. Information can be obtained through interviewing, asking questions, performing a physical examination, and laboratory work, radiography and other tests. A physical assessment should follow the "head-to-toe" method, which evaluates each body system systematically.

Other data can be gathered by interviewing family and close friends, obtaining documents and information from other previous health care providers involved with the client, and reviewing old bedside charts.

Information is separated into two categories of data—subjective and objective. Subjective data include information that depends on the perceptions of the individuals interviewed, such as health history, descriptions of symptoms, and reporting of behavioral changes. Objective data obtained during assessment of the nursing process generally include factual and unbiased information such as temperature, blood pressure and pulse measurements, laboratory, radiography, and electrocardiographic (ECG) reports, skilled observations made by the nurse about the client's condition, and discoveries gained through the review of other health care providers' records about the client.

The goal of all assessments is to obtain data about the client's health care needs that help the nurse, client, and client's family identify underlying health care problems. In addition, nursing assessment can point out strengths and coping mechanisms that the client has used in the past to deal with similar situations. In general, the more information that is gathered through a systematic and thorough assessment, the higher the quality of the care plan developed by the nurse to meeting the client's needs will be.

Analysis

This is referred to as either the analysis or the diagnosis step. An insightful analysis of the data obtained must be conducted before a diagnosis can be made. Analysis is the process of sifting through all the information gained during the assessment, categorizing it according to the client's needs, and then formulating these needs into specific statements of need.

Nursing diagnosis represents the conclusions the nurse has made about the client's needs as deduced from the analysis of the data gained during the assessment (Carpenito, 1989). The nursing diagnosis specifically identifies those areas of client need that professional nurses can treat independently in the health care setting.

Planning

Planning for client care always begins with the process of formulating and establishing goals, or outcomes, for the client. Goal setting ideally involves the nurse, the client, and sometimes the client's family working together to plan achievable outcomes for meeting health care needs as identified by the nursing diagnosis. Well-planned goals should have three important characteristics—they should be client-centered, time-oriented, and measurable.

Depending on the health care situation, goals are often written with two time frames in mind. **Short-term goals** are those that a client would reasonably expect to achieve in several hours to several days. For example, a client with a myocardial infarction having severe chest pain will experience relief within 1 hour. Long-term goals are those that can be achieved in a week, to several weeks, months, or even years. A reasonable long-term goal for the client with a myocardial infarction would be to return to work in 6 to 8 weeks. Time limits provide criteria to help the nurse evaluate the success of interventions.

Goals established during the planning step of the nursing process should be stated in measurable terms. A behavioral objective specifies a particular behavior that can be observed and measured in the fulfillment of the goal. By assessing whether or not the behavior has been achieved, the nurse can evaluate if the goal has been met. For example, a 3-day post–myocardial infarction client will walk 50 ft without chest pain, shortness of breath, or increased heart rate and blood pressure.

After goals have been decided, the next phase of the planning step involves making a decision about which goals can be achieved by nursing interventions alone (independent actions), and which goals require cooperative interventions from other health care providers such as physicians, physical therapists, or dietitians (interdependent actions). Often, in the acute health care setting, many of the goals involve interdependent actions. In settings such as community health and psychiatric clinics, nurses function with a higher degree of independence. Goals that nurses can help the client to achieve without involving other health care providers can often be met sooner than those goals where other health care personnel are involved. For example, postoperative clients are at high risk for respiratory complications. Although respiratory therapy is helpful in preventing these complications, many independent nursing actions, such as frequent turning, ambulation, and encouraging the client to deep-breathe and cough, can also achieve this goal without having to wait for the respiratory therapy (RT) department.

Prioritizing. Establishing an order for achieving goals is also an important aspect of the planning step of the nursing process. There are different ways of prioritizing goals. First, the goals should be ordered according to the problem's immediate effect on the client's general health care status and viability as identified by the nursing diagnosis. These needs generally follow Maslow's Hierarchy of Needs (Box 3–1), that is to say the physiologic and safety needs must be met before higher-level needs, such as love and belonging, can be met. The physiologic needs include food, water, and elimination. In other words, the needs that are crucial for the maintenance of life receive the highest priority. These are usually categorized according to the airway, breathing, and circulation (**ABCs**) procedure that is taught in basic cardiopulmonary resuscitation (CPR) classes. Any nursing diagnosis and subsequent goal that includes airway maintenance should receive the highest priority. Nursing diagnosis and goals that have breathing as an objective receive second priority. Third priority goes to those nursing diagnoses and goals that deal with the maintenance of normal circulation.

Goals can also be prioritized according to the possibility of achievement. It soon becomes evident during the planning step that some *goals* are more likely to be achieved than others. Goals change. As higher-priority goals are met, lesser ones become more important. An elderly client who has been in an automobile accident and sustained neck injury may initially have high-priority goals of maintenance of airway and maintenance of neurologic functioning, but chronic constipation problems may also be present. In the immediate period after the accident, the airway and neurologic goals would have the highest priority. After the client is stabilized, and beginning to recover, the goal of maintenance of normal bowel function will become more important.

The planning step of the nursing process is completed when specific actions are designated, again in collaboration with the client, to achieve the established goals. When the key assessment factors, the nursing diagnoses, and the goals are

---

Box 3–1   MASLOW'S HIERACHY OF NEEDS

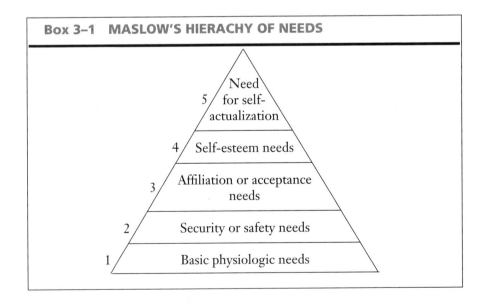

written down, they become the primary elements in the nursing care plan. The written nursing care plan is the road map of care that directs the actions the client and the nurse should take to achieve the proposed health care goals. As the saying goes, "If you don't know where you are going, it is difficult to tell when you get there." The nursing care plan tells nurses where they are going in the care of the client.

Implementation

When the actions necessary to achieve the client goals are initiated and completed, implementation has taken place. As in the other steps of the nursing process, it is important to involve the client in implementation.

Depending on which nursing model is being used, the implementation phase involves identical actions that are viewed as having different purposes. For example, in the Roy Adaptation Model, giving a client a bath is an action that *alters the focal stimuli*, and thus produces a change in behavior, or expressed symptomatology. In the Neuman Model, the same bath is viewed as a reinforcement of one of the concentric lines of defense, thereby reducing an external stressor, and re-establishing the client's internal steady state or balance. The bath, as a nursing implementation, has as an ultimate goal the maintenance of the client's health and comfort.

Evaluation

Evaluation looks at the behavior of the client to see if the goals have been met. If the goals are met, the nurse is successful in carrying out the plan of care. If the goals have not been met, the nurse needs to look at the care plan again to decide why they are unmet. Perhaps not enough information was obtained during the assessment step. Maybe the nursing diagnosis did not really pinpoint the major health care needs of the client, or the goals that were established for the client may have been unrealistic and not achievable from the start. Finally, there may have been a problem with the nursing actions taken during implementation.

Evaluation makes the nursing process circular and ties all the elements together. Nurses, historically, were not good at evaluating nursing care. Before the nursing process with its five steps became widely accepted, nurses tended to concentrate more on the action-oriented steps of assessment and implementation. Evaluating how the care affected the client was informal and disorganized. Very few criteria existed against which nursing care, as an independent health care entity, could be measured. With the recent development of standards of care, peer review, and quality assurance programs, nurses, like all health care providers, are now being measured against criteria established for the profession by other professionals. As health care professionals, nurses are expected and required to evaluate their actions and services in order to demonstrate that they have met the required minimum levels of care (Yura, 1988).

Evaluation does not just take place at the conclusion of the nursing process. It should be an activity that occurs throughout the nursing process.

NURSING DIAGNOSIS

Diagnosis has long been viewed as the sole responsibility of the physician. Dictionary definitions of **diagnosis** often describe the term as the art or act of identifying a disease from its signs and symptoms. And indeed, this is what physicians do when they make a diagnosis.

Another way of looking at diagnosis is as a process of conducting a careful examination and analysis to understand or explain something better, and then making a succinct statement about it. Although nurses have long been identifying clients' problems at an intuitive level, it was not until the early 1970s that nursing diagnosis became officially recognized as an activity that nurses could do independently (Gordon, 1992).

The initial steps in defining and formulating nursing diagnosis were met, as might be expected, with resistance from the medical community. Many physicians viewed it as a fundamental encroachment on their exclusive domain of medical diagnosis. Partially because of this fear and resistance, and partially also because of the pressure to make it something distinct from medical diagnosis, nursing diagnosis has developed into the rather cumbersome and often wordy enterprise it is today. This tendency toward wordiness may actually obscure rather than clarify the identification of client problems (Clark, 1992).

Nevertheless, nursing diagnosis is now accepted as one of the essential elements in the nursing process as well as a key activity conducted by professional nurses, important for identifying a client's nursing-care problems.

Although there are several definitions and descriptions of what nursing diagnosis is, the most widely accepted definition is the one adopted by the North American Nursing Diagnosis Association (NANDA) (Box 3–2), which began its work on nursing diagnosis in 1973 (Carroll-Johnson, 1991). NANDA describes nursing diagnosis as a clinical judgment about individual, family, or community response to actual or potential health problems or life processes. Nursing diagnosis also forms the basis for selecting certain nursing interventions for which the nurse is accountable. Despite its brevity, this statement implies several important elements that distinguish nursing diagnosis from medical diagnosis and reflect the true nature of nursing as a profession.

Nursing diagnosis is concerned with both health and illness, and with both the client's strengths and weaknesses. Medical diagnosis, on the other hand, deals almost exclusively with disease, illness, and injury. Nursing diagnosis takes a more holistic view on health and health care, and includes not only actual health care problems caused by disease and illness but also elements in the client's life, lifestyles, or activities that produce a healthy state or may cause health problems in the future.

Box 3–2   NURSING DIAGNOSES APPROVED BY THE NORTH AMERICAN NURSING DIAGNOSIS ASSOCIATION (11th Conference, 1995)

Activity intolerance
Activity intolerance, risk for
Adaptive capacity, intracranial decreased
Adjustment, impaired
Airway clearance, ineffective
Anxiety
Aspiration, risk for
Body image, disturbance
Body temperature, risk for altered
Breastfeeding, effective
Breastfeeding, ineffective
Breastfeeding, interrupted
Breathing pattern, ineffective
Caregiver role strain
Caregiver role strain, risk for
Communication, impaired verbal
Community coping, ineffective
Community coping, potential for enhanced
Confusion, acute
Confusion, chronic
Constipation
Constipation, colonic
Constipation, perceived
Decisional conflict (specific)
Decreased cardiac output
Defensive coping
Denial, ineffective
Diarrhea
Disuse syndrome, risk for
Diversional activity deficit
Dysfunctional ventilatory weaning response (DVWR)
Dysreflexia
Energy field disturbance
Environmental interpretation syndrome, impaired
Family coping: compromised, ineffective
Family coping: disabling, ineffective
Family coping: potential for growth

Continued on following page

Box 3–2 (Continued)

Family processes: altered
Family processes: alcoholism, altered
Fatigue
Fear
Fluid volume deficit
Fluid volume deficit, risk for
Fluid volume excess
Gas exchange, impaired
Grieving, anticipatory
Grieving, dysfunctional
Growth and development, altered
Health maintenance, altered
Health-seeking behaviors (specific)
Home maintenance management, impaired
Hopelessness
Hyperthermia
Hypothermia
Incontinence, bowel
Incontinence, functional
Incontinence, reflex
Incontinence, stress
Incontinence, total
Incontinence, urge
Individual coping, ineffective
Infant behavior, disorganized
Infant behavior, potential for enhanced organized
Infant behavior, risk for disorganized
Infant feeding patterns, ineffective
Infection, risk for
Knowledge deficit (specify)
Loneliness, risk for
Management of therapeutic regimen: community, ineffective
Management of therapeutic regimen: families, ineffective
Management of therapeutic regimen: individual, ineffective
Management of therapeutic regimen: ineffective
Memory, impaired
Noncompliance (specify)
Nutrition, less than body requirements, altered
Nutrition, more than body requirements, altered
Nutrition, potential for more than body requirements, altered

Continued on following page

Box 3–2 (Continued)

Oral mucous membrane, altered
Pain
Pain, chronic
Parental role conflict
Parent/infant/child attachment, risk for altered
Parenting, altered
Parenting, risk for, altered
Perioperative positioning injury, risk for
Peripheral neurovascular dysfunction, risk for
Personal identity disturbance
Physical mobility, impaired
Poisoning, risk for
Post-trauma response
Powerlessness
Protection, altered
Rape-trauma syndrome
Rape-trauma syndrome: compound reaction
Rape-trauma syndrome: silent reaction
Relocation stress syndrome
Role performance, altered
Self-care deficit, bathing/hygiene/dressing/grooming/feeding/
    toileting
Self-esteem, chronic low
Self-esteem, disturbance
Self-esteem, situational low
Self-mutilation, risk for
Sensory/perceptual alterations (specify):   visual/auditory/kines-
    thetic/gustatory/tactile/olfactory
Sexual dysfunction
Sexuality patterns, altered
Skin integrity, impaired
Skin integrity, risk for impaired
Sleep pattern disturbance
Social interaction, impaired
Social isolation
Spiritual distress
Spiritual well-being, potential for enhanced
Suffocation, risk for
Sustain spontaneous ventilation, inability to
Swallowing, impaired

Continued on following page

Box 3–2 (Continued)

Thermoregulation, ineffective
Thought process, altered
Tissue integrity, impaired
Tissue perfusion, altered (specify type)   renal/cerebral/
    cardiopulmonary/gastrointestinal/peripheral
Trauma, risk for
Unilateral neglect
Urinary elimination, altered
Urinary retention
Violence: self-directed or directed at others, risk for

Nursing diagnosis is limited to those actual or potential problems that nurses are qualified and licensed to treat independently. Diagnosing medical problems is not the function of professional nurses. Nurses need to diagnose those problems that can be treated with nursing interventions.

When diagnosing client strengths, the nurse looks for those internal biologic, psychologic, social, and spiritual characteristics that make the client unique. The purpose of identifying these inner qualities is to help the client use his or her resources in coping with health care problems or in achieving personal goals for health. Although these strengths are inherent in each client, nurses can help the client understand and develop them through appropriate interventions. A true therapeutic nursing intervention must include a realization and use of the client's own resources in dealing with health care problems.

Most time and effort spent in making nursing diagnosis is focused on client problems or needs. For most purposes, the terms **problems** and **needs** are used interchangeably when talking about nursing diagnosis. Nursing diagnosis divides client problems or needs into three relatively distinct categories: (1) actual problems, (2) potential problems, and (3) possible problems.

Actual problems are those that are affecting the client's health and well-being at that moment, and those that the nurse is able to identify from the data gathered during the assessment phase of the nursing process. For example, a client with a fractured femur would have actual nursing care problems such as alterations in comfort (pain), impaired mobility, and disturbed body image.

Potential problems are those that the client is at risk for developing because of a particular health care situation. Currently, potential problems are usually stated as "at risk for" problems. For the client with a fractured femur, potential problems might include a risk for altered tissue perfusion in the affected leg, risk for impaired tissue integrity if long-term immobility from traction was indicated, and risk for respiratory infection due to immobility.

The **possible problems category** for nursing diagnosis is used much less extensively than the first two categories. Possible problems are those that the nurse has identified from limited data and that constitute only a conjecture about a problem that may occur in the future. The client with the fractured femur may indicate that his insurance will take care of most of the hospital bills for several weeks, but expresses a concern that a longer hospitalization could lead to loss of income and creat a financial crisis for his wife and children. Possible ineffective family coping is a nursing diagnosis for this particular problem.

CONCLUSION

Nursing diagnosis, like much of professional nursing, is still in development. Many nursing students, as well as most nurses who were educated before the 1980s, initially find nursing diagnosis complicated and cumbersome to use, mostly because, to some degree, it *is* complicated and cumbersome. But it is an important step in the delineation of nursing as an independent profession. Through nursing diagnosis, nurses are beginning to be able to demonstrate that they perform important, independent functions in the health care system. By

CRITICAL THINKING EXERCISES

Use the steps in the nursing process to provide a plan of care, including at least two nursing diagnoses, for the following client situation:

> Mr. Y is 49 years old and has been complaining of chest pain starting in the center of his chest and radiating to his left arm and hand for 2 hours. He is having trouble breathing, is very pale, and has cool and moist skin. His pulse is 134 bpm and irregular, his blood pressure is 92/50 mmHg, and his respiratory rate is 24 bpm. He is very anxious, and expresses concern about having to leave his job as an accountant because of these symptoms. He is diagnosed as having an acute anterior myocardial infarction, and is admitted to the intensive care unit.

- What key assessment does the nurse need to identify as essential to this client's problem?
- What problems does this client have that a nurse can treat independently? Write nursing diagnoses for these problems.
- What can be accomplished in the nursing treatment of this client's problems (goals)?
- What type of activities can the nurse undertake to achieve the goals (intervention)?
- What does the nurse need to look for to see if the interventions have worked (evaluation)?

moving away from a task-oriented mentality and toward a philosophy based on the development of nursing treatment concepts, nurses are demonstrating that they can be accountable for the care they provide and meet the ever-increasing demands for high-quality care that a consumer-oriented client population seeks.

Nursing diagnosis will continue to change and develop as health care moves into the next century. Almost daily, categories and specific nursing diagnosis statements are increasing in number. As its acceptance by the medical community increases, the terminology and wording of nursing diagnosis is also undergoing change. Nurses have one of two choices regarding nursing diagnosis. They can choose to resist its use and continue to provide nursing care based on decisions made instinctively about client needs, or they can choose to work with nursing diagnosis and contribute to its refinement and validation as a skill that will guide nursing practice into the future. As a dynamic profession, nursing requires change and the ability to manage an ever-increasing array of complex client needs. Nursing diagnosis is a framework that can guide nurses in dealing with these changes.

ISSUES IN PRACTICE
Clarifying a Nursing Diagnosis

If it is unclear which nursing diagnosis is most appropriate for a particular client problem, the following three questions should be asked:
1. What are the most important health concerns for this client?
2. What can be done about the problem?
3. Which nursing intervention can best resolve the problem?
For example: In the client with a myocardial infarction, chest pain is a major concern, but does a nursing diagnosis such as alterations in comfort deal with the problem adequately?
- What are the most important health concerns about chest pain?
  It is a stressor that increases the heart rate, blood pressure, and overall workload of the heart, thereby placing the client at risk for more cardiac damage.
- Can anything be done about the chest pain?
  It can be relieved to reduce the level of stress, and reduce the workload of the heart.
- What are the nursing interventions that can be used to reduce the chest pain?
  In addition to using prescribed medications, and oxygen, positioning, and teaching comfort measures will help relieve the chest pain, thereby decreasing the stress on the heart and decreasing the risk for further damage to the cardiac tissues.
  Conclusion: An appropriate nursing diagnosis for this situation is Risk for Injury. A complete statement of the diagnosis might be: Risk for Injury: extended myocardial damage risk factor of prolonged and severe pain.

ISSUES IN PRACTICE
Errors to Avoid in Making a Nursing Diagnosis

1. Incomplete or inaccurate assessment may lead the nurse to miss a problem completely, or fail to recognize its seriousness.

   Example: A client with arthritis complains of lower leg pain. The nurse notes that the leg is tender to touch, but fails to notice that there is a warm, reddened area in the calf region indicating a possible thromboembolism. The client is not restricted to bed rest, and as a result develops a pulmonary embolus that requires emergency treatment.

2. Insufficient data, even with a thorough nursing assessment, is a chronic problem in health care that results in the misdirection of care.

   Example: An inebriated client comes into the emergency room complaining of chest pain. Due to his inebriation, he is unable to describe the characteristics of the pain, rate it on a scale, or state whether it is radiating. He is given nitroglycerine, and sent to the cardiac care unit. Later, it is determined that he has a hiatal hernia which often produces pain in the chest area.

3. Generalizations and stereotyping of clients and client problems may lead to inappropriate nursing diagnosis.

   Example: The belief that all elderly clients have difficulties with constipation may lead to the excessive use of cathartics and laxatives.

Modified from Sparks, S.M. & Taylor, C.M.: Nursing Diagnosis Reference. Springhouse, Springhouse, PA, 1993.

BIBLIOGRAPHY

Avant, K: The art and science in nursing diagnosis. Nurs Diag 1:51–56, 1990.

Benner, P: From Novice to Expert. Addison-Wesley, Menlo Park, CA, 1984.

Carpenito, LJ: Nursing Diagnosis: Applications to Clinical Practice. McGraw Hill, New York, 1989.

Carroll-Johnson, RM: Classification of Nursing Diagnosis: Proceedings of the Ninth Conference. JB Lippincott, Philadelphia, 1991.

Clark, MJ: Nursing in the Community. Appleton & Lange, Norwalk CT, 1992

Doenges, ME, Moorhouse, MF and Burley, JT: Application of Nursing Process and Nursing Diagnosis: An Interactive Text for Diagnostic Reasoning. FA Davis, Philadelphia, 1995.

Gordon, M: Manual of Nursing Diagnosis 1991–1992. CV Mosby, St. Louis, 1991.

Hildeman, TB and Ferguson, GH: Registered nurses' attitudes toward the nursing process and written printed care plans. Nurs Admin 22:5, 1992.

Iyer, PW, Taptich, BJ and Bernocchi-Losey, D: Nursing Process and Nursing Diagnosis. WB Saunders, Philadelphia, 1995.

Maslow, AH. Motivation and Personality. Harper & Row, New York, 1971.

McFarland, GK and McFarlane, FA: Nursing Diagnosis and Interventions. CV Mosby, St. Louis, 1989.

Moritz, P: Innovative nursing practice models and patient outcomes. Nurs Outlook, 39:111–114, 1991.

Weber, C: Making nursing diagnosis work for you and your client: A step by step approach. Nurs Hlth Care, 12:424–430, 1991.

Yura, H and Walsh, MB: The Nursing Process. Appleton Century Crofts, New York, 1988.

HISTORICAL PERSPECTIVES

Health Care in North American Colonies before the Revolutionary War

Health care in the New World varied somewhat from region to region depending on which nation or group was settling that particular area of the country. It also lacked resources to match even the minimal standards of the mother countries.

Mortality rates among these early settlers were extremely high. Quickly spreading diseases, infections, simple complications from pregnancy and delivery, and starvation frequently devastated whole villages. The five hospitals that existed in North America before the Revolutionary War were really no more than houses for the homeless and poor with rudimentary infirmaries attached to them. There were no identifiable groups of nurses for these infirmaries, and care of the sick was provided by other homeless people who had no health care training at all. The primary modes of nursing care consisted of prayer and folk remedies.

In 1658, the Dutch East India Company, one of the major trading companies of that time, founded Bellevue Hospital in Manhattan. It provided care for the newly arrived African slaves, and for sailors who had become sick at sea. With mortality rates ranging between 50% and 75%, Bellevue, the best of the early hospitals, soon became known as the "house of horrors."

Without any formal medical or nursing education, nor any system of registration or licensure to guarantee even minimal levels of competency, anyone with a strong back and a willingness to work long hours was hired as a nurse. Any man with even a high-school level education would be pressed into service as a physician, and quacks provided a large amount of the medical care. Women were considered subordinate to men, and usually were prevented from working outside the home.

After the initial period of exploration, conquest of the natives inhabiting the lands, and establishment of settlements, Europeans imported the same type of health care found in the mother countries. Health care in the regions settled by France and Spain was primarily provided by the religious nursing orders. An early French hospital, the Hotel Dieu, was established and staffed by the Sisters of St. Augustine. An early school of nursing was established in 1640 by the Sisters of St. Ursula in Quebec. Because of their religious orientation and the belief that care of the sick was an important element in living a Christian life, more Spanish and French religious orders established hospitals in the new world over the next 100 years. This care continued unchanged for many years, and religious hospitals can still be found in these areas today.

THE PROCESS OF EDUCATING NURSES

Learning Objectives

After completing this chapter, the reader will be able to:

1. Describe the process of educating nurses in early societies.
2. Compare the advantages and disadvantages of nursing education as conducted by the religious nursing orders.
3. Analyze the key elements that made the Nightingale School of Nursing unique for its time.
4. Contrast the major differences among the diploma, associate degree nursing, and bachelor of nursing science educational programs.
5. Discuss the origins and development of practical-vocational nursing education.
6. Discuss at least three types of advanced degrees that nurses may obtain.
7. Distinguish between the different types of doctoral degrees available to nurses.
8. Explain the concept of "Advanced Practice For Nurses."

Unlike many other professions, nursing has several related, but unique, educational pathways that lead to licensure and professional status. Indeed, the current system of nursing education creates a great deal of confusion about nursing, not only among the public, but even among nurses themselves. Perhaps the belief that "a nurse is a nurse is a nurse" developed from the fact that even though registered nurses may be prepared in educational programs that vary in length, orientation, and content, they all take the same licensing examination, and, superficially, all seem to be able to provide the same type of care.

The origins of the present diversity in nursing education can be traced to its historic roots. Although nursing education has changed, remnants from educational practices of the past are still found in even the most modern nursing education programs. Some of these have proven themselves over time and are valuable additions to current educational practices. Others are merely vestigial remnants that add little of importance to current nursing education.

THE APPRENTICE SYSTEM

In the earliest societies, nursing care was provided, but it usually took the form of care of the sick at home by one or more of the female members of the family. Through trial and error, these women discovered over the course of time which practices helped and which ones did not, and this information was handed down.

In other early societies where specific groups could be identified as health care providers with practices separate from those of the home setting, it was often difficult to distinguish between nurses and physicians. The primitive nature of medical practice even until the early part of this century made the separation of nursing practice and medical practice all but impossible. Much of what physicians did during these early times would be viewed as low-level nursing skills by today's standards. Most of what physicians did was being done at the same time by nurses.

Even though the skills were minimal and the knowledge requirements meager, some sort of educational system was required to prepare practitioners. The main form of education for nurses during this time was the apprentice system. A person who wanted to become a practitioner of nursing obtained the knowledge and learned the skills of the profession by becoming an apprentice to a nurse who was knowledgeable and skilled in nursing practice. The apprentice nurse became an unpaid assistant to the practicing nurse, often performing the less-glamorous duties the practicing nurse did not have the time or a willingness to perform. In exchange, the apprentice nurse got an education and usually free bed and board. This system formed the model for nursing education for many years.

NURSING EDUCATION IN RELIGIOUS ORDERS

The religious nursing orders that developed during the Middle Ages in Europe quickly spread throughout the known world at that time. The monks and nuns who organized and ran the monasteries and convents of that period believed that a key element in attaining salvation was to provide care for the sick and poor, in conjunction with prayer and lives of self-denial. The underlying belief that nurses should be selfless, totally dedicated to their clients with little regard for their own welfare, and morally incorruptible still exists to some degree today; and where it does, it can be traced back to the philosophical underpinnings of the medieval religious nursing orders.

When an individual entered a religious nursing order, the person first studied and learned what it meant to be a member of that order, and then learned how to care for clients. On completion of studies, the new religious (novice) took religious vows and became an official member of the order. Although there may have been a minimal amount of theoretic education, most of the nursing education was still obtained through a rigorous hands-on apprentice-type program that demanded equal amounts of prayer, study, and physical labor. The religious orders of the medieval period produced very dedicated, and very caring nurses, both male and female, who were highly skilled in basic nursing care techniques. This level of education was more than adequate during the Middle Ages when the advances in medical and health care practices over those of earlier days remained minimal. Later, during and after the Renaissance, when great strides were being made in health care–related knowledge, the rather inflexible nature of the religious orders' nurse preparation techniques caused them to lag behind these developments.

NIGHTINGALE INFLUENCE ON NURSING EDUCATION

Much of Florence Nightingale's early nursing education was obtained under the auspices of the religious nursing orders. During her formative years, she was also exposed to the secular health care practices of her native England, as well as the Protestant countries of Europe. She quickly became aware of the shortcomings of both forms of education for nurses. Although well-organized and sincere, the religious nursing orders were having difficulty keeping up with advances in health care. Many of these nurse training programs were only 3 months long. In the nonreligious health care sector, Nightingale noted the poor education and low quality of nurses, including their degraded social status (i.e., many were prostitutes) and dismal moral character.

After her work in the Crimean War, Nightingale established a school of nursing that sought to retain the best elements of the religious and secular programs, and to eliminate those elements that were detrimental to a nurse's education. The goal of the Nightingale School of Nursing was to educate nurses in a 1-year program to practice in both hospital and home settings, and also to prepare nurses who could themselves educate other nurses.

She accepted only women of good character and high moral standards into her school. These students attended lectures about theory in the classroom as well as practicing their nursing skills under close supervision in the hospital or home settings. Included in Nightingale's curriculum of study were topics such as preventive nursing measures, nutrition, hygiene and health promotion, mental health nursing, community nursing, and family nursing. She insisted on the scrupulous cleaning of all articles associated with patient care, and a clinical environment with sunlight and fresh air.

The major contribution that Nightingale made to nursing education, however, was her belief that nursing was both an art that required dedication and skill and a science that required an organized, systematic program of education to obtain the knowledge necessary to practice nursing competently (Seymer, 1954). One key to the success of her school was that it was run by nurses and was separate from, and therefore not under, the control of the hospital and the physicians who ran the hospital. A second key to her school's success was her belief that the primary goal of the school was the education of nurses, and not the provision of free labor for the hospital. She taught her students that the nurse's primary responsibility was to care for clients, not to carry out menial tasks that less-educated individuals could do. She emphasized the need for lifelong learning and education, one of the essential elements in the definition of a profession (Seymer, 1954).

After a rocky start, the Nightingale School of Nursing became a great success. Many of its first graduates went on to establish their own nursing schools based on the Nightingale philosophy, and became important leaders in nursing in their own right.

Florence Nightingale was one of the first nurses to recognize that formal, systematic education, both theoretic and practical, was essential for the preparation of high-quality nurses. During subsequent years, some of her key principles for nursing education were forgotten, or ignored for short periods, with negative effects on professional nursing. In recent years, the principles of education that she so strongly professed have again been recognized as important in nursing education.

HOSPITAL-BASED DIPLOMA SCHOOLS

The Nightingale School of Nursing was a **diploma school** in the strict use of the term. When nurses graduated from this school they were given a diploma, not an academic degree. The first Nightingale School graduates soon began establishing their own schools of nursing based on the Nightingale model and adhered to her philosophy of nursing education. These were also diploma schools. After an initial period of uncertainty and trepidation, both physicians and hospital administrators began to recognize that when the quality of nurses was improved, so was the overall quality of their hospitals. They also understood that these types of schools that were closely associated with hospitals could provide a source of free, or inexpensive, labor. Diploma schools sprang up throughout Europe so that, in time, each hospital had its own school of nursing. Many of Nightingale's principles and concerns about nursing education were abandoned during this period of growth.

In the United States, developments in nursing education, as with health care in general, lagged behind those in Europe. It was not until the middle 1870s that the first school of nursing was established in the United States. This was a diploma school that was attached to the New England Hospital for Women

(Jamieson, 1968). As in Europe, the idea of diploma schools quickly caught on, and within 10 years almost every large hospital in the United States had its own diploma school of nursing. These schools had very little in common with the Nightingale School of Nursing. There was no uniformity in curriculum, length of program, or requirements. To guarantee adequate enrollment, candidates were again being recruited from the lowest levels of society.

The hospitals used the student nurses as the major source of labor for their facilities. There was little or no classroom or theoretic study. The students learned exclusively by hands-on experience during their 12- to 14-hour work shifts. Most of the students consisted of young, single women recruited just after high school. The students were confined to dormitories on the hospital property. The dormitories were closely monitored by a house mother who enforced the rigorous rules of behavior, dismissing students for even minor infractions of the many rules. The early diploma schools of nursing were organized and administered on a model that was similar to the strictest of the religious orders.

The nurses who graduated from these schools were proficient in basic nursing skills, and could assume positions in the hospital where they were trained without any additional orientation or education. Because of the 24-hour-a-day, 7-day-a-week socialization process administered by these schools, diploma graduate nurses tended to be very submissive to authority, and willing to carry out any duty to please the physician, administrator, or head nurse. Before the advent of licensure examinations, and standardization of practice, nurses from diploma schools were often limited to employment in their own training institutions.

Diploma schools of nursing remained relatively unchanged in the United States until 1949 when the National Nursing Accrediting Service, working under the guidance of the National League for Nursing Education, became the licensing body for all schools of nursing who sought accreditation. The first formal accreditation of nursing schools occurred in the early 1950s. In 1952, the National League for Nursing (NLN) assumed accrediting responsibilities for all schools of nursing (Hegner & Caldwell, 1995).

In order to be accredited by the NLN, schools of nursing had to meet specific criteria, and to teach specific content in their curriculums. Many of the diploma schools of nursing could not or would not comply with these criteria, and eventually closed. Some of the requirements for those schools that did choose to comply with the NLN included a 3-year course of study meeting the criteria established by the state board of nursing, using only faculty with baccalaureate or higher degrees in nursing, developing a unique philosophy for their school, and demonstrating how that philosophy was implemented through learning objectives, course objectives, and outcome criteria, and by showing an adequate pass rate on the State Board, or National Council Licensure Examination (NCLEX).

One of the key factors that all state boards of nursing were concerned about was that the school should be able to demonstrate that the students were not being used as unpaid hospital personnel while they were in their education and training programs. When students could no longer be used as free labor, diploma nursing schools went from being virtually free to the hospital to being very expensive. Not only did they still have to pay for the room and board of the students, but they now had to hire and pay additional staff because the students could no longer be included in the overall staff numbers. Even more diploma schools closed due to the financial burdens to the hospitals. The ones that stayed open began increasing their tuition rates to the point where they were as expensive as programs granting academic degrees.

The 1960s and 1970s brought an increased awareness that for nursing to be considered a full profession, its members should be educated in institutions of higher education and should receive academic degrees and not just diplomas. Many diploma schools during this period became associated with universities and converted their curricula into degree-granting programs. According to the 1993–1994 statistics published by the NLN, there are only 128 accredited diploma programs still functioning. They are of universal high quality and meet all the standards necessary for NLN accreditation. The main emphasis remains on preparing nurses who are highly competent in the technical nursing skills through extensive hands-on practice in the clinical setting, but elements of leadership, humanities, and general sciences are also included in the classroom setting (NLN, 1990).

BACCALAUREATE EDUCATION IN NURSING

The development of schools of nursing in the university and college setting was a gradual process that extended over several decades. Only a few collegiate nursing programs were established during the years when the diploma programs were flourishing. Some of these early collegiate programs were a hybrid mixture of college-level classes and diploma school clinical experiences that still only granted a diploma, rather than an academic degree. Early attempts at college-level nursing programs sometimes took the form of "pre-nursing" courses over a 1- or 2-year period that prepared young women to enter schools of nursing. Generally acclaimed as the first university program to be completely conducted in the higher education setting, the University of Minnesota School of Nursing was opened in 1909. In 1923, the Yale School of Nursing began accepting students and is considered the first autonomous college of nursing in the United States.

The number of university-based nursing programs gradually increased over the years, and by the beginning of World War II (WW II) there were some 76 programs granting baccalaureate degrees in nursing. These programs tended to specialize in preparing nurses for public-health nursing, teaching, administration, and supervisory positions in hospitals. Although all these programs included a clinical component, the stress was more on theoretic knowledge, development of decision making skills, and leadership. Universities in general enjoyed rapid growth immediately following WW II, and higher education nursing programs expanded along with the universities. Many military nurses prepared by the Cadet Nurse Corps during WW I went back to school under the G.I. bill to complete their baccalaureate degrees.

During this rapid growth period, these baccalaureate degree programs were plagued with problems similar to those found in the diploma programs during their own rapid expansion period. Primarily, the lack of uniformity in content, curriculum, and even length of programs was problematic. It was difficult to find qualified faculty because most of the nurses up to this time had received their education in diploma programs. No doctorate degrees existed in nursing, few had master's degrees, and only a smattering of nurses had baccalaureate degrees. During the late 1940s and early 1950s, awareness began to develop that there was a need to stratify nursing education programs into technical levels and professional levels. It became apparent that all professionals should have, at minimum, a baccalaureate degree (O'Neal & Hare, 1990).

The NLN began to develop strict criteria for the accreditation of baccalaureate nursing programs. These criteria included courses in general education, general sciences, humanities, and language as well as specific nursing courses. They required a certain number of hours to be spent in the clinical setting practicing nursing skills, a faculty prepared at the master's degree level, and the availability of laboratory and library facilities for the students. Faculty-to-student ratios were to be limited, particularly in the clinical setting, and outcomes criteria for the students were required (NLN, 1991).

Although the concept of *Professional Nurse* had been around for many years, the American Nurses Association (ANA), the practice-oriented nursing organization, published an official position paper in 1965 recommending that the baccalaureate degree be the minimal educational level accepted in academic preparation for professional nurses. It further outlined what it felt were the key elements of professional nursing practice. The ANA believed that professional nursing was theory oriented, and involved the prevention of illness and the maintenance of health in conjunction with caring for and curing the sick or injured. Nurses who practiced professional nursing, according to the ANA, should be educated to supervise, teach, and provide direction to all who give nursing care.

As might be imagined, this position paper by a major nursing organization created a maelstrom of controversy and resentment. Diploma nurses, in particular, felt threatened, and became defensive about their form of nursing education. Physicians, who already felt that nurses were overeducated, criticized the plan. Hospital administrators had visions of rapidly increasing nursing wages as more and more baccalaureate nurses were employed, and so they also disputed the ANA's position. Greatly outnumbered by these opposing forces, the move toward professional-level education for nurses was quickly pushed into the background, although the number of university-based nursing programs continued to increase gradually. A similar resolution proposed by the ANA in 1985 also met strong opposition and was never enacted. This controversy remains unresolved today.

Although all university-level baccalaureate degrees in nursing have the same number of required credit hours and educational requirements for baccalaureate degrees, there are three avenues for attaining this degree. The bachelor of nursing science (BSN) degree fulfills the criteria to be known as a professional degree. It meets the overall requirements for a college baccalaureate degree (124 credit hours, 65 hours of nursing major, and most of the general education requirements), but does not meet all the general education requirements for an academic bachelor of science (BS) degree. Although this degree is usually obtained in a traditional college setting, it can also be obtained through an external degree program where the student has to meet the criteria for the BSN.

The second approach is found in programs that offer a bachelor of science degree with a major in nursing (BS-Nursing). This degree is the full academic college degree, and guarantees that the person holding it has met *all* of the general education, science, and major subject requirements. According to statistics published by the NLN for academic year 1993–1994, there are 526 accredited programs offering baccalaureate degrees in nursing.

A third avenue that may be pursued is sometimes called the *career-ladder* concept. These are individuals who are already licensed as registered nurses (RNs), but who have only either a diploma or associate degree (AD). There are a number of specialized schools, or departments within schools, that offer baccalaureate degrees specifically to students who are already RNs. These *Upper Division* colleges tailor their programs to meet the specific learning needs of RNs who may have many years of experience. Other programs may accept RN students and allow them to take examinations to prove proficiency (challenge out) in specific classes, thus giving them credit for their nursing experience. The RNs then take advanced-level nursing courses such as *Community Health, Leadership, Critical Care*, among others, that are not commonly found in diploma or AD programs. In either case, upon completion of the degree requirements, these nurses are granted a baccalaureate degree. There are 418 such programs accredited by the NLN (NLN, 1992).

PRACTICAL NURSING FILLS A GAP

The practical nurse, in one form or another, has been a part of the health care system in this country for well over 100 years. Although the earliest formal schools of practical nursing were started around 1890, informal training programs for this type of nurse probably existed well before this time, for example in the Young Womens' Christian Associations (YWCA), particularly in New York City. These programs took uneducated girls who had migrated from rural areas and farms to the cities in search of employment, and taught them a useful trade with which they could support themselves. With no regulation or accreditation for the early practical nurse programs, there were wide variations in the quality, length, and focus of what was being taught. Generally, these young women were taught to provide home care, similar to that given by private duty nurses for patients ranging from new borns to the elderly and invalid.

The number of practical nursing programs gradually increased over the next 50 years. Graduates of these 3-month programs were beginning to find employment in hospitals and nursing homes, as well as in areas of private duty. During the nurse shortage after World War I, many hospitals found that these relatively under educated nurses, after receiving on-the-job training in the hospital, could function at a fairly high level of skill, and at a much reduced cost. The word got around, and soon the number of these unlicensed nurses grew.

By the late 1930s, the ANA saw the need to regulate the quality of the practical nursing programs in order to protect public safety. It was not until 1938 that the state of New York took seriously the ANA's recommendation for compulsory licensure for practical nurses and enacted the first law requiring such licensure. About 20 years later, in 1960, all practical nurses were required to pass a licensure examination before they could practice. These nurses are now referred to as Licensed Practical Nurses (LPNs) (Licensed Vocational Nurses ([LVNs] in Texas and California).

Although education for LPNs or LVNs varies somewhat from state to state, there are some common characteristics. Most of the programs are from 9 months to 12 months long and are measured in clock hours rather than academic hours. They are often offered in hospitals, high schools, vocational schools, or trade schools, although a small number of programs are conducted in community colleges, or even universities. Orientation of the curricula in these programs is highly technical, and stresses the learning of skills in the setting of a hospital or nursing home with less emphasis on theoretic knowledge. It is much more important for practical nurses to learn *how* to do something than *why* it is being done.

The stated scope of practice for the practical nurse involves providing care for clients in hospitals, nursing homes, or the home setting for those who have stable conditions. These LPNs are to be under the supervision of an RN or a licensed physician. However, in the real world, LPNs are often required to provide care well outside of their scope of practice, often functioning in leadership roles, or by providing care in acute settings with highly unstable clients. LPNs are often hired when there are shortages of registered nurses to fill the gaps in client care. Many associate-degree RN programs have developed a ladder curriculum whereby an LPN can go back to school for a shorter period, often receiving credit for years of experience, complete the program in 1 year, and then take the RN licensure examination.

ASSOCIATE DEGREE NURSING

The nursing shortage after WW II created a crisis for the health care establishment in the United States. Even with the increased numbers of BSN and LPN programs, the hospitals, with their new technologies and expanded services, were seriously understaffed. The associate degree nursing (ADN) program was developed by Mildred Montague as a short-term solution to this problem (Kete-fian, 1993).

Originally designed to be technical, the 2-year ADN programs were offered through community colleges with an emphasis on developing the skills necessary to provide high-quality bedside care with less preparation time than it took for BSN programs. A successful pilot program for ADNs was conducted by Montague at Teacher's College in Columbia University in New York City in 1952. It demonstrated that community college–based programs could attract large numbers of students, prove cost effective, and produce skillful technical nurses in half the time required for BSN programs (Calhoun, 1993).

Some heated debate took place concerning licensure and titling for this group of nurses. The technical orientation of the curriculum was, and is, very similar to that of the LPNs, but the location of the programs in the community-college setting and the increased theoretic orientation seemed to elevate these programs to a higher educational plane. It was finally decided that the ADN graduates should take the RN licensure examination, rather than the LPN examination.

The emphasis on technical skills of the ADN programs met a need in the health care system of the 1960s and 1970s. By the early 1980s, there were over 800 ADN programs across the United States; the current number is 874, with over 64,000 students attending (NLN, 1992). Graduates from these programs soon exceeded the number of graduates from all the BSN and LPN programs combined. But as the nature of health care has become more complex during the last two decades, the original intention of the ADN programs to emphasize technical nursing skills has changed.

Gradually, ADN programs have incorporated more of the general education and theoretic courses of BSN programs. As the content in the ADN programs has increased, so has the length of the programs. Although it is possible to complete the requirements in 2 academic years, most ADN programs, in reality, take at least 3 years to complete for a new student who has no prior college credit (NLN, 1991).

ADN graduates, although generally well accepted by the health care establishment, are coming under increased scrutiny in some states due to the increasing complexity of health care needs. ADN graduates can provide safe bedside care for patients from the first day they are hired. They function well as team members, and after a period of orientation can assume responsibility for the care of patients who are more acutely ill. Yet, as ADNs attempt to move into leadership and management positions, the gaps in their education become more noticeable. Most of the ADN programs do not provide the theoretic basis for subjects of this type (NLN, 1992).

The most important question to be considered is whether or not an individual prepared in a technical course of study has enough knowledge to be a provider of professional nursing care in today's more complex health care system. If the answer is no, then something needs to be done with the ADN programs: either to upgrade them, or to reclassify them as producing people less skilled than professional nurses. If the answer is yes, then the BSN schools need to be closed down or converted into the more cost-effective ADN programs.

MASTER'S AND DOCTORAL LEVEL EDUCATION

The baccalaureate degree is considered a *generalist* degree that exposes a student to a wide range of subjects during the 4 years spent in college. The master's degree, on the other hand, is a specialist's degree (Forni, 1987). Students who pursue a master's degree concentrate their study in one particular subject area and become expert in that given particular area.

Master's-degree nursing programs have been in existence almost from the time baccalaureate-level nursing programs were started. These early master's degree in nursing programs were designed for students who had baccalaureate degrees in other majors, such as biology, who wanted to become nurses. After completion of an additional 36 to 42 credit hours in nursing courses only, these students were awarded the master's degree, and could then take the licensure examination for registered nurses.

Today, most master's degree in nursing programs are restricted to registered nurses who already have baccalaureate degrees. These programs require at least 1 year of clinical practice after the BS, and range anywhere from 36 to 46 college credit hours in length. Most students who enter master's-degree programs attend classes on a part-time basis while they are working, and may take up to 5 years to complete the requirements. Many universities have recognized this trend and have tailored their programs to meet the needs of these part-time students, offering courses in the evening, on weekends, or 1-day-a-week programs. There are 290 accredited master's-degree programs across the United States (NLN, 1992).

There are a number of available areas of study for those pursuing master's degrees in nursing. Some of the more popular areas include nursing administration, community health, psychiatric-mental health, adult health, maternal-child health, gerontology, rehabilitation care, nursing education, and some more advanced areas of practice, such as anesthesiology, pediatric nurse practitioner (PNP), family nurse practitioner, and OB-GYN nurse practitioner (Lipman & Deatrick, 1994). Most of these programs require the student to pass a comprehensive written or oral examination, and in some courses, to write an extensive research thesis before graduation.

There are two basic types of master's degrees in nursing. The masters of science in nursing (MSN) is the professional degree, and the master of science with a major in nursing degree (MS-Nursing) is the formal academic degree (Kalish, 1995). In practice, however, little differentiation is made between the two. Almost all master's programs accredited by the NLN require the applicant to have at least a 3.0 grade point average (GPA) and to demonstrate academic proficiency by achieving a satisfactory score on the Graduate Record Examination (GRE), or the Miller's Analogy Test, before admission. The GRE is also used to recommend remedial course work needed to correct deficiencies before the master's program is undertaken. There are a growing number of universities that are offering the RN to MSN degree to nurses who hold associate degrees and who now wish to increase the level of their education.

In the evolution of the various levels of education, the baccalaureate degree is a generalist's degree, the master's degree is a specialist's degree, and the doctoral degree is a generalist's degree, although at a much higher academic level than that of the baccalaureate degree. Actually, the major purpose of early doctoral degrees was to prepare the individual to conduct advanced research in a particular area of interest.

Currently there is a wide range of available doctoral degrees for nurses. The doctor of philosophy (PhD) degree is the most accepted academic degree and is designed to prepare individuals to conduct research. The doctor of education (EdD) degree is considered to be at a professional level, although in many programs there is little difference between the courses of study taken by the EdD and PhD candidates.

Since the 1970s, other doctoral programs for nurses have been developed that stress the clinical rather than academic nature of nursing (AACN, 1987). These include the doctor of nursing science (DNSc) and the doctor of science in nursing (DSN), which is a clinically oriented nursing degree. The doctor of nursing (DN or ND) degree is for the person with a BS or MS in a field other than nursing who wants to pursue nursing as a career. It is a generalist's degree at a basic level of education. In addition, for nurses who wish to pursue a career in higher education, the doctor of nursing education (DNEd) degree is available.

Despite the wide range of doctoral degrees in nursing, there are relatively few programs across the United States that offer these degrees. Many nurses who seek them may obtain them in fields such as higher education, psychology, college teaching, and adult education.

The requirements for doctoral education are similar, even though the specific degrees being sought are different. The student must have attained a master's degree, and again must have achieved a satisfactory score on the GRE. Often there is an admission interview and preprogram examination that must be passed before the candidate can be formally admitted to the program. Doctoral programs are at least 60 college credit hours in length, require many statistics and research courses, and often have a residency requirement. Before the doctoral degree can be granted, the student must successfully complete both oral and written comprehensive examinations, as well as write a doctoral dissertation explaining the conduct of a major research project.

Some individuals pursuing doctoral degrees do so on a part-time basis while they are working full-time, whereas others attend classes full-time while working full-time, often completing the program in 3 to 4 years. Many programs require that the individual complete all the requirements within a 10-year time period. Although this may seem like a long time, it is not unusual for the dissertation process itself to take 2 to 3 years.

Nurses with master's or doctoral degrees are looked upon as leaders in the profession of nursing. Many of the larger hospitals across the United States require their head nurses and supervisors to have master's degrees, and their directors of nursing to have doctorates. Of course, in higher education, the minimal requirement for teaching is the master's degree, with the doctorate preferred. Nurses with these advanced degrees provide direction and leadership for the profession though their publications, research, and theory development. As health care delivery becomes more complicated, larger numbers of nurses with advanced degrees will be required.

EDUCATION OF NURSES

ANA Position Paper on Education for Nursing (1965)

After evaluating changes in the health care system and studying the projected educational needs for nurses, the ANA published a paper in 1965 that took a stand on an issue that was, and still is, highly controversial.

For full appreciation of the significance of this paper, it must be examined from a historic perspective. The overall purpose of the ANA has always been to ensure high-quality nursing care to the public by fostering high standards of nursing practice. In addition, the ANA was concerned with furthering the professional and educational advancement of nurses as well as protecting the occupational welfare of nurses. To achieve these goals, the ANA took responsibility for establishing the scope of practice for nurses and for guaranteeing the competence of those who claim the title of nurse.

After WW II, there was an explosion of scientific and technologic knowledge used in health care. The educational level of the population was also increasing, thus resulting in greater public demand for more and better health care. In re-evaluating the nature and scope of nursing practice, and the type and level of quality of education needed to meet these new demands, the ANA reached the conclusions that are presented in its position paper.

Since 1965, the ANA has upheld the belief that baccalaureate education should be the basic level of preparation for professional nurses. Specifically, the ANA concluded that:

> The education for all those who are licensed to practice nursing should take place in institutions of higher education; minimum preparation for beginning professional nursing practice at the present time should be the baccalaureate degree education in nursing; minimum preparation for beginning technical nursing practice at the present time should be associate degree education; education for assistants in the health care service occupations should be short, intensive pre-service programs in vocational education institutions rather than on the job training (ANA Position Paper on Education, 1965).

There were a number of assumptions on which the ANA based this position paper. These included:

1 Nursing is a helping profession and, as such, provides services that contribute to the health and well-being of people.
2 Nursing is of vital consequence to the individual receiving services; it fills needs that cannot be met by the person, by the family, or by other persons in the community.
3 The demand for the services of nurses will continue to increase.
4 The professional practitioner is responsible for the nature and quality of all nursing care that clients receive.
5 The services of professional practitioners of nursing will continue to be supplemented and complemented by the services of nurse practitioners who will be licensed.
6 Education for those in the health care professions must increase in depth and breadth as scientific knowledge expands.
7 The health care of the public, in the amount and to the extent needed and demanded, requires the services of large numbers of health-occupation workers, in addition to those licensed as nurses, to function as assistants to nurses. These workers are presently designated nurse's aides, orderlies, assistants, and attendants.
8 The professional association must concern itself with the nature of nursing practice, the means for improving nursing practice, and the standards for membership in the professional association (ANA Position Paper on Education, 1965).

The rationale for taking such a strong stand on the future of nursing education derived from recognition by the profession of its heritage, its immediate problems, the emerging social issues and trends, the nature of nursing practice, and the extent to which nurses could realistically enact changes for continued professional progress. The ANA drew upon Florence Nightingale's vision of nursing and nursing education, which stressed the value of education for the development of the profession. It was important to Nightingale that schools of nursing be independent of hospitals, and that they have a strong theoretic component to undergird clinical practice.

By recognizing the increasing complexity of society, the ANA realized that nursing was not only becoming more specialized but also moving toward greater interdependence with other groups in society. One of these key groups was the U.S. federal government. As the government began increasing aid for nursing education, educational facilities expanded, providing greater opportunities for professional advancement. Larger numbers of students with more varied backgrounds were recruited into the profession, requiring greater flexibility in nursing education programs to accommodate their needs. Schools of nursing were, at the same time, also hard pressed to meet the attendant demands of science and technology, which were changing the traditional role of nurses. In addition to expanding roles for nurses, greater consumer awareness and expectations were placing new demands on the abilities of nurses.

As long ago as 1965, the ANA recognized that nurses were required to master a very large and extremely complex body of knowledge. Added to this was the demand that nurses be able to make critical and independent decisions about client care.

Effects of the ANA Paper on Education

The implications of this paper were far reaching, and highly controversial. It affected many different elements of society and the health care industry.

Hospitals recognized that they would no longer retain their traditional role of preparing nurses for practice. Even though pressure to move nursing education from hospital-based diploma schools to institutions of higher education had been building for some time, in the mid-1960s, a full 75% of the graduating nurses were awarded diplomas (Fitzpatric, 1983).

Colleges and universities were hard pressed to develop undergraduate and graduate programs quickly for nursing majors. The relatively few and small baccalaureate programs in existence at the time were called on to expand their programs rapidly. It also became evident that a clear distinction between technical and professional programs needed to be made.

To this day, the ANA remains firmly committed to its stand that all nursing education should be housed in institutions of higher learning. Even 30 years after this statement was made, the profession of nursing is still trying to reach a consensus on the issue of basic educational preparation for entry into practice. Continuing discussion and efforts to bring about collaborative agreement on nursing education is a goal that the profession must work toward. Only after the issue of basic entry-level education for professional nursing is resolved, and when nurses, like all other professionals, obtain their knowledge from recognized schools of higher education, will nursing as a profession be able to resolve its other important problems. Advancement of clinical practice, preparation for advanced practice roles, and increasing the body of nursing knowledge all depend on baccalaureate entry-level education for professional nurses.

EDUCATION FOR ADVANCED PRACTICE

Advanced practice is one of those often misused terms in nursing that adds to the public's confusion about educational levels of those in the profession. Sometimes referred to as involved in expanded practice, nurses who obtain certification in these areas are allowed to practice on a higher and more independent level depending on the nurse practice act of their individual state. Advanced practitioners diagnose illnesses, prescribe medications, conduct physical examinations, and refer clients to specialists for more intensive follow-up care. These nurses practice nursing under their own licenses, but often work closely with a physician, so that they can quickly refer clients' medical problems that lie outside their scope of practice.

The nurse practitioner levels of nursing are most widely accepted as advanced practice areas for nursing. These include the pediatric nurse practitioner (PNP), the neonatal nurse practitioner (NNP), the geriatric nurse practitioner (GNP), the OB-GYN nurse practitioner, the family nurse practitioner (FNP), rehabilitation nurse practitioner (RNP), the psychiatric nurse practitioner, and the nurse midwife. The certified registered nurse anesthetist (CRNA) is the oldest of the advanced practice certificates for nurses, and is already well accepted in the medical community.

In the past, nurses with baccalaureate degrees could attend highly concentrated courses of study for 1 to 2 years, and become increasingly proficient in a particular specialty area without, however, obtaining any specific academic degree. They could then take the certification examination and become certified as nurse practitioners. Currently nurse practitioner programs are offered in major universities, which require the student to complete a master's degree before allowing them to take the certification examination.

One job classification of nursing that falls under the umbrella of advanced practice is the **clinical nurse specialist.** Although there are a few schools that offer specific clinical nurse specialists curricula, more often these nurses are self-classified as clinical nurse specialists after completing a master's degree, or some additional education, in a particular clinical area. They are usually hired by hospitals, and often function as in-service educators for the hospital. Recently, the state of New York passed a law that prevents the use of the title of clinical nurse specialist. All advanced practice nurses in New York are now to be termed **nurse practitioners.** As can be imagined, this change has produced a great deal of confusion concerning what the scope of practice of these clinical nurse specialists/nurse practitioners is to be. The resulting debate about this issue will lead to a clearer definition and understanding of the term **advanced practice nurses.**

The opportunities for advanced practice nurses are vast. Although many nurse practitioners work for county health departments, rural clinics and on Native-American reservations, others work in hospitals, with physicians in private practice, in rehabilitation centers, or have even established their own independent clinics. They provide primary health care services in areas where there is a lack of primary care physicians. Although many of these areas are traditionally rural, today inner-city areas also often have need for this type of health care.

In addition, a common element of the several proposed national health care plans is the requirement that a client seeking entry into the health care system be evaluated by a primary health care practitioner before referral to any specialized health care practitioner. Although the family practice physician, or general practitioner, would be the most common primary health care provider to evaluate the client, the nurse practitioner could also meet this requirement. If any of these proposed health care plans are adopted on a national level, the demand for nurse practitioners will increase tremendously.

A Closer Look

CRITICAL THINKING: A STRATEGY FOR SOLVING PROBLEMS

Nurses have always been called upon to make clinical decisions that are based on a strong body of knowledge. Nurses have constantly been challenged to use their reasoning ability to recognize and choose appropriate courses of action for patients in changing situations. These are exercises in critical thinking. Why then all the renewed current emphasis being placed on critical thinking?

The critical thinking skills that nurses have long used informally in patient care are even more crucial in a rapidly changing consumer-oriented health care system. The ability to use logical and analytical skills, in conjunction with intuitive and creative problem-solving abilities is required to survive the vagaries of the current health care system. For example, nurses frequently deal with controversial ethical issues such as the right to die. By using a critical thinking approach to this type of issue, nurses can identify the essential elements and work toward a satisfactory resolution of the dilemma. In addition, nurses who can integrate logical elements with the more intuitive have a much better chance to provide care in a flexible, individualized way.

Nurses have been traditionally educated in a system that stressed logical and systematic approaches to solving patient problems. Emphasis was placed upon didactic knowledge and manual skill perfection as the measures of a nurse's success in the health care system. This approach worked perfectly well in a system where patients viewed themselves as the mere recipients of care. In today's society, more and more patients insist on taking an active part in their care, participating at all levels ranging from the actual physical care to the final decision-making process. Nurses who were professionally prepared under the old system are finding it difficult to adjust to the new consumer-focused health care system.

Although critical thinking has a number of different definitions, the key elements common to many of the definitions include the ability to solve problems creatively by both processing technical information logically, and by using intuition to guide the application of that information. The ability to use intuition in conjunction with a logical approach to problems allows nurses to make fast and accurate decisions about care, while helping the patient deal with the patient's emotions and physical needs. This type of thinking is much more difficult to teach than simple logical problem solving.

An important first step in learning real critical thinking is the identi-
Continued on following page

CRITICAL THINKING: A STRATEGY FOR SOLVING PROBLEMS (Continued)

fication and recognition of the nurse's style of processing information. Many nurses rely on a logical and analytical approach to do this. Once a nurse's personal style is identified, allowing or even requiring that nurse to use a different approach expands her or his ability to adapt to different situations.

Critical thinking in the current health care system is an ex-tremely important skill. Nurses who can use creative methods to solve problems at the beside are essential for the survival of the profession. Nurses who share those experiences with other nurses in which critical thinking was used to solve problems increases the insight of both participants into the process. Nursing, can only be strengthened when nurses understand that creative problem solving is the key to meeting the needs of future health care consumers.

Brookfield, S: On impostorship, cultural suicide, and other dangers: How nurses learn critical thinking. J Cont Educ Nurs 24:197–205, 1993.

Snyder, M: Critical thinking: A foundation for consumer-focused care. J Cont Educ Nurs 24:206–210, 1993.

 ## CRITICAL THINKING EXERCISES

1 Discuss why the current educational system for nurses leads to confusion over the role and scope of practice for nurses.

2 Develop an *ideal* educational program for nurses that would include all the key aspects of a required curriculum.

3 What historic factors had an important influence on the development of nursing education as it is currently conducted in the United States?

4 What should the minimum level of education be for the professional nurse—ADN, BSN, MSN? Defend your position.

5 The current over-supply of nurses and health care reform are likely to produce changes in nursing education. Identify possible changes that may occur in nursing education because of this over-supply. Will these changes be beneficial or harmful to the profession of nursing?

A Closer Look

DELEGATION—ESSENTIAL ELEMENT IN THE RN ROLE

With the recent trend in health care toward increasing the use of unlicensed assisting personnel (UAP), the ability to make decisions about what responsibilities can be delegated and to whom has become a major responsibility of RNs. Delegation involves the transfer of authority to a competent individual to do a selected nursing task in a specific situation. When the nurse delegates a task or series of tasks to a UAP, the UAP is responsible for performing the task; however, the RN retains the ultimate responsibility and accountability for the total nursing care of the client. Although delegation of tasks is not a new role for RNs, its sudden increase has made many RN uncomfortable, particularly if their education program has not prepared them for assuming this responsibility.

Guidelines for delegation were established by the National Council of State Boards of Nursing in 1990. According to these guidelines, the decision to delegate should be based upon:

1 Determination of the task, procedure or function that is to be delegated
2 Staff available
3 Assessment of client needs
4 Consideration of the potential delegatee's abilities
5 Consideration of the level of supervision available and a determination of the level and method of supervision required to assure safe practice

Schools of nursing need to include classes on delegation as the requirements for nurses to develop the skill of delegation increases in importance. Making a decision about whether or not to delegate a nursing task based upon UAP job description, client circumstances, difficulty of the task, and staffing patterns involves a high level of decision-making skills. In making this sort of decision, the RN often places her license, career, and future on the line.

Modified from National Council of State Boards of Nursing, Inc. (1995).

ACUTE CARE NURSE PRACTITIONER—SUPPORTED BY AACN

A new category of nurse practitioners has developed in recent years—Acute Care Nurse Practitioners. These nurse practitioners practice advanced nursing in the hospital setting, often in the critical care unit. As might be imagined, difficulties about their scope of practice, role, and functions have arisen.

The American Association of Critical-Care Nurses (AACN) supports this role of advanced nursing practice. The AACN views this new role for nurses as an integral element in the development of a health care system driven by the needs of patients and their families rather than the needs of hospitals and physicians.

Among other efforts, the AACN is collaborating with other nursing organizations, such as the National Organization of Nurse Practitioner Faculty, the Oncology Nursing Society, and so forth on advanced practice issues, building a state and national data base on advanced practice nurses, promoting the development of educational guidelines, and planning continuing education for advanced practice nurses. One of the most important undertakings of the AACN is to support legislation that eliminates restrictions and regulations on advanced practice nurses. Some of the long-term goals include gaining prescriptive authority, allowing hospital privileges, and supporting reimbursement mechanisms for all advanced practice nurses.

Although the current numbers of acute care nurse practitioners remain small, efforts to define and widen their scope of practice promote the role. Nurses who are interested in practicing acute or critical care at an advanced level should seek educational programs that would prepare them for this role.

Modified from Caterinicchio, MJ: Advanced practice. AACN News, February 1995, p 3.

CRITICAL CARE MEETS HOSPICE CARE

My friend Marjorie was within days of dying of colon cancer. Two years before, after her initial surgery, she had told me that the high point of her hospital stay was when a private duty nurse gave her a "wonderful, wonderful bath." Since it was Thanksgiving and her hospice team wouldn't be providing services, I offered to come to her home and bathe her.

I felt a bit intimidated because I've never been known to give a "wonderful" bath. I'm a critical care nurse, not a hospice nurse. When you give a bath in the ICU, you have to sandwich it in between giving meds, doing Swan-Ganz readings, and answering phone calls from relatives. You're always on guard for other things. Right in the middle, you have to peek outside the curtain to make sure another patient isn't falling out of bed. Or you may have to slap the washcloth back into the basin if you hear the cardiac monitor alarm across the aisle.

Marjorie's bathroom was near her bed, so I put some warm, soapy water in the sink. I spread soft towels over and under her. I noticed her lips were flaking and sent her husband to the convenience store for Vaseline. I was relieved he wouldn't be there to watch me.

As I washed Marjoire's chest, I noticed her respirations were rather slow. They weren't labored, but she was breathing only seven times a minute. My initial reaction was: *Hold the morphine! This woman's respirations are only seven!* But I'm a critical care nurse, and this was hospice care.

I went on to bathe her abdomen. She hadn't eaten for days. Her colostomy bag was bone dry, but she wasn't hungry. I looked down at her Foley. There was about 120 mL of urine in the bag. "How long since that's been emptied?" I asked her. "Day before yesterday," she replied. I thought: *She needs to be hydrated! Sink an IV! Give her fluids!* But this wasn't critical care.

I finally finished washing her front and dried her, trying to keep her cold body from losing heat. Apologizing, I said, "Marjorie, I've never been able to give a bath that's a work of art."

"You're doing fine," she said very slowly. "You're doing just fine."

Turning her onto her side, I wondered: *Percussion and postural drainage? No. She's comfortable, she's dying, I'm not going to bother her. I wish I could squelch that critical care in me.*

I massaged the reddened areas—stage I decubiti—on her heels and sacral area, even though maybe you're not supposed to. I asked her if she had any powder, and she said, "Well, the hospice nurse said powder isn't good for me." I rummaged through her bureau drawer and found some,

Continued on following page

CRITICAL CARE MEETS HOSPICE CARE (Continued)

figuring that if you like powder, you're entitled to it during your last few days of life. I finished the bathing, put on lotion, and sprinkled the powder liberally around.

By then her husband had returned and we put Vaseline on her lips and propped her up on some pillows. I gave her a kiss and said good-bye. I'd never kissed a patient before.

That night in the ICU I took care of a man who was a "full code." He too was dying of cancer. He'd had chemotherapy a few days before. He was in pain and disoriented but I had to withhold pain medication because his blood pressure was low. He had a tracheostomy and was on a respirator. I suctioned and turned him. I restrained his hands because he was grabbing at his trach tube.

I checked his feeding tube to make sure no residual remained in his stomach. The feeding had gone through him, all right. I cleaned him up for diarrhea five times during the 12-hour shift. His urine output was getting low, so I called the doctor for an order to increase IV fluids and for something to quell his diarrhea. And I gave him a bath—with many interruptions.

Both Marjorie and he died the following Tuesday—she at home in her own bed, powdered and comfortable; he, his hands tied down, with discarded vials of epinephrine at his bedside.

Her choice . . . his choice. No problem. Just a little discomfort in the mind of a critical care nurse who masqueraded one day as a hospice nurse.

BIBLIOGRAPHY

American Association of Colleges of Nursing: Indicators of quality in doctoral programs in nursing. J Prof Nurs 3:72–74, 1987.

American Nurses Association: Position Paper on Education. American Nurses Association, Kansas City, MO, 1965.

Calhoun, J: The Nightingale pledge: A commitment that survives the passage of time. Nurs Hlth Care 14:130–136, 1993.

Fitzpatrick, ML: Prologue to Professionalism. Brady, Bowie, MD, 1983.

Forni, PR: Nursing's diverse master's programs: The state of the art. Nurs Hlth Care 8:770–775, 1987.

Hegner, BR and Caldwell, E: Nursing Assistant: A Nursing Process Approach. ed. 6. Delmar Publishers, Albany, NY, 1995.

Jamieson, EM, Sewall, MF and Suhrie, EB: Trends in Nursing History. WB Saunders, Philadelphia, 1968.

Kalish, PA and Kalish, BJ: The Advance of American Nursing, ed 3. JB Lippincott, Philadelphia, 1995.

Ketefian, S: Moving beyond traditional boundaries. J Prof Nurs 9:25–31, 1993.

Lipman, TH and Deatrick, JA: Enhancing specialist preparation for the next century. J Nurs Educ 33:53–58, 1994.

National League for Nursing: Characteristics of Associate Degree Education in Nursing. Council of Associate Degree Programs, National League for Nursing, New York, 1992.

National League for Nursing: Characteristics of Baccalaureate Education in Nursing. Council of Baccalaureate and Higher Degrees, National League for Nursing, New York, 1987.

National League for Nursing: Criteria and Guidelines for Accreditation of Associate Degree Programs, ed 7. Council of Associate Degree Programs, National League for Nursing, New York, 1991.

National League for Nursing: Education Outcomes of Associate Degree Programs Roles and Competencies. Council of Associate Degree Programs. National League for Nursing, New York, 1990.

O'Neal, EH and Hare, DM: Prospectives on Health Care Professions. Duke University Press, Durham, NC, 1990.

Seymer, LR: Selected Writings of Florence Nightingale. Macmillan, New York, 1954.

 HISTORICAL PERSPECTIVES

Health Care in Early America

It was perhaps inevitable that the colonies of Great Britain in North America, established on the principle of freedom of religion, would eventually attempt to break away from the mother country. Life as a colonial soldier was dangerous and deadly, perhaps less because of English and Hessian musket balls than from starvation, hypothermia, and disease. Especially during the winters, dysentery, scarlet fever, and smallpox devastated whole camps. There was no organized medical or nursing corps for this rag-tag army, but small groups of untrained volunteers cared for the wounded and sick in their own homes, or in large buildings such as churches.

Before the Revolutionary War, Benjamin Franklin founded the Pennsylvania Hospital in 1751, which was the first hospital in the British Colonies dedicated to treatment of the sick. This hospital had separate areas for the sick, the insane, and those who were afflicted with moral defects, that is, those considered morally degenerate. Another facility, the Philadelphia Dispensary, was founded in 1786 under the auspices of the Society of Friends (Quakers) to provide free outpatient care for the poor, as well as surgical, obstetric, and medical services for those who could not pay.

New York Hospital was established in 1791. It offered classes in basic health, the biologic sciences, and even child delivery and child care. With wider religious freedom after the conclusion of the Revolutionary War, religious nursing orders such as the Dominicans, Sisters of Mercy, Lutheran deaconesses (Germany), and the Sisters of Charity began to establish hospitals based on their European prototypes. Through the influx of these religious nursing orders, the standards of health care in the United States improved markedly between the Revolutionary War and the American Civil War (1783–1861).

Early schools of nursing, usually under the control of the religious nursing orders, were being developed at this time. Despite rapid increases in the number and quality of hospitals, most nursing care was still given at home by family members. Hospitals were considered places of last resort, when home care failed or was insufficient to effect a cure. Until the early 1900s, only people who were at death's door went to the hospital. Mortality rates were very high in these institutions.

5

ETHICS IN NURSING

Learning Objectives

After completing this chapter, the reader will be able to:

1   Discuss and analyze the difference between law and ethics.
2   Define the key terms used in ethics.
3   Discuss the important ethical concepts.
4   Distinguish between the two most commonly used systems of ethical decision making.
5   Apply the steps in the ethical decision-making process.

Nurses who practice in today's health care system soon realize that making ethical decisions is a common part of every day nursing care. However, experience shows that in the full curricula of many schools of nursing, the teaching of ethical principles and ethical decision making gets less attention than the more pressing topics of nursing skills, pathophysiology, and nursing care plans. As health care technology continues to advance into the 21st century, making these ethical decisions will become more and more difficult. This leaves many nurses feeling the need to be better prepared to understand and deal with the complex ethical problems that keep evolving as they attempt to provide care for their clients.

Ethical decision making is a skill that can be learned by any nurse. The ability to make sound ethical decisions is based on an understanding of underlying ethical principles, ethical theories or systems, a decision-making model, and the profession's Code of Ethics. And like all skills, learning it involves mastering the theoretical material, and practicing the skill itself.

This chapter will present the basic information required to understand ethics, the code of ethics, and ethical decision making. It will also highlight some of the important bioethical issues that nurses face in today's health care system.

IMPORTANT DEFINITIONS

In Western cultures, the study of ethics is a specialized area of philosophy the origins of which can be traced to ancient Greece. In fact, certain ethical principles articulated by Hippocrates still serve as the underpinning of many of today's debates. Like most specialized areas of study, ethics has its own language and uses terminology in precise ways. The following are some key terms encountered in studies of health care ethics.

Values are ideals or concepts that give meaning to the individual's life. Values are most commonly derived from societal norms, religion, and family orientation and serve as the framework for making decisions and taking certain actions in everyday life. Values are usually *not* written down, but, at some time in their professional careers, it may be important for nurses to make a list of their values. This **value clarification process** requires that the nurse assess, evaluate, and then determine a set of personal values and in what priority they are to be ranked. This will help the nurse to make decisions when confronted with situations in which the client's values are different from the nurse's.

Value conflicts that often occur in everyday life can force an individual to select a higher priority value over a lower. For example, a nurse who values both her career and her family may be forced to decide between going to work and staying home with a sick child.

Morals are the fundamental standards of right and wrong that an individual learns and internalizes, usually in the early stages of childhood development. An individual's moral orientation is generally based on religious beliefs, although societal influence plays an important part in this development. Moral behavior is often manifested as behavior in accordance with a group's norms, customs, or traditions. In Church of Latter Day Saints' (Mormon) tradition, for example, polygamy was an accepted practice and therefore considered morally correct, whereas most other Christian religions consider polygamy immoral (Aiken, 1994).

Laws can generally be defined as man-made rules of social conduct that protect society and are based on concerns about fairness and justice. The goals of laws are preserving the species and promoting peaceful and productive interactions between individuals or groups of individuals by preventing the actions of one citizen from infringing on the rights of another. Two important aspects of laws are that they are enforceable through some type of police force, and they should be applied equally to all persons.

Ethics are declarations of what is right or wrong, and of what ought to be. Ethics are usually presented as systems of value behaviors and beliefs; they serve the purpose of governing conduct to ensure the protection of an individual's rights. Ethics exist on several levels, ranging from the individual or small group to the society as a whole. The concept of ethics is closely associated with the concept of morals in both their development and purposes. In one sense, ethics can be considered a system of morals for a particular group. There are usually no systems of enforcement for those who violate ethical principles.

Code of Ethics is a written list of a profession's values and standards of conduct. The code of ethics provides a framework for decision making for the profession and should be oriented toward the day-to-day decisions made by members of the profession.

Ethical Dilemma is a situation that requires an individual to make a choice between two equally unfavorable alternatives. When ethical dilemmas are reduced to their elemental aspects, conflicts of one individual's rights with those of another, or one individual's obligations with the rights of another, or a combination of one group's obligations and rights conflicting with anothers' obligations and rights usually forms the basis of the dilemma. By the very nature of an ethical dilemma, there can be no simple correct solution, and whatever decision is made often must be defended against those who disagree with it.

KEY CONCEPTS IN ETHICS

In addition to the terminology used in the study and practice of ethics, several important concepts, or principles, often underlie ethical dilemmas. Although the following list is by no means comprehensive, it does present several key principles that often serve as the underpinnings for ethical dilemmas.

1   **Autonomy** is the right of self-determination, independence, and freedom. Autonomy refers to the clients' right to make health care decisions for themselves, even if the provider does not agree with those decisions.

   Autonomy, as with most rights, is not absolute, and under certain conditions, limitations can be imposed on it. Generally these limitations occur when one individual's autonomy interferes with another individual's rights, health, or well-being. For example, a client generally can use his right to autonomy by refusing any or all treatments. In the case of contagious diseases that affect society, however, such as tuberculosis (TB), the individual can be forced by the health care and legal systems to take medications to cure the disease. The individual can also be forced into isolation to prevent the disease's contagious spread.

2   **Justice** is the obligation to be fair to all people. The concept is often expanded to what is called **distributive justice,** which states that individuals have the right to be treated equally regardless of race, sex, marital status, medical diagnosis, social standing, economic level, or religious belief. The principle of justice underlies the first statement in the American Nurses Association (ANA) Code of Ethics for Nurses: "The nurse provides services with respect for human dignity and the uniqueness of the client unrestricted by considerations of social or economic status, personal attributes, or the nature of health problems." (ANA, 1976). Distributive justice sometimes includes ideas such as equal access to health care for all. As with other rights, limits can be placed on justice when it interferes with the rights of others.

3   **Fidelity** is the obligation of an individual to be faithful to commitments made

to self and others. In health care, fidelity includes the professional's faithfulness or loyalty to agreements and responsibilities accepted as part of the practice of the profession. Fidelity is the main support for the concept of accountability, although conflicts in fidelity might arise from obligations owed to different individuals or groups. For example, a nurse who was just finishing a very busy and tiring 12-hour shift may experience a conflict of fidelity when she is asked by a supervisor to work an additional shift because of the hospital's being short staffed. The nurse would have to weigh her fidelity to herself against fidelity to the employing institution and against the fidelity to the profession and clients to do the best job possible, particularly if she felt that her fatigue would interfere with the performance of those obligations.

4 **Beneficence** is an old requirement for health care providers that views the primary goal of health care as doing good for clients under their care. In general, the term **good** includes more than providing technically competent care for clients. Good care requires that the health care provider take a holistic approach to the client, including the client's beliefs, feelings, and wishes as well as those of the client's family and significant others. The difficulty in implementing the principle of beneficence is in determining what exactly is good for another and who can best make the decision about this good.

5 **Nonmaleficence** is the requirement that health care providers do no harm to their clients, either intentionally or unintentionally. In a sense, it is the opposite side of the concept of beneficence, and it is difficult to speak of one term without referring to the other. In current health care practice, the principle of nonmaleficence is often violated in the short run to produce a greater good in the long-term treatment of the client. For example, a client may undergo painful and debilitating surgery to remove a cancerous growth in order to prolong the client's future life.

By extension, the principle of nonmaleficence also requires that health care providers protect those from harm who cannot protect themselves. This protection from harm is particularly evident in groups such as children, the mentally incompetent, the unconscious, and those who are too weak or debilitated to protect themselves. For example, very strict regulations have developed around situations involving child abuse and the health care provider's obligation to report suspected child abuse.

6 **Veracity** is the principle of *truthfulness*. It requires the health care provider to tell the truth, and to not deceive or mislead clients intentionally. As with other rights and obligations, limitations to this principle exist. The primary limitation is when telling the client the truth would seriously harm (principle of nonmaleficence) the client's ability to recover, or to produce greater illness. Many times, health care providers feel uncomfortable giving clients bad news, and have a tendency to avoid answering these questions truthfully. Feeling uncomfortable is not a good enough reason to avoid telling clients the truth about their diagnosis, treatments, or prognosis. Clients have a right to know this information.

7 **Standard of Best Interest** describes a type of decision made about a client's health care when the client is unable to make the informed decision for his or her own care. The standard of best interest is based on what health care providers and the family decide is best for that individual. It is very important to consider the individual client's expressed wishes, either formally in a written declaration (such as a living will) or informally in what may have been said to family members.

The standard of best interest should be based on the principle of beneficence. Unfortunately, in situations where clients are unable to make decisions for themselves, the resolution of the dilemma can be a unilateral decision made by health care provider(s). The making of a unilateral decision by health care providers that disregards the client's wishes implies that the providers alone know what is best for the client is termed **paternalism.**

8 **Obligations** are demands made upon an individual, a profession, a society, or a government to fulfill and honor the rights of others. Obligations are often divided into two categories:

a **Legal obligations** are those which have become formal statements of law, and are enforceable under the law. For example, a nurse has a legal obligation to provide safe and adequate care for clients assigned to him or her.

b **Moral obligations** are those based on moral or ethical principles, but are *not* enforceable under the law. For example, in most states no legal obligation exists for a nurse on a vacation trip to stop and help an automobile accident victim.

9 **Rights** are generally defined as something owed to an individual according to just claims, legal guarantees, or moral and ethical principles. Although the term **right** is frequently used in both the legal and ethical systems, its meaning is often blurred in everyday usage. Individuals tend to claim things as rights that are really privileges, concessions, or freedoms. Several classification systems exist for rights in which different types of rights are delineated. The following three types of rights seem to cover the range of definitions.

a **Welfare rights** (also called **legal rights**) are based on a legal entitlement to some good or benefit. These rights are guaranteed by laws (such as the Bill of Rights of the U.S. Constitution) and violation of such rights can be punished under the legal system. For example, citizens of the United States have a right to equal access to housing regardless of race, sexual preferences, or religion.

b **Ethical rights** (also called **moral rights**) are based on a moral or ethical principle. Ethical rights usually do not need to have the power of law in order to be enforced. Ethical rights are, in reality, often privileges allotted to certain individuals or groups of individuals. Over time, popular acceptance of ethical rights can give them the force of a legal right. For example, in the United States and South Africa, the access to health care is really a long-standing privilege, whereas in many other industrialized countries, such as Canada, Germany, Japan, and England, universal health care is a legal right.

c   **Option rights** are rights that are based on a fundamental belief in the dignity and freedom of human beings. Option rights are particularly evident in free and democratic countries such as the United States, and much less evident in totalitarian and restrictive societies such as Iraq. Option rights give individuals freedom of choice and the right to live their lives as they choose, but within a given set of prescribed boundaries, however. For example, people may wear whatever clothes they choose, as long as they do wear some type of clothing.

ETHICAL SYSTEMS

Every time a nurse interacts with a client in a health care setting, an ethical situation exists. Nurses are continually making ethical decisions in their daily practice, whether or not they recognize it. These are termed **normative decisions.** Normative ethical decisions deal with questions and dilemmas requiring a choice of actions where there is a conflict of rights or obligations between the nurse and the client, the nurse and the client's family, or the nurse and the physician. In resolving these ethical questions, these nurses often just use one ethical system, or perhaps a combination of several.

The two fundamental and predominant systems that are most directly concerned with ethical decision making in the health care professions are **utilitarianism** and **deontology.** Both systems apply to *bioethics,*—the ethics of life (or, in some cases, death). **Bioethics** and **bioethical issues** are terms that are in common use, that have become synonymous with health care ethics, and encompass not only questions concerning life and death but also questions of quality of life, life-sustaining and life-altering technologies, and biological science in general. It is in the context of bioethics that the following discussion of these two systems of ethics is undertaken.

UTILITARIANISM

Ethical Precepts

Utilitarianism (also called *teleology, consequentialism,* or *situation ethics*) is referred to as the ethical system of utility. As a system of normative ethics, utilitarianism defines *good* as happiness or pleasure. It is associated with two underlying principles. The first principle states: "The greatest good for the greatest number." The second principle is "The end justifies the means." Because of these two principles, utilitarianism is sometimes subdivided into *act utilitarianism* and *rule utilitarianism.* According to rule utilitarianism, the individual draws upon past experiences to formulate internal rules that are useful in determining the greatest good. With act utilitarianism, the particular situation in which a nurse finds himself or herself determines the rightness or wrongness of a particular act. In practice, the true follower of utilitarianism does not believe in the validity of any system of rules because the rules can change depending on the circumstances surrounding whatever decision needs to be made.

Situation ethics is probably the most publicized form of act utilitarianism. Joseph Fletcher, one of the best-known proponents of act utilitarianism, outlines a method of ethical thinking in which the situation itself determines whether the act is morally right or wrong. Fletcher views acts as good to the extent that they promote happiness and bad to the degree that they promote unhappiness. *Happiness* is defined as the happiness of the greatest number of people, yet the happiness of each person is to have equal weight. For example, abortion is considered ethical in this system in a situation where an unwed welfare mother with four other children becomes pregnant with her fifth child. The greatest good, and the greatest amount of happiness, is produced by aborting this unwanted child.

Because utilitarianism is based on the concept that moral rules should not be arbitrary but rather serve a purpose, ethical decisions derived from a utilitarian framework weigh the effect of alternative actions that influence the overall welfare of present and future populations. As such, this system is oriented toward the good of the population in general and the individual as the individual participates in that population.

Advantages

The major advantage of the utilitarian system of ethical decision making is that many individuals find it easy to use in most situations. Utilitarianism is built around an individual's needs for happiness in which the individual has an immediate and vested knowledge. Another advantage is that utilitarianism fits well into a society that otherwise shuns rules and regulations. A follower of utilitarianism can justify many decisions based on the *happiness principle.* Also, its utility orientation fits well into Western society's belief in the work ethic and a behavioristic approach to education, philosophy, and life.

For example, the follower of utilitarianism will support a general prohibition against lying and deceiving because ultimately, the results of truth telling will lead to greater happiness than the results of lying. Yet truth telling is not an absolute requirement to the follower of utilitarianism. If telling the truth will produce widespread unhappiness for a great number of people and future generations then it would be ethically better to tell a lie that will yield more happiness than to tell a truth that will lead to greater unhappiness. Although such behavior might appear to be unethical at first glance, the strict follower of act utilitarianism would have little difficulty in arriving at this decision as a logical conclusion of utilitarian ethical thinking.

Disadvantages

Some serious limitations to utilitarianism as a system of health care or bioethics exist. An immediate question is whether *happiness* refers to the average happiness of all or the total happiness of a few. Because individual happiness is also important, one must consider how to make decisions when the individual's happiness is in conflict with that of the larger group. More fundamental is the question of what constitutes happiness. Similarly, what constitutes the *greatest good for the greatest number?* Who determines what is good in the first place? Is it society in general, the government, governmental policy, the individual? In health care delivery and the formulation of health care policy, the general guiding principle often seems to be the greatest good for the greatest number. Yet where do minority groups fit into this system?

Also, the tenet of *ends justify the means* has been consistently rejected as a rationale for justifying actions. It is generally unacceptable to allow any type of action so long as the final goal or purpose is good. The Nazis in the 1930s and 1940s used this aphorism to justify many actions that may be viewed by others as considerably less than *good*.

The other difficulty in determining what is good lies in the attempt to quantify such concepts as **good, harm, benefits,** and **greatest.** This problem becomes especially acute when dealing with health care issues that involve individuals' lives. For example, an elderly family member has been sick for a long time, and that course of illness has placed great financial hardship on the family. It would be ethical under utilitarianism to allow this client to die, or even to euthanatize her to relieve the financial stress created by her illness.

The function of utilitarianism as an ethical system in the health care decision-making process requires use of an additional principle of distributive justice as an ultimate guiding point. Unfortunately, whenever an unchanging principle is combined with this system, it negates the basic concept of pure utilitarianism. Pure utilitarianism, although easy to use as a decision-making system, does not work well as an ethical system for decision making in health care because of its arbitrary, self-centered nature. In the everyday delivery of health care, utilitarianism is often combined with other types of ethical decision making in the resolution of ethical dilemmas.

DEONTOLOGY

Ethical Precepts

Deontology is a system of ethical decision making based on moral rules and unchanging principles. This system is also termed the **formalistic system,** the **principle system of ethics,** or **duty-based ethics.** A follower of a pure form of the deontological system of ethical decision making believes in the ethical absoluteness of principles regardless of the consequences of the decision. Strict adherence to an ethical theory, in which the moral rightness or wrongness of human actions is considered separately from the consequences, is based on a fundamental principle called the *categorical imperative*. It is not the results of the act that make it right or wrong, but the principles by reason of which the act is carried out. These fundamental principles are ultimately unchanging and absolute and derived from the universal values that underlie all major religions. Focusing on a concern for right and wrong in the moral sense is the basic premise of the system. Its goal is the survival of the species and social cooperation.

Rule deontology is based on the belief that standards exist for the ethical choices and judgments made by individuals. These standards are fixed and do not change when the situation changes. Although the number of standards or rules is potentially unlimited, in reality, and particularly in dealing with bioethical issues, many of these principles can be grouped together into a few general principles. These principles can also be arranged into a type of hierarchy of rules and include such maxims as: "People should always be treated as ends and never as means; Human life has value; One is always to tell the truth; Above all in health care, do no harm; Humans have a right to self-determination; and All people are of equal value;" among others. These principles echo such fundamental documents as the Bill of Rights and the Hospital Association's Patient's Bill of Rights (Box 5–1).

Advantages

The deontological system is useful in making ethical decisions in health care because it holds that an ethical judgment based on principles will be the same in a variety of given similar situations regardless of time, location, or particular individuals involved. In addition, deontological terminology and concepts are similar to the terms and concepts used by the legal system. The legal system stresses rights, duties, principles, and rules. Significant differences between the two exist, however. Legal rights and duties are enforceable under the law, whereas ethical rights and duties usually are not. In general, ethical systems are much wider and more inclusive than the system of laws which they underlie. It is difficult to have an ethical perspective on law without having it lead to an interest in making laws that govern health care and nursing practice. When nurses evaluate and change laws from an ethical perspective, they will no longer be placed in situations whereby their practice is unsupported by the legal system.

Disadvantages

The deontological system of ethical decision making is not free from imperfection. Some of the more troubling questions include: "What do you do when the basic guiding principles conflict with each other? What is the source of the principles? Is there ever a situation where an exception to the rule will apply?" Although various approaches have been proposed to circumvent these limitations, it may be difficult for nurses to resolve situations in which duties and obligations

---

Box 5-1   THE AMERICAN HOSPITAL ASSOCIATION'S PATIENT'S BILL OF RIGHTS

---

1   The patient has the right to considerate and respectful care.

2   The patient has the right to obtain from his doctor complete and current information about his diagnosis, treatment, and prognosis in terms the patient can be reasonably expected to understand. When it is not medically advisable to give such information to the patient, it should be made available to an appropriate person in his behalf. He has the right to know by name the doctor responsible for coordinating his care.

3   The patient has the right to receive from his doctor information necessary to give informed consent prior to the start of any procedure or treatment. Except in emergencies, such information for informed consent should include but not necessarily be limited to the specific procedure or treatment, the medically significant risks involved, and the probable duration of incapacitation. Where medically significant alternatives for care or treatment exist, or when the patient requests information concerning medical alternatives, the patient has the right to such information. The patient has the right to know the name of the person responsible for the procedure or treatment.

4   The patient has the right to refuse treatment to the extent permitted by law and to be informed of the medical consequences of his action.

5   The patient has the right to every consideration of his privacy concerning his own medical care program. Case discussion, consultation, examination, and the treatment are confidential and should be conducted discreetly. Those not directly involved in his care must have the permission of the patient to be present.

6   The patient has the right to expect that all communications and records pertaining to his care should be treated as confidential.

7   The patient has the right to expect that within its capacity a hospital must make reasonable response to the request of a patient for services. The hospital must provide evaluation, service or referral as indicated by the urgency of the case. When medically permissible, a patient may be transferred to another facility only after he has received complete information and explanation concerning the needs for and alternatives to such a transfer. The institution to which the patient is to be transferred must first have accepted the patient for transfer.

8   The patient has the right to obtain information as to any relationship of his hospital to other health care and educational institutions insofar as his care is concerned. The patient has the right to obtain information as to the existence of any professional relationships among individuals by name who are treating him.

Continued on following page

Box 5–1 (Continued)

9 The patient has the right to be advised if the hospital proposes to engage in or perform human experimentation affecting his care or treatment. The patient has the right to refuse to participate in such research projects.

10 The patient has the right to expect reasonable continuity of care. He has the right to know in advance what appointment times and doctors are available and where. The patient has the right to expect that the hospital will provide a mechanism whereby he is informed by his doctor or a delegate of the doctor of the patient's continuing health care requirements following discharge.

11 The patient has the right to examine and receive an explanation of his bill, regardless of the source of payment.

12 The patient has the right to know what hospital rules and regulations apply to his conduct as a patient.

Modified from American Hospital Association: A Patient's Bill of Rights. AHA Board of Trustees, 1973, revised 1992, with permission.

---

conflict, particularly when the consequences of following a rule end in harm or hurt being done to a client. In reality, there are probably few pure followers of deontology because most people will consider the consequences of their actions in the decision-making process.

THE APPLICATION OF ETHICAL THEORIES

Ethical theories do not provide recipes for resolution of ethical dilemmas. Instead, they provide a framework for decision making that the nurse can apply to a particular ethical situation.

At times, ethical theories may seem too abstract or general to be of much use to specific ethical situations. Without them, however, ethical decision making often becomes merely an exercise in personal emotions. Most nurses in attempting to make ethical decisions combine the two theories presented above.

NURSING CODE OF ETHICS

A code of ethics is generally defined as the ethical principles that govern a particular profession. Codes of ethics are presented as general statements and so do not give specific answers to every possible ethical dilemma that might arise. These codes do, however, offer guidance to the individual practitioner in making decisions.

Ideally, codes of ethics should undergo periodic review to reflect necessary changes in the profession and society as a whole. Although codes of ethics are not judicially enforceable as laws, consistent violations of the code of ethics by a professional in any field may indicate an unwillingness to act in a professional manner and will often result in disciplinary actions ranging from reprimands and fines to suspension and revocation of licensure.

Although similar, there are several different codes of ethics that nurses may adopt. In the United States, the American Nurses Association (ANA) Code of

---

Box 5–2   THE AMERICAN NURSES ASSOCIATION CODE OF ETHICS

1   The nurse provides services with respect for human dignity and the uniqueness of the client unrestricted by considerations of social or economic status, personal attributes or the nature of the health problems.

2   The nurse safeguards the client's right to privacy by judiciously protecting information of a confidential nature.

3   The nurse acts to safeguard the client and the public when health care and safety are affected by the incompetent, unethical, or illegal practice of any person.

4   The nurse assumes responsibility and accountability for individual nursing judgements and actions.

5   The nurse maintains competence in nursing.

6   The nurse exercises informed judgment and uses individual competence and qualification as criteria in seeking consultation, accepting responsibilities, and delegating nursing activities to others.

7   The nurse participates in activities that contribute to the ongoing development of the profession's body of knowledge.

8   The nurse participates in the profession's efforts to implement and improve standards of nursing.

9   The nurse participates in the profession's efforts to establish and maintain conditions of employment conducive to high quality nursing care.

10   The nurse participates in the profession's efforts to protect the public from misinformation and misrepresentation and to maintain the integrity of nursing.

11   The nurse collaborates with members of the health professions and other citizens in promoting community and national efforts to meet the health needs of the public.

From American Nurses Association: Code for Nurses. American Nurses Association, Kansas City, 1985, with permission.

Ethics (Box 5–2) is the generally accepted code. There is also a Canadian Nurses Association Code of Ethics (Box 5–3).

The ANA Code of Ethics has been acknowledged by other health care professions as one of the most complete. It is sometimes used as the benchmark against which other codes of ethics are measured. Yet, a careful reading of this code of ethics reveals only a set of clearly stated principles that the nurse must apply to actual clinical situations. For example, the nurse involved in resuscitation will find no specific mention of *no resuscitation* orders in the ANA Code of Ethics. Rather, the nurse must be able to apply general statements such as "The nurse provides services with respect for human dignity . . ." and "The nurse assumes responsibility and accountability for individual nursing judgments and actions" to the particular situation.

THE DECISION-MAKING PROCESS IN ETHICS

Nurses, by definition, are problem solvers, and one of the important tools that nurses use is the nursing process. The nursing process is, if nothing else, a systematic, step-by-step approach to resolving problems that deal with a client's health and well-being.

Although nurses deal with problems related to the physical or psychologic needs of patients, many feel inadequate when dealing with ethical problems associated with patient care. Nurses in any health care setting can, however, develop the decision-making skills necessary to make sound ethical decisions if they learn and practice using an ethical decision-making process.

An *ethical decision-making process* provides a method for the nurse to answer key questions about ethical dilemmas and to organize the nurse's thinking in a more logical and sequential manner. Although several ethical decision-making processes are in existence, the problem-solving method presented here is based on the nursing process. It should be a relatively easy transition for the nurse to move from the nursing process used in the resolution of a client's physical problems to the ethical decision-making process for the resolution of problems with ethical ramifications.

The chief goal of the *ethical decision-making process* is the determination of right and wrong in situations where clear demarcations either do not exist or are not readily apparent. This process presupposes that the nurse making the decision knows that a system of ethics exists, knows the content of that ethical system and knows that the system applies to similar ethical decision-making problems despite multiple variables. At some point, the nurse needs to undertake the task of clarifying his or her personal values, if this has not been done. The nurse also needs an understanding of the possible ethical systems that may be used in making decisions about ethical dilemmas.

The following five-step ethical decision-making process is presented as a tool for resolving ethical dilemmas:

Box 5–3 CANADIAN NURSES CODE OF ETHICS

Value I

A nurse treats clients with respect for their individual needs and values.

Value II

Based upon respect for clients and regard for their right to control their own care, nursing care reflects respect for the right of choice held by clients.

Value III

The nurse holds confidential all information about a client learned in the health care setting.

Value IV

The nurse is guided by consideration for the dignity of clients.

Value V

The nurse provides competent care to clients.

Value VI

The nurse maintains trust in nurses and nursing.

Value VII

The nurse recognizes the contribution and expertise of colleagues from nursing and other disciplines as essential to excellent health care.

Value VIII

The nurse takes steps to ensure that the client receives competent and ethical care.

Value IX

Conditions of employment should contribute in a positive way to client care and the professional satisfaction of nurses.

Value X

Job action by nurses is directed toward securing conditions of employment that enable safe and appropriate care for clients and contribute to the professional satisfaction of nurses.

Value XI

The nurse advocates the interests of clients.

Value XII

The nurse represents the values and ethics of nursing before colleagues and others.

Value XIII

Professional nurses' organizations are responsible for clarifying, securing and sustaining ethical nursing conduct. The fulfillment of these task requires that the professional nurses' organizations remain responsive to the rights, needs and legitimate interests of clients and nurses.

From Canadian Nurses Association: Canadian Nurses Association Code of Ethics for Nursing, 1985, revised 1991, with permission.

ISSUES IN PRACTICE
Withdrawing Informed Consent:
A Case Study

Mrs. Hobbs was a 52-year-old unemployed teacher who received minor injuries when she fell down the steps at a neighbor's house. She was intoxicated at the time, and had a long history of alcohol abuse. She was brought to the emergency department of a large city hospital and treated. She was also offered a chance for treatment in the alcohol dependency unit of the hospital at no charge if she agreed to participate in a study on the long-term effects of alcohol on the central nervous system. Dr. Wei, the chief investigator of the study, and Ms. Anderson, the nurse in charge of the unit, explained to Mrs. Hobbs that the study involved the administration of a medication that, over a period of time, might reduce the long-term effects of alcohol on the brain. The study required Mrs. Hobbs to be hospitalized and to be given an experimental medication intravenously for 45 days. She was also required to eat a well balanced diet and take supplemental vitamins. After the risks and benefits of the study were discussed, Mrs. Hobbs signed the consent form and was admitted to the chemical dependency unit.

During the first 20 days of the study, Mrs. Hobbs was cooperative with the nursing staff, participated actively in the group therapy, and had a positive attitude about the program. Her physical condition and her mental function continued to improve until the 25th day into the study. On that day, she awoke in the morning very agitated and slightly disoriented, and appeared somewhat depressed. She said she had "real bad cabin fever," and needed to "get out of this loony bin." She made the point that she was much, much better than when she was admitted, and should be permitted to go home. When she was reminded that she had signed a consent form for the study, and had agreed to participate for the full 45 days, she claimed that she did not remember signing it. Even after being shown the signed form, she denied it was her signature and stated she was going home, like it or not.

Upon closer examination of the document, Ms. Anderson (the nurse) noted that the signature looked like a poorly scribbled "H." The chart also noted that while Mrs. Hobbs had been in rather severe alcohol withdrawal from shortly after admission until about 48 hours into her hospitalization, she had not had any hallucinations and was generally oriented to person, place, and time.

Two questions arise from this case. First, because of Mrs. Hobbs' condition on admission, was the consent fully informed and valid? Second, if an informed consent is valid, can the person who signed it ever withdraw the consent, and if so, when?

Step 1: Collect, Analyze, and Interpret the Data

Obtain as much information as possible concerning the particular ethical dilemma. Unfortunately, such information is sometimes very limited. Among the issues important to know are the client's wishes, the client's family's wishes, the extent of the physical or emotional problems causing the dilemma, the physician's beliefs about health care, and the nurse's own orientation to issues concerning life and death.

For example, many nurses face the question of whether or not to initiate resuscitation efforts when a terminally ill client is admitted to the hospital. Physicians often leave instructions for the nursing staff indicating that the nurses really should not resuscitate the client but should, instead, merely go through the motions to make the family feel better. The nurse's dilemma is whether to make a serious attempt to revive the client or to let the client die quietly.

Important information that will help the nurse make the decision might include the mental competency of the client to make a no-resuscitation decision, the client's desires, the family's feelings, and whether the physician previously sought input from the client and the family. Many institutions have policies concerning no-resuscitation orders, and it is wise to consider these during data collection. After collecting information, the nurse needs to bring the pieces of information together into a manner that will give the clearest and sharpest focus to the dilemma.

Step 2: State the Dilemma

After collecting and analyzing as much information as is available, the nurse then needs to state the dilemma as clearly as possible. In this step, the nurse should also identify whether the problem is one that directly involves the nurse or is one that can be resolved only by the client, the client's family, or the physician.

Recognizing the key aspects of the dilemma helps to focus the nurse's attention on the important ethical principles. Most of the time, the dilemma can be reduced to a statement or two that encompass the key ethical issues. Such ethical issues often involve a question of conflicting rights, obligations, or basic ethical principles.

In the situation of a no-resuscitation order, the statement of the dilemma might be: "The client's right to death with dignity versus the nurse's obligation to preserve life and do no harm." In general, the principle that the competent client's wishes must be followed is unequivocal. If the client has become unresponsive before expressing his or her wishes, then the family members' input must be given serious consideration. Additional questions can arise if the family's wishes conflict with those of the client.

Step 3: Consider the Choices of Action

After stating the dilemma as clearly as possible, the next step is to attempt to list, without consideration of their consequences, all possible courses of action that can be taken to resolve the dilemma. This brain-storming activity in which *all* possible courses of action are considered may require input from outside sources such as colleagues, supervisors, or even experts in the ethical field. The consequences of the different actions are considered later in this chapter.

Some possible courses of action for the nurse might include the following: resuscitating the client to the nurse's fullest capabilities despite what the physician has requested, not resuscitating the client at all, just going through the motions without any real attempt to revive the client, seeking another assignment so as to avoid dealing with the situation, reporting the problem to a supervisor, attempting to clarify the question with the client, attempting to clarify the question with the family, or confronting the physician about the question.

Step 4: Analyze the Advantages and Disadvantages of Each Course of Action

Some of the courses of action developed during the previous step are more realistic than others. The identification of these actions becomes readily evident during this step in the decision-making process, when the advantages and the disadvantages of each action are considered in detail. Along with each option, the consequences of taking each course of action must be thoroughly evaluated.

The nurse should consider whether initiating discussion might anger the physician or cause distrust of the nurse involved. Both these responses may reinforce the attitude of submission to the physician, and either could make continuing to practice nursing at that institution difficult. The same result might occur if the nurse successfully resuscitates a client despite orders to the contrary. Failure to resuscitate the client has the potential to produce a lawsuit unless a clear order for no resuscitation has been given. Presenting the situation to a supervisor may, if the supervisor supports the physician, cause the nurse to be considered a troublemaker and thus have a negative effect on future evaluations. The same process could be applied to the other courses of action.

When considering the advantages and disadvantages, the nurse should be able to narrow the realistic choices of action. Other relevant issues need to be examined when weighing the choices of action. A major factor would be choosing the appropriate code of ethics. The ANA Code of Ethics should figure in many client-care decisions clouded by ethical dilemmas.

Step 5: Make the Decision

The most difficult part of the process is actually making the decision and living with the consequences. By their nature, ethical dilemmas produce differences of opinion and not everyone will be pleased with the decision.

In the attempt to solve any ethical dilemma, there will always be a question of the correct course of action. The client's wishes almost always supersede independent decisions on the part of health care professionals. Collaborative decisions made by client, physician, nurses, and family about resuscitation is the ideal and tends to produce fewer complications in the long-term resolution of such questions.

SUMMARY

Ethical dilemmas, by definition, are difficult to resolve. Rarely will a nurse find ethical dilemmas covered in policy, procedure, and protocol manuals, but nurses can develop the skills necessary to make appropriate ethical decisions. The key to developing these skills is the recognition and frequent use of an ethical decision-making model, and application of the appropriate ethical theories to the dilemma. As an orderly approach in solving the often disorderly aspects of ethical questions encountered in nursing practice, the decision-making model previously presented can be applied to almost every type of ethical dilemma. Although each situation is different, ethical decision making based on ethical theory can provide a potent means for resolving dilemmas found in client-care situations.

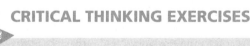

CRITICAL THINKING EXERCISES

1 Compare and contrast ethics with laws by delineating the purposes, scopes, and methods of enforcement of each.
2 Distinguish between the two types of obligations.
3 Distinguish between the three categories of rights.
4 Analyze the following ethical dilemma case study using the ethical decision-making process:

What are the important data in relation to this situation?

State the ethical dilemma in a clear, simple statement.

CRITICAL THINKING EXERCISES (Continued)

What are the choices of action and how do they relate to specific ethical principles?

What are the consequences of these actions?

What decision can be made?

CASE STUDY

Bill L., a veteran emergency room (ER) nurse, called the resident physician about a client just admitted to the ER after a fall from a ladder. The client, a 52-year-old man, had been fixing his roof when the accident occurred. He had suffered a minor head injury, a twisted ankle, and a badly bruised arm. He also had a long history of asthma and heavy smoking. Shortly after admission to the ER, the client became cyanotic, dyspneic, and semiconscious. By the time the resident physician arrived, Bill had the client prepared for endotracheal intubation, and had already notified the personnel in the medical intensive care unit (MICU) that they would be receiving this client.

After a hasty evaluation of the client, the resident decided to perform an emergency tracheostomy before transporting the client to the MICU. While performing the tracheostomy, the physician severed a major blood vessel and the client hemorrhaged profusely. After several tense minutes, the endotracheal tube was inserted, and the client was quickly transported to the MICU but remained cyanotic and had great difficulty breathing. Shortly after leaving the ER, the nurse realized that the oxygen tank the client had been connected to was empty. The client never regained consciousness, and died 3 days after admission. His death was due to respiratory failure and not to the injuries sustained in his fall.

When the client's wife came to the unit to collect the deceased's belongings, nurse Bill is torn between telling her about the mistakes that were made in the treatment of her husband and remaining silent. What are the key ethical principles involved in this situation? Are there any statements in the ANA Code for Nurses that may help resolve this dilemma? What would be the consequences of informing the client's wife of the truth? What are the consequences of not informing her?

A Closer Look

THE NEW DISEASE: PERSISTENT VEGETATIVE STATE

The term **persistent vegetative state** (PVS) describes a condition wherein a client is awake, but shows no awareness of self or environment, and has no voluntary movements, emotional responses, or cognitive ability. Unlike brain death, clients in PVS do have reflex responses, brain-stem activity, eye movements, and cycles of sleep and wakefulness. Medical science is not sure what causes PVS, has no specific tests or criteria to diagnose it, and finds similar symptoms in conditions such as coma, dementia, and unconsciousness.

Clients who have PVS have only an even chance of regaining some degree of normal functioning, and may live, with artificial hydration and nutrition, for as long as 5 years in this state. The ages of the 5000 to 10,000 PVS clients in the United States range from very young to very old. Many are institutionalized in long-term care facilities, whereas an increasing number are cared for at home by family members with the assistance of home health care nurses. The cost of maintaining one of these clients for 1 year is estimated to approach $100,000.

Some medical experts have suggested that the definition of brain death be expanded to include clients who have PVS. These experts argue that loss of the higher brain functions, especially of the cerebral cortex as is seen in PVS, should suffice as a legal definition of death. By expanding this definition of brain death, clients in PVS could be allowed to die by the withdrawal of intravenous fluids and tube feedings, thereby saving the health care system upwards of $1 billion per year. PVS clients also could be designated as organ donors, thereby saving the lives of many people who need organ transplants. In today's health care system, even without this expanded definition of death, many clients with PVS are allowed to die through dehydration and starvation. The cases of Nancy Cruzan and Christine Busalacchi demonstrates the courts' willingness to accept PVS as a form of brain death.

Yet many ethical questions persist. Nurses, as the health care providers most immediately involved with the care of PVS clients and those most directly responsible for the withholding of fluids and feedings, are placed in a particularly sensitive ethical position. If PVS clients are indeed alive, then nurses have a strong ethical obligation to provide the same type of care they would for any other client. The ethical obligations become even more complicated if PVS clients are considered dead.

Strictly speaking, clients who are dead have no rights; therefore basically no obligations on the part of the health care provider can be thought

THE NEW DISEASE: PERSISTENT VEGETATIVE STATE
(Continued)

to exist. Yet, PVS clients do breathe, do have a heartbeat, and can absorb nutrients and fluids. In addition, these clients may have expressed some wishes or desires about treatment to be given or not given if they were ever to become unable to make decisions about their care. These wishes may have been expressed in the formal manner of a living will, but may also take the form of a designated decision maker (i.e., one with *durable power of attorney*), or through an informal declaration to a relative of the client. Often living wills of either the written or oral type do not cover situations such as PVS; they therefore may not be an accurate indication of the client's wish to die, particularly where there is a chance they may recover.

The ethical principle of beneficence (doing good for the client) must take precedence in situations when the expressed wishes of the client are not clearly known. In these situations, nurses have the ethical and legal duty to care for the client and assume that the client's desire is to obtain the treatments necessary to live. Nurses are obligated to care for these clients until ordered to stop either by the clients themselves or by any person authorized to speak for them. The most serious ethical dilemma arises when the person who has ordered the care stopped does not, in fact, have the legal authority to make that type of decision.

Nurses have a general prohibition against participating in executions. The key question is whether or not withholding liquids and nutrition from clients is a form of execution. The ANA Code of Ethics is rooted in the tenets regarding respect for people, the noninfliction of harm, and faithfulness to the clients being cared for. Nurses are not, however, required to prolong life (or death) at all costs, particularly in the case of obviously terminally ill clients. An ethical dilemma arises for many nurses because PVS patients are not necessarily terminal, and because fluids and nutrition are not really death-delaying treatments.

Like many ethical issues, the care and destiny of PVS clients have no perfect solution. Although the courts have attempted to deal with this dilemma, the decisions handed down have been inconsistent and seem arbitrary. Some states have enacted *conscience clauses* in their nursing practice acts that would allow nurses to refuse to participate in procedures that would lead to the death of PVS clients. Although conscience clauses demonstrate legislative concern for nursing's ethics and morals, they may open the door to lawsuits against nurses for participating in death-causing procedures because nurses can no longer claim that they had no choice. In any case, nurses need to carefully consider how and when they participate in withholding care to clients who are not yet dead, in a legal sense.

Modified from Hall, JK: Caring for corpses or killing patients. Nurs Management 25:81–89, 1994.

ISSUES IN PRACTICE
Drug Experimentation and Informed
Consent

Picture yourself in this situation. You are in the terminal stages of an incurable dis-ease. Your physicians have used all the conventional and approved treatments that are normally used for this disease, but you are still getting progressively worse. Then, one morning, a new physician you have never seen before enters your room and begins to tell you about an experimental drug that has been used on a few other clients who have the same disease as you do. This therapy has shown some promise for improvement or even a cure. He then offers to give you this drug, free of charge, if you are willing to participate in the experiment. You will have to sign a six-page form that prevents you, or your family, from suing either the physician or the drug company if the experiment does not prove to be successful. What would you do?

If you are like most clients who find themselves in this situation, you would prob-ably take the risk and try the new drug. But do you really understand what you are agreeing to? Is the consent you give thus really *informed* consent?

Although this is a common method for testing new drugs, recent reports of drug trials that went wrong have brought the whole process under question. When 5 out of 15 clients died after receiving an experimental drug for hepatitis B, attention be-gan to focus on how well the participants were prepared for the risks incurred when receiving experimental drugs. The basic question is whether the consent given by any critically ill client can ever be considered informed.

Consent forms used for trial medications need to explain the nature of the ex-periment and the risks of the trial. The difficulties for the experimenters preparing these forms to determine how much information to provide and to word the form in such a way that the average client can understand it. Obviously if the form is too de-tailed or complicated, some clients may refuse to undergo the treatment. On the other hand, if the form is too simple, the client may be agreeing to something for which full information has not been given. The six-page consent form used for the new hepatitis B drug listed fatigue, nausea, skin rashes, bone marrow suppression, seizures, pain, and numbness in the arms and legs as the only major risk factors. A general disclaimer at the end of the form stated: "This is a new medication, and its side effects have not been completely described." It is interesting to speculate about how many patients would have taken this medication if "death" had been listed as one of the possible side effects.

Another factor that enters into the question of informed consent is coercion. Al-though the experimenters are not physically *forcing* these clients to take the trial med-ication, desperately ill clients tend to grasp at any glimmer of hope and may sign the consent form without understanding it, or even without reading it. And, of course, the physician who is explaining the new medication is going to try to put the med-ication and test in as positive a light as possible.

In new guidelines for experimental medication forms, it has been suggested that no mention of benefit or cure from the drug be made. It would be much more honest to let the client know that they are involved in research whose primary goal is to obtain new knowledge. If the medication should produce a benefit or cure, then it will have been successful and everyone is happy. But the client also needs to realize that the drug may produce worse symptoms, or even death, and those results are also of benefit to the experimenter.

Modified from Altman, L.K.: Fatal drug trial raises questions about informed consent. New York Times, October 5, 1993, C-3.

ISSUES IN PRACTICE
A Question of Distributive Justice

Jessica B. was diagnosed with acute lymphocytic leukemia at age 4. She is now 7 years old and has been treated with chemotherapy for the past 3 years with varying degrees of success. She is currently in a state of relapse, and a bone marrow transplant seems to be the only treatment that might improve her condition and save her life. Her father is a day-laborer who has no health insurance, so Jessica's health care is being paid for largely by the Medicaid system of her small state in the Southwest.

The current cost of a bone marrow transplant at the state's central teaching hospital is $1.5 million, representing about half of the state's entire annual Medicaid budget. Although bone marrow transplants are an accepted treatment for leukemia, this therapy only offers a slim chance for a total cure of the disease. The procedure is risky with a chance that it may cause death, will involve several months of post-transplant treatment and recovery in an ICU many miles from the family's home, and many years of costly antirejection medications.

The family understands the risks and benefits. They ask the nurse caring for Jessica what they should do. How should the nurse respond? Does the nurse have any obligations toward the Medicaid system as a whole?

BIBLIOGRAPHY

Aiken, TD and Catalano, JT: Legal, Ethical, and Political Issues in Nursing. FA Davis, Philadelphia, 1994.

Altman, LK: Fatal drug trial raises questions about informed consent. New York Times, October 5, 1993, C-3.

American Nurses Association: Code for Nurses with Interpretive Statement. American Nurses Association, Kansas City, 1976.

Bullough, UL: The Emergence of the Modern Nurse, Macmillan, New York, 1969.

Catalano, JT: Critical care nurses and ethical dilemmas. Crit Care Nurse 11:16–21, 1991.

Catalano, JT: Systems of ethics. Crit Care Nurse 12:91–96, 1992.

Davis, AJ and Aroskar, MS: Ethical Dilemmas and Nursing Practice. Appleton-Century-Crofts, New York, 1978.

Doheny, M, Cook, C and Stopper, C: The Discipline of Nursing. Appleton & Lange, Norwalk, CT, 1987.

Fiesta, J: The Law and Liability: A Guide for Nurses. John Wiley & Sons, New York, 1988.

Fletcher, J: Situation Ethics. Westminister, Philadelphia, 1966.

Ford, RD (ed.): Nurse's Legal Handbook. Springhouse Springhouse, PA, 1985.

French, PA: The Spectrum of Responsibility. St. Martin's Press, New York, 1991.

Jameton, A. Nursing Practice: The Ethical Issues. Prentice Hall, Englewood Cliffs, N.J. 1984.

Mappes, TA and Zembaty, JS: Biomedical Ethics ed 3. McGraw-Hill, New York, 1991.

Quinn, CA, and Smith, MD: The Professional Commitment: Issues and Ethics in Nursing. WB Saunders, Philadelphia, 1987.

Sawyer, LM: Nursing code of ethics: An international comparison. Int Nurse Rev 36:145–148, 1989.

Thompson, JE and Thompson, HO: Bioethical Decision Making for Nurses. Appleton-Century Crofts, Norwalk, CT, 1985.

Thompson, JE and Thompson, HO: Teaching ethics to nursing students. Nurs Outlook 37:84–88, 1989.

 # HISTORICAL PERSPECTIVES

Health Care During and After the Civil War in the United States

The Civil War was the most costly for the United States in numbers of American dead and injured. Existing health care services were soon overwhelmed by large numbers of the wounded and dying. Neither side had any organized first-aid battlefield services, nor any medical or nursing corps. Medical supplies were often impossible to obtain, particularly on the Confederate side, and many surgeries, such as amputations and removal of bullets, were performed under filthy battlefield conditions without anesthesia. Infections after injury killed as many on both sides as the actual wounds did.

As in all wars where there are large numbers of wounded and sick, the demand for nurses increased dramatically. Some of the sisters from the religious nursing orders attempted to meet these needs, but their numbers were inadequate. Shortly after the war started, it became the practice for large numbers of female volunteers to follow the armies as they went from battlefield to battlefield, providing some basic nursing care. The Union forces had as many as 6000 mostly untrained volunteers at the height of the war, and the Confederates had about 1000. What little nursing knowledge they had was derived by trial and error and from observing and mimicking the care provided by the few religious nursing sisters who were among them. These volunteers cleaned and dressed wounds, prepared food and fed wounded soldiers, gave what few medications they had, and tried to keep the temporary hospitals, which were set up in requisitioned churches and schools, as clean as possible. Their services generally went unappreciated or were even ridiculed by the few medical doctors that the opposing armies had pressed into service.

Several major advances in medical and nursing care did occur during the Civil War. The origin of nurses in the U.S. Navy can be traced to this period when a transport ship, the *Red Rover*, was converted to a hospital ship, staffed by the Sisters of Mercy. The American Red Cross and the Army nurse corps also began during this period, under the guidance and planning of individuals who would later become important leaders in nursing. Among the volunteers in the Union forces was a group of African-American women. In general, the Civil War allowed large numbers of women out of the home and into the hospitals who never would have been there without war. Despite the slurs and derogatory remarks of some army medical officers, the public image of nurses improved markedly during the Civil War, because of the selfless efforts of the volunteers (Bullough, 1969).

6

BIOETHICAL ISSUES

Learning Objectives

After completing this chapter, the reader will be able to:

1 Discuss the key ethical principles involved in:
   a Abortion
   b Genetic research
   c Fetal tissue research
   d Organ transplantation
   e Use of scarce resources
   f Assisted suicide
   g AIDS
2 Discuss the nurse's role in these ethical dilemmas.
3 Analyze and make a thoughtful ethical decision in a complex situation.

If recent history has brought nothing else to nursing, it has introduced a flood of biomedical and ethical dilemmas. Historically, nurses have been concerned with moral responsibility and ethical decision making. The early development, frequent revision, and high degree of refinement found in the nursing code of ethics demonstrate the profession's concern and feeling of responsibility for providing ethical health care. The earliest of the codes of ethics made obedience to the physician the nurse's primary responsibility. The present code recognizes that the primary responsibility of the nurse is the client's well-being. This altered sensibility reflects the profession's increased self-awareness, independence, and growing accountability. Unfortunately, this new attitude has also heralded an era of increased tension, self-doubt, and ethical confusion. By examining the issues, and by identifying the key moral and ethical conflicts, nurses will be able to accept their moral responsibilities and make sound ethical decisions successfully.

COMMON ETHICAL DILEMMAS IN NURSING

In the course of their careers, nurses are likely to face ethical dilemmas. Although a complete analysis of every issue is beyond the scope of this book, some of the more common situations and their important ethical features will be presented as examples of ways to analyze such dilemmas and to make informed decisions. Resolving ethical dilemmas is never an easy task, and it is likely that someone will be displeased by the decision, no matter how carefully and thoughtfully it is made.

ABORTION

Few issues evoke as strong an emotional reaction as abortion. Because of its religious, ethical, social, and legal implications, the abortion issue touches everyone in one way or another. There seems to be very little "middle ground." People are either strongly in favor of abortion or oppose it completely.

Elective (therapeutic) abortion is described as the voluntary termination of a pregnancy before 24 weeks of gestation. In the case of *Roe v. Wade* in 1973, the Supreme Court changed the legal status of therapeutic abortion in the United States, but its ethical basis and moral status remain controversial.

A careful reading of the decision in *Roe v. Wade* reveals that the court made no decision about the ethics or morality of elective abortion. Rather, the court said that, according to the U.S. Constitution, all people have a right to determine what they can do with their bodies (right to self-determination) and that such a right includes terminating a pregnancy.

The fundamental issues at the heart of the abortion debate center on the right of freedom of choice, which the court recognized, and the question of when life begins. Those who argue against abortion believe life begins at the moment of conception and therefore hold that abortion is a killing act. Proponents of abortion argue that the fetus is not really human until it reaches the point of development where it can live outside the mother's body, that is, the age of viability. From a deontologic standpoint, abortion represents a basic conflict of rights.

On the one hand is the women's right to privacy and the right to self-determination and freedom of choice. In the United States, these rights are fiercely held and are considered issues of public policy and constitutional law. Indeed, these are the rights that form the basis of the *Roe v. Wade* decision.

On the other hand, the conflicting right from the antiabortion side of the dilemma is the very basic right to life of the fetus. In most Western civilizations, particularly those that are based on Judeo-Christian beliefs, strong prohibition exists against the casual and intentional taking of a human life. Life is the most basic good because without it there can be no other rights. In general, the right to life is considered the most profound of the rights, and is absolute in most situations.

When one is attempting to resolve the ethics and morality of abortion, these two conflicting rights need to be weighed against each other. Nurses are often placed in situations where they must help clients make decisions about abortion. Just as frequently, they are asked to participate in the procedure itself. In practice, ethical issues are always affected by the health care provider's moral values. In the dilemma over abortion, nurses must analyze their own values and perceptions of their roles in order to make the best decisions. As a client advocate, should a nurse be for or against abortion? How can a nurse avoid influencing the woman's decision about abortion? Can a nurse ethically and legally refuse to assist at abortions? Ought the client's reason for wanting an abortion or stage of pregnancy (first or second trimester) have any influence on the nurse's decision? These questions are not easily answered, but understanding the underlying principles involved in the issue may help lessen some of the emotional impact that often surrounds its discussion. As in all complicated ethical dilemmas, the nurse needs to remember that the client must receive competent, high-quality care regardless of the nurse's own personal values or moral beliefs.

GENETIC RESEARCH

The ability to alter genetic material in such a way as to produce organisms that differ greatly from their original form is now a reality. Current scientific and popular literature is filled with reports of new ways to identify and change the genetic material of all types of living creatures. Currently, genetically altered bacteria, such as *Escherichia coli*, are used to produce a variety of medications, including a purer form of insulin. Genetically altered corn is now growing in very hot, dry places, and is resistant to most insects. Abnormal genes that signal individuals who are at risk for various types of cancer, Alzheimer's disease, and Down's syndrome have been identified.

Society in the 20th century has become so accustomed to the idea that science should be allowed to do whatever it is capable of doing that very few questions have been asked about the ethics of genetic engineering and research. As with most scientific research and techniques, the techniques of genetic engineering are ethically neutral. Procedures such as refining recombinant DNA, gene therapy, altering germ cells, and cloning other cells, in themselves, are neither good nor bad. Potential for misuse of these procedures is so great, however, that it may permanently alter or even destroy the human race entirely.

Several ethical issues need to be considered when genetic engineering and research are being conducted, including those involved with the safety of genetic research, the legality and morality of genetic screening, and the proper use of genetic information. Recently proposed laws will attempt to regulate genetic research to prevent the production of a supervirus or superbacteria that could exterminate the entire human population of the earth.

With current technology, it is possible to detect genetic patterns in newborn infants that are linked to breast and colon cancer, heart disease, and Huntington's and Parkinson's diseases. The advantage to insurance companies, which could screen individuals as early as infancy for costly and potentially lethal diseases, is obvious—these individuals could be excluded from health and life insurance coverage, saving the insurance companies a great deal of money. Although this practice would most likely be unethical, the specter of mandatory genetic screening is not unrealistic. Because it requires just one blood sample from a person sometime during that person's life, it is possible that this type of screening could even be done without the knowledge or consent of the individual.

Informed consent is discussed in Chapter 8 of this book. Confidentiality is at great risk of being violated by genetic screening. The confidentiality that exists between the health care provider and the client has been the bedrock of the therapeutic relationship. Information obtained through genetic screening *can* be used to benefit clients and to prepare them for future problems or it can be released to insurance companies to give them a basis for refusal of coverage. In some cases, individuals may be denied employment based on the results of genetic testing. In this age of the information superhighway and vast computerized databases, very little of a client's health history remains confidential.

An important ethical implication for nurses is the emotional impact that genetic information may have on the client. Knowing the possible long-term outcome of one's health, particularly if that knowledge is negative, may cause a client to become depressed or suicidal. Nurses must further hone their teaching and counseling skills to assist clients to deal with implications of this type of information.

Obstetric nurses have been involved with genetic screening procedures for years. Some of the most important information obtained from amniocentesis deals with the genetic composition of the fetus. It is important that the mother understand the procedure and the type of information it may yield, and that she give informed consent for it.

A strict ethical obligation exists for nurses to refuse to participate in mandatory, involuntary screening programs, as well as a strict prohibition about revealing genetic test results to unauthorized individuals. Forcing clients who are strongly opposed to finding out information about their genetic status to be tested is clearly a breach of those clients' right to self-determination. Yet, much as the current practice of routine screening for diseases such as tuberculosis, hepatitis, and blood lead levels promotes the general health of the population, so does the screening for genetic diseases. Clients who are strongly opposed to such genetic screening must be allowed the option to refuse it to maintain their right to self-determination.

USE OF FETAL TISSUE

Although it has just recently become the news in the popular media, fetal tissue research has been going on for at least 10 years. Traditional fetal tissue research has been generally limited to taking living cells from aborted fetus and transplanting them into other human beings with chronic or severe diseases. The procedure has been found to be helpful to a limited extent in the treatment of Alzheimer's and Parkinson's diseases.

During the past several years, a new twist has been added to this research. Rather than using tissue from aborted fetuses, scientists are now growing their own fetal tissue in the lab through in vitro fertilization procedures. These *test-tube* fetuses are then dissected. Various tissues from them are used for genetic and other types of research. The legal system has become aware of abuses of these procedures and has proposed legislation to control its use, including limiting the age of in vitro fetuses to 6 weeks. After 6 weeks, such fetuses will have to be destroyed.

Fetal tissue is highly desirable for research and transplantation because it lacks some of the genetic material that makes more mature tissues and organs more likely to cause rejection in the host. These fetal tissues are also in a rapid-growth mode and naturally develop more quickly than tissues from other sources. Scientists involved in this research see fetal tissue as one of the most important means of curing diseases, both now and into the future.

Yet even a superficial consideration of these procedures necessarily raises many important ethical issues. Basic to the ethics of this type of research is the source of the research material. In the past, most of the material came from elective abortions. Because of the immaturity and lack of differentiation of cells during the first trimester of pregnancy, however, the best fetal tissue comes from fetuses aborted during the second trimester. Most scientists agree that second-trimester fetuses have well-developed nervous, cardiovascular, gastrointestinal, and renal systems and are capable of feeling pain. Even though fetal tissue research has not led to an increase in abortions, the potential for abuse is tremendous.

It is also not definite whether the fetal tissue research scientists are paying others for these aborted fetuses. If they *are* paying for aborted fetuses, it seems to violate the laws that prevent payment for organs used in transplantation. Questions also arise concerning who is giving permission for the use of fetuses in transplantation procedures. Does anyone really own them?

Another important ethical issue concerns the use of in vitro fertilization as a sourse for fetal tissue. Many religious groups question the morality of the procedure itself. Even if in vitro fertilization is considered ethical for procedures such as surrogate motherhood, is it ethical to create fetuses that are going to be used *only* for research and transplantation? From whom are the ova and sperm coming? Have the people from whom these have been obtained given permission for such use of their tissues? What about the rights of a fetus who was created in a test-tube without ever having a hope of a normal life?

Despite a 1988 directive, which was extended indefinitely in 1990, to prevent the Department of Health and Human Services from using federal money for fetal tissue research, such research continues. Recent administrations have unofficially lifted the ban by allowing local biomedical ethical panels to make decisions about this type of research. Composed largely of research scientists, many of these panels have come out in favor of continued research.

Nurses may have an important role to play in issues involving fetal tissue research. Although they will not likely be involved in direct research itself, nurses often are employed in facilities were elective abortions are performed. Nurses employed in such places must become aware of the issues involved in abortion. They also should know where the aborted fetuses are taken and how they are disposed of. Nurses should also remain informed about developing procedures and techniques regarding fetal tissue research; they should support legal and ethical efforts to control its abuses.

ORGAN TRANSPLANTATION

Despite widespread public and medical acceptance of organ transplantation as a highly beneficial procedure, ethical questions still remain. Whenever a human organ is transplanted, many people are involved, including the donor, the donor's family, medical and nursing personnel, as well as the recipient and the recipient's family. Society in general could also be added to this mix because of the high cost of organ transplantation, which is usually paid from tax monies directly, or indirectly in the form of increased insurance premiums. Each one of these persons or groups has rights that may conflict with the rights of others.

Most institutions that perform transplants or organizations that are involved in obtaining organs have developed elaborate, detailed, and involved procedures to help deal with the ethical and legal issues involved in transplantation. Despite these efforts, some ethical uncertainties remain whenever the issue of organ transplantation is raised. One particularly sensitive issue is exemplified when a child donates an organ, for example, a kidney transplant for a sibling, a procedure that poses some risk. Although parents are usually required to give consent for medical procedures for their children, by legal definition, a child under the age of 18 cannot give informed consent to such a procedure. It can be argued, however, that ethically, the donor child, as a participant, should have a voice in such a decision. At what age can a child have a say in the decision? Can a child be forced, for example, to donate a kidney even if he or she refuses?

One situation that illustrates this dilemma is that of a teenaged girl who developed leukemia. The only way to save her life was to find a bone-marrow donor who matched her genetic type. When no donor could be found, the parents decided to have another baby in the hopes that the bone marrow of the second child would match that of the first child. After the baby was born, it was found that the bone marrow did indeed match and when the child was old enough to donate safely, the bone marrow was taken and transplanted into the older child.

Despite the best efforts of the medical and legal community to establish criteria for death, some ethical questions still linger about what constitutes death. Because organs such as hearts, lungs, and livers need to come from a beating-heart donor, some clinicians fear a tendency to declare death before it actually occurs. The most widely accepted criterion for death is brain death. Some researchers, however, question whether the death of the brain necessarily means that a person ceases to exist as a human being. Or are there some other criteria that ought to be examined?

One of the most difficult ethical issues involved in organ transplantation is the selection of recipients. Because many fewer organs are available than people who need them, the potential ethical dilemmas are great. The national organ recipient list attempts to list and rank all people who need organs in a nondiscriminatory manner. Some important criteria include need, length of time on the list, potential for survival, prior organ transplantation, value to the community, and tissue compatibility.

Nurses can be, and often are, involved in some aspect of the organ-donation process. Many states have passed laws that require the health care workers to ask the family members of potential organ donors if they have ever thought about their dead or dying loved one being used for organ donation. Many nurses, particularly those who work in critical care units, provide care for clients who may potentially become organ donors. Nurses in operating rooms may help in the actual surgical procedures that remove organs from a cadaver and transplant them into a recipient's body. Many general-care nurses provide the post-operative care for clients who have received a transplanted organ. Home health care nurses give the follow-up care to such clients at home.

Nurses working with organ transplantation need to be sensitive to the potential for manipulation. Most people who are seeking organ transplantations are desperately ill or near death. They, and their families, can be very easily manipulated or themselves become very manipulating. On the other side, the families of potential organ donors are usually distraught about the sudden and traumatic loss of a loved one. They too are vulnerable to psychologic manipulation. Because of the emotionally fragile state present in the family of a trauma victim, they are vulnerable to guilt and grief. Health care providers should avoid appealing to these emotions when obtaining permission to harvest organs for transplantation.

As a general rule, neither the donor nor his or her family should play any part in the selection of a recipient. Nurses need to avoid making statements or giving nonverbal indications of their approval or disapproval of potential recipients.

USE OF SCARCE RESOURCES IN PROLONGING LIFE

In these days of restructuring and down-sizing, money for health care is in short supply. It is recognized that most public money allocated for health care is spent during the last year of life for many elderly clients (Macklin, 1987). Expensive procedures, therapies, technologies, and care are provided to terminally ill individuals to extend their lives by a few days or even a few hours. It is not unusual to spend as much as $5000 a day on a client receiving care in an intensive care unit.

The traditional belief has been that life should be preserved at all cost and by any means available. Health care providers feel uncomfortable when cost considerations are mentioned regarding treatments for terminally ill clients. Yet, in the context of current problems in society, such considerations are both economic and ethical realities. The necessity of conserving resources has forced society, through governmental action, to face this issue. All of the present proposed health care plans take into consideration some type of cost-control measures related to restricting payment for client care.

In reality, the current health care system is already rationing care to some degree. Many people who are not covered by health care insurance do not seek health care. Groups such as the poor, who are covered by massive governmental programs, shy away from seeking health care because of the many restrictions placed on it. Individuals who *are* covered by insurance often have restrictions placed on them by the insurance companies.

The use of public funds for health care is an ethical issue that revolves around the principle of distributive justice. In this context, distributive justice requires that all citizens have equal access to all types of health care, regardless of their income levels, race, sex, religious beliefs, or diagnosis. Many complex issues are involved in this dilemma.

These issues go far beyond the questions of who gets what type of care and where and how the care take place. Some type of universal health care is likely to be mandated for all Americans, sometime in the future. Is it fair that some individuals (taxpayers) pay for the health care of others? Should individuals who contribute to their own poor state of health by smoking, drinking, taking illicit drugs, or overeating be provided with the same type of care as those who do not put themselves at risk? And who is going to make the decisions about who gets expensive treatment such as organ transplantations, experimental medications, placement in intensive care units, or life-extending technologies?

Using criteria such as age, potential for a high-quality life, and availability of resources for determining who receives life-extending technologies is gaining wider acceptance. But is this a valid ethical position? Nurses are often involved in situations where terminal clients are brought to the hospital for end-of-life care. They need to play an active role in helping to formulate policies concerning the issues they face everyday.

RIGHT TO DIE

The right-to-die issue is an extension of the right to self-determination issue discussed in Chapter 8. It also overlaps with the dilemma about euthanasia and assisted suicide. Health care providers often become involved in the decision-making process when clients are irreversibly comatose, vegetative, or suffering from a terminal disease. The choices the families of such clients often face are death or the extension of life using painful and expensive treatments.

One of the difficulties in resolving right-to-die issues is understanding the terminology used. Often clients who have living wills state that they want no extraordinary treatments if they should become comatose or unable to make decisions about their care. But what actually constitutes extraordinary treatments? A general definition of ordinary treatments includes any medications, procedures, surgeries, or technologies that offer the client some hope of benefit without causing excessive pain or suffering (Fromer, 1981). Using this definition, extraordinary treatments, sometimes called heroic measures, become those treatments, medications, surgeries, and technologies that offer little hope for curing or improving the client's condition. Although these general definitions provide some guidelines for making decisions about ordinary and extraordinary treatments, discerning the nature of the specific modalities remains difficult. For example, a ventilator is a machine that assists a client's respiration. In intensive care units (ICUs), it is a common mode of treatment for many types of clients, including post-operative clients, clients with cardiac and respiratory diseases, and victims of trauma. Does its widespread and frequent use make the ventilator an ordinary mode of treatment? Many would say yes, whereas others would say it is still extraordinary due to its invasive nature and complicated technology.

Another issue often included under the right-to-die issue is that of "codes" and "do not resuscitate" (DNR or no code) orders. Cardiopulmonary resuscitation (CPR) is widely taught to both health care providers and the general public. It is often used to treat clients who have suffered heart attacks and have gone into cardiac arrest, as well as clients suffering from electrical shock, drowning, and traumatic injuries. In the hospital setting, the nursing staff is obligated to perform CPR on all clients who do not have a specific DNR order. This leads to situations where terminally ill clients may be subjected to CPR resuscitative efforts several times before they die.

As an issue of self-determination, it is essential that the client's wishes about health care be followed. All client communication to the nurse about desires for future care should be documented. If at all possible, the client should be encouraged to designate an individual to act as a surrogate decision maker should the client become unable to make his or her own decisions. The expressed desires about future medical care are known as advanced directives. They are the best means to guarantee that a client's wishes will be honored.

Advanced directives, in the form of a living will or durable power of attorney, can and should specify which extraordinary procedures, surgeries, medications, or treatments can or cannot be used. These directives are often in the form of formal documents that need to be witnessed by two individuals who are not related to the client. As useful as advanced directives are in helping the client decided on future care, clients often are unable to anticipate all the possible types of treatments used. For example, an elderly client with a long history of cardiovascular disease specified in his living will that he did not want CPR performed and did not want a ventilator. When his heart developed a potentially lethal dysrhythmia that rendered him unresponsive, his physician made the decision to cardiovert* the client using the electric cardioverter because this mode of treatment was not specifically forbidden by the client's living will. Strictly speaking, the physician did not violate the letter of the living will, but did he violate its spirit?

Nurses can help clients plan ahead for their care should they become unable to make decisions for themselves. Although the nurse should not *make* the decisions for the client, the nurse should provide important information and explanations of what is involved in the various treatment modalities that the client is considering. The nurse can also help clients clarify their wishes and guide them through the process in formulating an advanced directive.

EUTHANASIA AND ASSISTED SUICIDE

The term **euthanasia** generally means killing or refusing to treat a client to allow a painless or peaceful death. A distinction is often made between passive and active euthanasia. **Passive euthanasia** usually refers to the practice of allowing an individual to die without any extraordinary intervention. Under this umbrella definition, such practices as DNR orders, living wills, and withdrawal of ventilators or other life support are usually included. **Active euthanasia,** on the other hand, usually describes the practice of speeding an individual's death through some act or procedure. This practice is also sometimes referred to as mercy killing and takes many forms ranging from using large amounts of pain medication for terminal cancer clients to using poisons, guns, or knives to end a person's life.

Assisted suicide, recently brought to public attention by Dr. Jack Kevorkian, a Michigan physician, who has publicly practiced it, is really a type of active euthanasia or mercy killing. The central issue that has been publicized by Dr. Kevorkian is whether it is ever ethically permissable for health care personnel to assist in taking a life. In most states the practice is illegal. The definition of homicide, bringing about a person's death or assisting him to do so, seems to fit the act of assisted suicide. There is still a great deal of hesitation on the part of the legal system to prosecute persons who are involved in assisted suicide.

The fundamental ethical issue is the right to self-determination. In almost every other health care situation, a client, as long as the person is mentally competent, can make decisions about what care to accept and what care to refuse. Yet, when it comes to the termination of life, this right becomes controversial. Supporters of the practice of assisted suicide hold to the belief that the right to self-determination remains intact, even to the decision to end one's life. It is the last act of a very sick individual to control his or her own fate. Many feel medical personnel should be allowed to assist these clients in this procedure, just as they are allowed to assist clients in other medical and nursing procedures.

Those who oppose assisted suicide find these arguments unconvincing.

---

*Cardioverting is a procedure in which electrical shock is used to change the heart rhythm from ventricular tachycardia or other rhythms to normal sinus rhythms.

Legally, ethically, and morally, suicide in the society of the United States has never been an accepted practice. Health care staff go to great lengths to prevent clients who are identified as suicidal from injuring themselves. In addition, it would seem that individuals in the terminal states of a disease who are overwhelmed by pain and depressed by the thought of prolonged suffering might not be able to think clearly enough to give informed consent for assisted suicide. Also, because the termination of life is final, it does not allow for spontaneous cures, or the development of new treatments or medications.

Nonmaleficence is the term that describes the obligation to do no harm to clients. Whether assisting in or causing the death of a client is a violation of this principle is most likely an issue that will continue to be debated for some time.

HUMAN IMMUNODEFICIENCY VIRUS AND ACQUIRED IMMUNODEFICIENCY SYNDROME

Human immunodeficiency virus (HIV) and acquired immunodeficiency syndrome (AIDS) have evoked strong emotions both in the public and in the medical community. Nurses, who for years held strongly to the ethical principle that all clients regardless of race, sex, religion, age, or disease process should be cared for equally, are now questioning their obligation to take care of clients who have AIDS.

Several ethical issues underlie the AIDS controversy. One of the most important is the right to privacy. Although there is a general requirement to report infection with HIV/AIDS to the Centers for Disease Control (CDC), many states have strict laws regarding the confidentiality of the diagnosis. Revealing the diagnosis of HIV/AIDS brings the possibility of a lawsuit against the health care provider or institution. But the right to privacy is not absolute. Diseases such as tuberculosis, gonorrhea, syphilis, and hepatitis that are highly contagious and sometimes fatal must be reported to public health officials. If the right to privacy can be violated when the public welfare is at stake, does AIDS represent this type of threat? Is it unjust to ask health care providers to care for clients with this disease without knowing that the client has it? Is it just to violate a client's privacy when the disease carries with it a potential for social stigma and isolation? Does the client have a right to know that a health care provider is infected with HIV/AIDS?

Another important ethical issue is the right to care. Can a nurse refuse to care for an AIDS client? Obviously, a fundamental right of a client is to receive care, and a fundamental obligation of a nurse is to provide care. The first statement of the American Nurses Association (ANA) Nurses Code of Ethics states that a nurse must provide care unrestricted by any considerations. Surely, though, there are some exceptions, for example if the nurse is pregnant, or is receiving chemotherapy, or has had other immunity problems. In most situations, however, the nurse is obligated to provide the best nursing care possible for all clients, including those with AIDS.

What about the tremendous cost involved in treating individuals who have

AIDS? Recent studies estimate that the medical cost of treating an AIDS client from the time of diagnosis to the time of death will be in the neighborhood of $750,000 (Catalano, 1992). In the face of this crisis, governmental agencies, who bear the brunt of paying for AIDS treatment, will have to make some hard decisions concerning this issue. With over 1 million people already infected with this disease, the cost to society is astronomic. Nurses have the obligation to care for all clients, including those with AIDS, but ought physicians, hospitals, or governmental agencies also be held to this same precept? Should our society regard health care as a right or a privilege?

SUMMARY

Ethical issues and ethics are a factor in the day-to-day practice of all nurses. Any time a nurse comes in contact with a client, a potential ethical situation exists. In today's world, with rapidly advancing technology and unusual health care situations, ethical dilemmas are proliferating. Nurses can be prepared to deal with most of these dilemmas if they keep current with the issues and are able to follow a systematic process for making decisions about them. Hiding from ethical issues is not a solution. At some point, difficult decisions must be made. One of the worst elements of ethical decision making is that it is very unlikely that everyone involved in the dilemma will be happy with the decision. If the decision is made after an analysis of the situation and is based on sound ethical principles, however, it usually can be defended.

 ## CRITICAL THINKING EXERCISES

Analyze the following case study using the ethical decision-making process:

What data are important in relation to this situation?

State the ethical dilemma in a clear, simple statement.

What are the choices of action and how do they relate to specific ethical principles?

What are the consequences of these actions?

What decisions *can* be made?

CASE STUDY

Lisa, a registered nurse in the ICU, is caring for a 52-year-old male client with a gunshot wound to the head. The client is comatose, is on

CRITICAL THINKING EXERCISES (Continued)

life support, and has an extremely poor prognosis. The physician in charge doubts the client will live more than 72 hours. The client was shot with a .22 rifle, allegedly by his 12-year-old daughter, whom he reportedly tried to molest sexually. The client has a wife and two other daughters, one aged 18 who still lives at home, and another aged 22, who is married and lives in another town. The whole family is present in the client's room around the clock.

Lisa spends a great deal of time providing care for this client because of the complexity of the treatments involved. There are a ventilator, pulmonary artery catheter, arterial line, intercranial pressure monitor, central venous line, and a number of potent vasoactive medications being infused, all of which require close attention. Lisa, normally a very quiet person, is in the room so much that the family generally pays little attention to her. To them, she has become another of the room fixtures. Over the course of her 12-hour shift, Lisa learns from overhearing the family talking among themselves that the father had also sexually molested the two older daughters when they reached ages 12 or 13. In addition, it becomes evident to Lisa that it was not the 12-year-old daughter who shot the father, but rather the 18-year-old daughter. Apparently, the 18-year-old had made an agreement with her father that he could do whatever he wanted to her, so long as he left the youngest daughter alone. When he violated that agreement and attempted to molest the youngest daughter, the 18-year-old shot him. The girls had agreed among themselves to blame it on the 12-year-old because she would be much less likely to be prosecuted for the shooting.

The father died during the night shift the following day. Lisa was in a quandary about what to do. Should she report what she had learned while in the room caring for this man, or should she just let it go? The District Attorney had already made public the fact that the 12-year-old was not going to be charged or prosecuted.

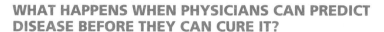

WHAT HAPPENS WHEN PHYSICIANS CAN PREDICT DISEASE BEFORE THEY CAN CURE IT?

The sciences' headlong rush into genetic research has led to the identification of some 900 genes that are related to, or may cause, genetic diseases. Unfortunately, there are no cures or even very effective treatments for many of these diseases. In practice, a sample of fetal blood subjected to genetic analysis can tell if an unborn fetus will, at some point in its life, develop breast cancer, Parkinson's disease, or Alzheimer's disease; have a heart attack or high cholesterol; develop neurofibromas or a variety of other conditions that may not become evident until the person is middle-aged or older.

Given this knowledge and the lack of cure for these diseases, should children be tested for potential genetic disorders? And if they are tested, should they, or their parents, be given this information? Should this information be made available to insurance companies?

There are no clear guidelines for making these types of decisions. On the one hand, it is a generally accepted principle that patients have a right to information about their diseases and treatments. Collateral to that right is the right of parents to have medical information about their children. Yet, of what advantage is it for a child to know that he or she is likely to develop tumors along the nerves (neurofibromatosis) for which there is no treatment and some of which would likely be malignant?

However, there would seem to be some advantage in knowing that a child was at high risk for some diseases. For example, if it is known that a child is at high risk for high cholesterol, diet modifications could help keep the cholesterol at a lower level. In the case of breast or colon cancer, knowing about the predisposition for these diseases could prompt a person to seek more frequent screening at an earlier age. It is well proven that early detection and treatment of cancer greatly increases the chance of survival.

Testing for, and use of, genetic, information will remain an unsettled issue in the future. As more and more disease-causing genes are identified, the problem will only become more complicated.

Modified from Kolata, G: Should children be told if genes predict illness? The New York Times (national edition), September 26, 1994, A-1.

ISSUES IN PRACTICE
Case Study—Determining the Greatest Good

Sherry is an RN who works for a rehabilitation center that deals primarily with developmentally delayed children. For several years, Sherry has been following the case of Margie N., who is now 8 years old and has Down's syndrome and moderate retardation. Margie has made steady, if slow, progress in achieving basic motor and cognitive skills but still requires close supervision of all activities and care for all basic hygiene needs. Margie is still not advanced enough to participate in group activities at the center's day clinic.

Mrs. N., Margie's mother, a 42-year-old widow, has been providing a high level of care for Margie at home, as well as meeting the child's demands for love and attention. Recently, Mrs. N. has been diagnosed with systemic lupus erythematosus (SLE), which has displayed as its primary symptoms severe joint pain and stiffness. During the past several months, Mrs. N. has been finding it increasingly difficult to care for Margie because of the progressive nature of the SLE.

Mrs. N. is trying to make a decision about long-term care for Margie. She trusts Sherry's judgment completely and often relies on the information and teaching given by the nurse to make changes in Margie's care. Sherry is unsure about what advice she should give. She recognizes that the high level of care and comfort provided by Mrs. N. has been an essential part in the advances Margie has made up to this point, but she also recognizes that Mrs. N. may soon reach a point where that care can no longer be provided. It seems that to do what is good for Mrs. N. (i.e., placing Margie in an institution) would be harmful to Margie, whereas doing what is good for Margie (i.e., leaving her at home) would be harmful to Mrs. N. What is the best course of action in this situation? Are there any alternative solutions to this dilemma?

A Closer Look

ORGAN DONATION
What Families Need to Know

Seven Questions Families Often Ask About Organ Donation—and How You Should Answer Them

Many families refuse to donate a loved one's organs simply because they don't fully understand organ donation. By being prepared to address their concerns, you can help them make a decision they're comfortable with.

Here are the most common questions families ask about organ donation. Review them—and the answers—so you're prepared the next time you need to counsel a family on this sensitive issue.

1. *Whose consent is needed to allow organ donation?*
   Consent must come from the patient's legal next of kin, even if the patient has a signed donor card or an organ donation sticker on his driver's license.

2. *How can you ask us to make this decision at such a tragic time?*
   I know this is a very stressful time for you, but I need to ask that you think about organ donation. Is it what your loved one would have wanted?

   I understand that you may not be able to say yes right now, and that's okay. However, if you decide to donate, we need to know as soon as possible so that any tissues or organs may be removed in time to help another person.

3. *What does brain death mean?*
   Brain death is an irreversible condition that occurs when blood no longer flows to the brain and the brain tissue dies. Although the brain is dead, other organs and tissues can function if supported by artificial means. A doctor will pronounce brain death only after everything possible has been done for your loved one and he has no chance of survival.

4. *Is the body disfigured when the organs are removed?*
   Surgeons use as few incisions as possible to recover the donated organs or tissues. Donation shouldn't interfere with an open-casket funeral, if that's what you've planned.

5. *Will we be charged for donation costs?*
   No. All costs related to removal of the organs are covered by the donor program. However, you'll still be responsible for the funeral, burial arrangements, and related costs.

6. *How are recipients chosen?*
   Recipients are chosen from the United Network of Organ Sharing, a national computer registry. They're selected according to degree of need,

ORGAN DONATION (Continued)

how long they've been on the waiting list, and certain medical criteria, such as blood type compatibility, tissue matching, and body size.

7. *We're not sure if our religion allows organ donation. What should we do?*
Many religions support organ donation, but if you're concerned, speak with your religious leader.

—TERESA M. ODELL, RN,C
Coordinator
Nursing Staff Education
Cobb Hospital and Medical Center
Kennesaw, Ga.

From Odell, T.M., Organ donation. What families need to know. Nurs 94, December 1994, p. 321, with permission.

ISSUES IN PRACTICE
Treatments Not Specifically Listed in the Living Will: The Ethical Dilemmas

PART 1: THE ETHICAL CASE
Joseph T. Catalano, RN, PhD, CCRN

Because of publicity regarding living wills and laws on required request, the number of patients with them has increased. Consequently, related ethical dilemmas are also becoming more common. One example of such an ethical dilemma occurs when a living will fails to describe the current patient situation. The following case illustrates this type of problem, one which critical care nurses are likely to encounter more often over the next few years.

Sharon has worked as an RN in the 15-bed medical intensive care unit (MICU) of a rural 250-bed hospital for 5 years. She is concerned with the ethical and legal obligations of nurses who care for patients with living wills. During her tenure at this facility, several patients entered the hospital with living wills. Recently, however, Mr. K was admitted to the MICU with congestive heart failure, and he brought along his living will. The presence of the living will created problems for Sharon, Mr. K's primary nurse, and the MICU staff.

Mr. K was 72-years-old and had a long history of smoking and emphysema. He had recently developed congestive heart failure and angina. Because of his poor pulmonary function, his condition was inoperable. Mr. K was one of the MICU's "regulars;" he was admitted to the unit whenever he had an exacerbation of his pulmonary

Continued on following page

condition, usually once or twice a year. He chose to be treated aggressively with medications and respiratory therapy, excluding the use of a ventilator. Mr. K usually responded well to treatment and was generally discharged within a week of admission.

Mr. K's family consisted of a three adult children by a first wife, his current wife, their two adult children, plus several elderly brothers and sisters. His extended and immediate family were actively involved with his care and were aware of the living will he had executed two years previously after one of his hospitalizations. Based on Mr. K's living will, the physician classified him as a "no code" upon his most recent admission.

His living will was one of the general, standard-form documents consistent with the laws of his home state. The living will stated that should Mr. K become unable to make decisions about his care, he should be allowed to die and not be kept alive by artificial means.

The only specific stipulation in the living will was, "I am not to be placed on a ventilator." He had talked with Sharon, his primary nurse, several times about his fear of being kept alive on a ventilator when there was little or no hope of survival, or when he would be unable to return to his prior level of functioning. Mr. K's living will did not, however, address tube feedings, cardiopulmonary resuscitation (CPR), or life sustaining medications.

Upon Mr. K's most recent admission to the MICU for acute respiratory distress and chest pain, the electrocardiogram showed changes that might indicate a myocardial infarction, but the enzyme studies were inconclusive. He responded well to the prescribed treatments and medication therapy, and on the evening of his second day after admission Sharon helped Mr. K into a chair. Shortly thereafter, however, he suffered a sustained run of multiform ventricular tachycardia. During the dysrhythmic event, he became unresponsive and cyanotic. Four family members who were visiting at the time came running out of the room yelling, "Do something, Daddy's passed out!"

Simultaneously, one of Mr. K's physicians was making his evening rounds in the unit. The physician and Sharon quickly went into the room. The nurse quietly reminded the doctor that Mr. K had a living will and was ordered to be a "no code." The physician ordered that a code be initiated anyway. Mr. K was returned to his bed, intubated with an oral endotracheal tube, and resuscitated, including full CPR, electro-cardioversion, and chemical resuscitation using lidocaine and dopamine. The code produced a life sustaining cardiac rhythm, blood pressure, pulse, and spontaneous respirations, but Mr. K remained unresponsive and intubated for two more days, connected to a T-tube at 60%. His prognosis was extremely poor, and Mr. K lived only one day after extubation.

After the code, the nurse asked the physician why they had resuscitated Mr. K when he had a living will and was classified as a "no code"? The physician answered that a patient in Mr. K's condition was highly unlikely to file a law suit for violating the living will, whereas the family members might easily file a suite for wrongful death, especially if Mr. K had been allowed to die in the chair before their eyes. He also said that the spirit of the living will was followed by not placing Mr. K on a ventilator. The physician stated that Mr. K's living will was more oriented towards respiratory problems than cardiac dysrhythmias.

PART 2: ETHICAL ANALYSIS

Advance directives, which include living wills, are now a required part of the health care of all patients. The Omnibus Budget Reconciliation Act of 1990 requires that all hospitals, nursing-care facilities, home health-care agencies, and care givers ask patients about advance directives and provide information concerning living wills and Durable Power of Attorney (DPOA) to help patients make informed health-care decisions. However, the federal law mandates only the requirements and not the directives to implement the law. The actual implementation of the law is left to the individual states. Because of the vagueness of the law, a great deal of confusion exists, particularly with regards to living wills.

Nurses play an important role in insuring that patients understand the implications of their choices pertaining to decisions that may prolong their lives during medical emergency. Because of their "front-line" position as care givers within the health-care system, nurses must understand this role, specifically as it pertains to living wills.

This case study illustrates some of the difficult issues that nurses encounter when they care for patients with living wills. Some difficult legal and ethical questions need to be considered, for example:

- Dilemma 1: What legal and/or ethical implications do living wills have if families or physicians act against the patient's expressed wishes?
- Dilemma 2: Does the nurse have any ethical obligation to refuse to participate in the case of resuscitation efforts that are inconsistent with the patient's living will?
- Dilemma 3: If the physician had not been present to initiate the code, should the nurse have allowed Mr. K to die in the presence of his emotionally involved family?

Ethical Considerations

The questions formulated above address many practical concerns related to the execution of a living will. The living will, however, covers only very specific instances. There are always grey areas in ethically complex situations, such as the one presented here, that make a living will alone inadequate or which it is unable to address.

Identifying The Ethical Issues

Living wills are generally defined as "a directive from a competent individual to medical personnel and family members regarding the treatment he or she wishes to receive when he or she is no longer able to make the decision for himself or herself."[1] Although living wills have been present in the health-care setting, in one form or another, for as long as 20 years, they first attained the status of a legal document in 1976 when California passed the "Natural Death Act."[2] Since that date, 44 States have adopted a "Natural Death Act" in some form, although it varies widely from state to state. Also, the form that the living will may take varies, and no single form is acceptable in all states.[3] Some living wills are very specific as to what treatments

Continued on following page

are to be excluded, other living wills are general and non-specific about treatments. Each state has its own particular regulations determining the exact format and number of signatures required to make a living will valid.[1]

The nurse needs to be able to identify potential problems in the living will and get ethical analysis before situations like the one above occur. Look closely at the patient's living will to identify some of the key components (Figure 1 [pp. 137–139]). If the will is not signed, not witnessed or notarized, or is very old, be sure to call that to the attention of the patient and/or ethics committee. If the will is not clear on the types of treatments to use or not, ask the patient what he or she meant by certain sections or requests in the will and record his or her comments.

The concept of and need for living wills developed during the late 1960s as a response to the rapid advances in bio-science technology that allowed nurses and other health-care personnel to artificially prolong the lives of patients who would otherwise have died naturally.[4] This technology has progressed even further in the past fifteen years. However, both the legal and ethical systems have not been able to keep pace with these technological advances. For some patients, the technology available for resuscitation and prolonging life does result in their active return to society as productive persons who are able to function at their prior state of health. For a large number of patients, however, resuscitation methods and advanced life support technology merely extend the physiological existence of the person even though their cognitive or conscious activity is diminished.

The key ethical issue nurses need to be aware of when involved with living wills is the principle of autonomy, the person's right to self-determination. Living wills protect the patient's right to self-determination by clearly stating what the person desires while he or she is competent to decide. This document communicates patient preferences should that person become incompetent and therefore unable to make his or her own decisions.[2]

Nurses need to be aware of a second important ethical issue that is closely related to self-determination in the execution of a living will; this is the person's right to refuse treatment. In general, if a person is determined to be competent, then that person has a right to refuse any and all treatments.[5] From this particular view point, a living will can be seen as a directive for the refusal or withdrawal of treatment at some future time. However, the principle of self-determination does have societal limitations. For example, if a person refuses treatment for a highly contagious disease, that person poses a threat to the needs of society as a whole. Consequently, public health agencies are required by law to report and treat communicable diseases such as sexually transmitted diseases, hepatitis, and tuberculosis.

Ethical Difficulties of Living Wills

While a living will seems to be a simple solution to a complex care situation, there are some ethical difficulties inherent in their use that nurses need to know about. Primary among these ethical difficulties is the question of the person's level of knowledge of

Continued on following page

Fig 1A. Checklist for Evaluating a Patient's Living Will Document

✓ 1.   Statement of intention states the document was written freely when the patient was competent.

✓ 2.   Statement of when the document goes into effect. This is usually when the patient is no longer able to make decisions for him/her self.

✓ 3.   A section specifies general health care measure to be excluded from care.

✓ 4.   Open section for specific measures (ventilators, pacemakers, etc) and any other specific instructions concerning care.

✓ 5.   Proxy statement (sometimes called Durable Power of Attorney) which is optional, but a strong addition. Allows another person to make decisions in situations that may not have been anticipated in the living will. (Check your state law concerning details of proxy selection.)

✓ 6.   Substitute proxy. This section is optional. Specifies who can make decisions, if first choice proxy is not available.

✓ 7.   Legal statement that the proxy(s) may make decisions.

✓ 8.   Witness selection statement. Many states require that witnesses not be related nor members of the health care team.

✓ 9.   Signature and date. Must be signed and dated by the patient. Some states have very specific regulations concerning how long the will is valid. It may range from a few months to 5 years.

✓ 10. Legal signatures of witnesses are required.

✓ 11. Notary seal, if required by state law. State laws differ on notary seal requirement. It is usually required, if a proxy is selected.

Figure 1. Key elements in most living wills. A) Check list of items the nurse should look for in a patient's living will. State laws vary widely concerning advance directives, but the elements listed here are common and should be present in most states' living wills. B) Sample advance directive. Numbers show where each point listed in Figure 1A appears on pages from a generic advance directive which was created by the Choice In Dying Legal Committee. Because the laws on advance directives vary widely from state to state, there is no standard advance directive whose language conforms exactly with all states' laws. (Part B reprinted with permission of Choice In Dying, formerly Concern for Dying/Society for the Right to Die, 200 Varick Street, New York, NY 10014, 212-366-5540).

Continued on following page

INSTRUCTIONS	# PENNSYLVANIA DECLARATION

<table>
<tr>
<td>PRINT YOUR
NAME</td>
<td>I, _____, being of sound mind, willfully and voluntarily make this declaration to be followed if I become incompetent. This declaration reflects my firm and settled commitment to refuse life-sustaining treatment under the circumstances indicated below.

I direct my attending physician to withhold or withdraw life-sustaining treatment that serves only to prolong the process of my dying, if I should be in a terminal condition or in a state of permanent unconsciousness.

I direct that treatment be limited to measures to keep me comfortable and to relieve pain, including any pain that might occur by withholding or withdrawing life-sustaining treatment.</td>
</tr>
<tr>
<td>CHECK THE
OPTIONS WHICH
REFLECT YOUR
WISHES</td>
<td>In addition, if I am in the condition described above, I feel especially strongly about the following forms of treatment:
    I ( ) do ( ) do not want cardiac resuscitation.
    I ( ) do ( ) do not want mechanical respiration.
    I ( ) do ( ) do not want tube feeding or any other artificial or invasive
              form of nutrition (food) or hydration (water).
    I ( ) do ( ) do not want blood or blood products.
    I ( ) do ( ) do not want any form of surgery or invasive diagnostic tests.
    I ( ) do ( ) do not want kidney dialysis.
    I ( ) do ( ) do not want antibiotics.

I realize that if I do not specifically indicate my preference regarding any of the forms of treatment listed above, I may receive that form of treatment.</td>
</tr>
<tr>
<td>ADD PERSONAL
INSTRUCTIONS
(IF ANY)</td>
<td>Other instructions:</td>
</tr>
</table>

© 1994
CHOICE IN DYING, INC.

Figure 1B.

Continued on following page

APPOINTING A SURROGATE	Surrogate decisionmaking:
	I ( ) do ( ) do not want to designate another person as my surrogate to make medical treatment decisions for me if I should be incompetent and in a terminal condition or in a state of permanent unconsciousness.
PRINT THE NAME, ADDRESS AND PHONE NUMBER OF YOUR SURROGATE	Name: _____ Address: _____ Phone: _____
PRINT THE NAME, ADDRESS AND PHONE NUMBER OF YOUR ALTERNATE SURROGATE	Name and address of substitute surrogate (if surrogate designated above is unable to serve): Name: _____ Address: _____ Phone: _____
PRINT THE DATE	I made this declaration on the _____ day of _____. 　　　　　　　　　　　　　　　　*(day)*　　　　　　*(month, year)*
SIGN THE DOCUMENT AND PRINT YOUR ADDRESS	Declarant's signature: _____ Declarant's address: _____
WITNESSING PROCEDURE	The declarant, or the person on behalf of and at the direction of the declarant, knowingly and voluntarily signed this writing by signature or mark in my presence. Witness's signature: _____ Witness's address: _____
YOUR TWO WITNESSES MUST SIGN AND PRINT THEIR ADDRESSES	Witness's signature: _____ Witness's address: _____

Courtesy of Choice In Dying　1/94 200 Varick Street, New York, NY 10014 1-800-989-WILL

© 1994
CHOICE IN DYING, INC.

PAGE 2

Continued on following page

potential and future health-care problems at the time the will was formulated. Because living wills are often formulated long before they are to be used, there may later be serious questions about how informed the person was about the disease states and treatment modalities that might later affect care. If there is any indication that the person did not understand the full implications of future therapies or potential medical problems, then the validity of the living will is in question.[2]

A second ethical difficulty for nurses encompasses the principles of beneficence and nonmaleficence. The principle of beneficence states that a health-care professional's primary duty is to benefit or do good for the patient. The principle of nonmaleficence states that the patient should be protected from harm by health-care providers.[6] It is sometimes difficult to determine if the primary duty is to produce benefit or prevent harm. Generally, most health-care providers think that the duty to avoid harming the patient outweighs the concerns for providing benefit. When evaluated from the beneficence and nonmaleficence view points, living wills seem to violate the principle of providing benefit to the patient. This perception makes many health-care providers ethically uncomfortable. In some situations, the implementation of a living will might actually involve the termination of some modes of treatments already in use. Termination seems to constitute actual harm to the patient. In either case, respecting a living will might often appear to health-care providers to be a violation of their duty to help patients and preserve life.

Nurses, as well as other health-care providers, often experience a sense of frustration when they are not allowed to use all the skills they have learned to preserve life. In the case of Mr. K, the physician obviously felt that intubation and clinical resuscitation were consistent with his living will, while the nurse perceived the situation in a different light.

A third difficulty nurses and other health-care workers may have with living wills is their formulation and legal enforcement. In general, the language used in the standard living will document is broad and vague. Living wills are often not specific enough to include all the forms of treatments that are possible for the many types of illnesses that might render a person incompetent to make decisions. Health-care providers may have little direction as to the care they are to give if the circumstances at the time the living will is to be honored are significantly different from the declared wishes of patient.[1]

Furthermore, unless the particular state has enacted into law a special type of living will called a "natural death act," the living will has no mechanism of legal enforcement.[1] Currently, 44 states plus the District of Columbia have natural death laws.[8] In states without this legislation, there is no obligation to accept the living will as a valid legal document.

Even in some states that do have a natural death act, it is considered only advisory and the physician has the right to comply with the living will or treat the patient as the physician deems most appropriate. There is no protection for nurses or other health-care practitioners against criminal or civil liability in the execution of living wills in states without a natural death act. Once a valid living will exists, it only becomes effective when the person who formulated it meets the qualifications for the natural death act. In most states, the individual must be diagnosed as having a terminal condition where the continuation of treatment and life-support would only prolong the patient's dying process.[2] But, there is no clear consensus on the definition of "terminal condition."

Despite all these difficulties, living wills are still a good way for a patient to make health-care wishes known to health-care providers. Documents that are specific about treatment modalities, are written in a "legal" format, and signed by two or more witnesses, tend to be treated with an increased level of respect by health-care providers.

Case Discussion

These principles regarding living wills can be used to analyze the ethical dilemmas in this case. Here are discussions of the three dilemmas introduced previously.

Dilemma #1. Living wills have more ethical implications than legal weight. Although many states have statutes that recognize living wills, the regulations are variable and even in states with "strong" living will legislation, the final decision as to whether to honor a living will is often left up to the physician and/or patient's family.

Ethically, there is a fairly strong obligation for nurses and other health-care workers to carry out the patient's wishes as a part of that patient's right to self-determination. However, because patients often do not understand all the implications of "not being kept alive by artificial means" or the various levels of the many treatments available, there is almost always some question about the validity of the living will based on the principles of informed consent. Given the circumstances of the situation involving Mr. K, the physician may have believed that he followed the only reasonable option of action available to him. "No code" order status varies considerably from hospital to hospital. Mr. K's primary physician wrote the "no code" order on the basis of the requests in Mr. K's living will. More detailed delineation of the aspects of the "no code" order and how the decision is made would be helpful in clarifying its meaning.

Dilemma #2. Nurses always have a right and even an ethical obligation to refuse to perform procedures that they firmly believe to be unethical and/or harmful to patients. However, there are several factors that must be considered when refusing to carry out procedures requested by physicians. Although Mr. K's living will was not specific about the kind of resuscitation, intubation, and ventilation desired, performing a code on him seems to be a violation of his wishes. If the ventricular tachycardia had been terminated quickly with lidocaine or a precordial thump, Mr. K might have recovered without requiring further treatment or suffering any long-term complications.

Patients with living wills, like Mr. K, are not automatically "no codes." Living wills that make reference to specific treatments, such as "no ventilator," do not necessarily mean that the patient is not to be resuscitated. It is important to discuss exactly what the patient with a living will wishes to have done in a variety of circumstances.

Continued on following page

It is also important to clarify these wishes with all the physicians involved in the case. The family members also need to be informed of the patient's wishes. The nurse needs to support the family while simultaneously carrying out the patient's . wishes.

A second consideration the nurse needs to keep in mind in refusing to carry out a physician's request is the consequences of that refusal. A nurse who refuses to act in an emergency situation such as a code, with a physician standing there giving orders is at risk for a variety of punitive if not legal consequences. If it could later be determined that the nurse failed to meet a standard of care by not following the physician's direct order, then the nurse might be open to a malpractice suit.[7]

Most likely, other nurses on the unit would have responded to the code so that any specific nurse's refusal to conduct the code would not have substantially changed the final outcome of the situation, but a blatant refusal to act in a code situation is unacceptable. However, if the nurse's ethical convictions about performing a code on a specific patient are so strong that he or she is unable to function, then the nurse should remove himself or herself from the situation.

While the family involvement complicates decision making, such as the decision to perform the code on Mr. K, a nurse's first obligation is to meet the needs of the patient. Although they might have been aware of the living will, Mr. K's family did not seem to understand the full consequences of the decisions it required. The death of a loved one is always a powerful, emotional experience for family members, so powerful that it usually clouds rational decision making. It is even more difficult to actually watch a loved one die, particularly if that patient seems to be on the road to recovery.

Similarly, there are very few nurses who are not affected by the death of a patient, but the education nurses receive helps place that event in a more rational context. The nurse needs to support the family emotionally while carrying out the wishes of the patient as stated in the living will. Education of the family members concerning the important aspects of the living will, prior to the time when the terms of the living will go into effect, may help prevent the type of response demonstrated by Mr. K's family.

Dilemma #3. Refusing to initiate a code on Mr. K is the ethically correct choice of action because the nurse is following his wishes as outlined in the living will. However, not initiating the code is difficult in a situation where a group of hysterical family members are demanding some type of action. Other possible courses of action might include gently but firmly ushering the family members out of the unit to a waiting room while Mr. K was returned to bed and allowed to expire without a code; allowing the family to stay in the room and attempting to explain what a living will really means while Mr. K expires in their presence; or calling a code but not pursuing it with a great deal of enthusiasm.

Also, a discussion between the physician, nurse, clergy, ethics committee, and other members of the health-care team to clarify the meaning of "no code" status and how to better uphold the patient's wishes may be valuable.

Understanding Terminology

Defining terminology becomes important when executing living wills. The word "artificial," for example, is likely to have a much different meaning to the patient than it does to the nurse. In the strictest sense, any type of technology or equipment, including intravenous infusions (IVs), monitors, antibiotics, feeding tubes, catheters, and even oxygen delivery equipment is "artificial."[4,8] Members of the health-care community use artificial technology so frequently that it is accepted as an ordinary part of patient care. Few patients are admitted without having IVs, oxygen, and some type of monitoring equipment attached to them. For health-care providers, the key term becomes "extraordinary" technology used to maintain life. Equipment such as ventilators, intra-aortic balloon pumps, external pacemakers, intracranial pressure monitors, and vasoactive pharmacologic agents may qualify as "extraordinary means." In some tertiary care settings, however, these advanced technologies may be classified as "ordinary means" for maintaining life.

The important question the nurse needs to ask concerning Mr. K's living will is did he mean "artificial" or did he say "artificial" but mean "extraordinary"? By allowing "aggressive treatment" (which likely included several "artificial" technologies, such as antibiotics, bronchodilators, intermittent positive pressure breathing treatments, and oxygen therapy) for his acute respiratory distress episodes, it seems that he meant "extraordinary" rather than "artificial" in the strictest sense of the word. Intubation, using an oral or nasal endotracheal tube, is always an "artificial" mode of treatment. Also, this mode of intubation is usually considered an "extraordinary" mode of treatment due to its highly invasive nature and potential for complications. This particular treatment modality would seem to be a clear violation of Mr. K's wishes as expressed in his living will, even if he did not understand the nuances of the terminology used. If Mr. K's resuscitation could have been accomplished through the use of a manual resuscitator and a mask and not an endotracheal tube, it is less clear that it would be a violation of his wishes as stated in his living will.

Summary

Because of the limitations inherent in living wills, critical care nurses should ask about the patient's personal preferences, values, and choices. Nurses need to ask about specific items that are life sustaining or life-saving. Most importantly, nurses must document any patient statements or discussions that clarify these wishes. Asking patients if they have a living will or advanced directive is not enough. As professionals, nurses must educate patients in the available treatments and help them communicate what measures they do or do not want. This will help prevent the problem of resuscitating patients who really do not want it.

Continued on following page

Clinical Research Questions

There are several questions still needing research in this area including:

■ How do critical care nurses feel about having patients in their units who have a living will or are designated "no code"?
■ How do critical care nurses feel about conducting codes on patients who have a living will or have been designated "no code"?
■ Do patients who enter the critical care unit have a full understanding of the therapies that are possible and what they involve?
■ What teaching methods used by critical care nurses are most effective in educating patients about living wills?

REFERENCES

1. Guido GW. Legal Issues in Nursing. Norwalk, CT: Appleton & Lange, 1988.
2. O'Rourke K, Brodeur D. Medical Ethics, St. Louis: Catholic Health Association of the United States, 1989.
3. Jameton A. Nursing Practice: The Ethical Issues. Englewood Cliffs, NJ: Prentice Hall Inc., 1984.
4. Catalano JT. Ethical and Legal Aspects of Nursing. Springhouse PA: Springhouse Corporation, 1991.
5. Davis AJ, Aroskar MA. Ethical Dilemmas and Nursing Practice. New York: Appleton-Century-Crofts, 1978.
6. Veatch RM, Fry ST. Case Studies in Nursing Ethics. New York: J.B. Lippincott Company, 1987.
7. New Law Requires Hospitals to Ask About Living Wills, Medical Ethics Advisor 1991;7(1):1–16.
8. Nurses Legal Handbook. Springhouse, PA: Springhouse Corporation, 1992.

BIBLIOGRAPHY

American Nurses Association: Code for Nurses with Interpretive Statement. American Nurses Association, Kansas City, 1976.
Catalano, JT: Critical care nurses and ethical dilemmas. Crit Care Nurse 11:16–21, 1991.
Catalano, JT: Systems of ethics. Crit Care Nurse 12:91–96, 1992.
Catalano, JT: The ethics of cadaver experimentation. Crit Care Nurse 14:82–85, 1994.
Eakes, GG and Lewis, JB: Should nurses be required to administer care to patients with AIDS? Nurse Educ 16:36–38, 1991.
French, PA: The Spectrum of Responsibility. St. Martin's Press, New York, 1991.

Fromer, MJ: Ethical Issues in Health Care. CV Mosby, St. Louis, 1981.

Mappes, TA and Zembaty, JS: Biomedical Ethics, ed 3. McGraw-Hill, New York, 1991.

Macklin, R: Mortal Choices: Ethical Dilemmas in Modern Medicine. Houghton Mifflin, Boston, 1987.

O'Rourke, KD and Brodeur, D: Medical Ethics: Common Ground for Understanding, Vol 1. Catholic Health Association of the United States, St. Louis, 1987.

O'Rouke, KD and Brodeur, D: Medical Ethics: Common Ground for Understanding, Vol 2. Catholic Health Association of the United States, St. Louis, 1987.

Pavalon, EI: Human Rights and Health Care Law. American Journal of Nursing, New York, 1980.

Perdew, S: Facts About AIDS: A Guide for Health Care Providers. JB Lippincott, Philadelphia, 1990.

Quinn, CA and Smith, MD: The Professional Commitment: Issues and Ethics in Nursing. WB Saunders, Philadelphia, 1987.

Thompson, JE and Thompson, HO: Bioethical Decision Making for Nurses. Appleton-Century Crofts; Norwalk, CT, 1985.

Thompson, JE and Thompson, HO: Teaching ethics to nursing students. Nursing Outlook 37:84–88, 1989.

Trought, EA and Moore, F (eds.): Guidelines for the Registered Nurse in Giving, Accepting or Rejecting a Work Assignment. Florida Nurses Association, Orlando, 1989.

Veatch, RM and Fry, ST: Case Studies in Nursing Ethics. Prentice-Hall, Englewood Cliffs, NJ, 1987.

 HISTORICAL PERSPECTIVES

Changes in American Society

The problems associated with population concentration in American cities were intensified by the 30,000,000 immigrants who arrived in the United States between 1800 and 1900. These immigrants, escaping from famine, wars, and the general poverty found in a number of European countries, initially settled in the growing port cities along the East Coast. As the rail system was completed, many immigrants migrated West, seeking a new life in the wilds of the Central Plains and the Rocky Mountains.

During the Industrial Revolution, factories, located in the cities, attracted rural migrants, who found horrid conditions. Because their poverty forced malnourished people to live in crowded apartments, disease quickly spread among the population. Wages were low. Child labor was a fact of life, with children as young as 7 and 8 years old working 18-hour days in hot, unventilated sweatshops. Alcoholism, drug addiction, and crime were rampant among factory workers.

Factory owners were concerned that the degenerating health conditions of their workers would reduce production and thereby affect profits. Although generally opposed to most reforms that dealt with their labor practices, many factory owners supported and even implemented forms of health care that would keep their workers on the job.

A form of community health nursing, in which nurses with various levels of knowledge and skill would visit the sick at home, grew out of the desire to keep

Continued on following page

workers healthy. It soon became evident that the cause of disease among this population derived from their living and working conditions. Without changing these conditions, no one could improve health care. As interest in reform grew, several groups were organized to help the poor, the sick, and the abandoned.

The Sisters of Charity, who were organized to provide nursing care in the city hospitals, expanded their services to include care in homes and orphanages for abandoned children. The Sisters also started an education program for unmarried and abandoned women to prepare them to work as care providers in hospitals. The Brothers of St. John of God, one of the few male nursing orders to survive the Reformation and Industrial Revolution, provided similar services. Several non-Catholic nursing orders were founded, including the famous Quaker Society of Protestant Sisters of Charity who provided care primarily for prisoners and children.

As the population grew, the need for health care increased. Hospitals sprang up in the cities to meet the needs of the urban population. Without external controls or standards, there was a noticeable range of quality in these institutions.

Many of the newly established hospitals instituted their own schools of nursing. Because much health care was still being given in the home, community health programs were developed and visiting nurse or in-home care became the preferred types of nursing of the period. Many of the early nursing leaders lived during this time and made major contributions to health care in general and to the profession of nursing in particular.

In the religious hospitals of predominantly Roman Catholic countries, the Industrial Revolution had little effect on the provision of health care. Strongly resistant to newly developing medical knowledge and technology, caregivers tended to stay with more traditional methods of medical and nursing care. Although predominantly Protestant countries were more open to new medical techniques, discoveries, and modes of treatment, the conditions in most of the secular hospitals was so poor that the quality of the health care remained low. Although this period has often been called the "Dark Ages of Nursing," many important contributions, including those of Florence Nightingale, occurred during the Industrial Revolution.

7

REALITY SHOCK IN THE WORKPLACE

Learning Objectives

After completing this chapter, the reader will be able to:

1 Describe the concept of reality shock.
2 Define burnout and list its major symptoms.
3 Discuss the key factors that produce burnout.
4 List the important elements in personal time management.
5 Analyze how the nurse's humanity affects nursing practice.
6 List at least four health care practices nurses can use to prevent burnout and to improve their professional performance.
7 Name three methods that can be used to "decompress."
8 Discuss how to conduct a successful employment interview.

The majority of nursing students, if asked what they wanted most in the world, would likely answer, "to graduate and practice real nursing in the real world." To some degree, they are correct in assuming that the world of nursing school and education is not the real world. Although nursing school is demanding physically, mentally, and emotionally and raises the anxiety levels of nursing students a great deal, it is also a place where the student is sheltered from the realities of the workplace and provided with relatively clear goals for advancement. Students are given a constant stream of reinforcement and always have someone to turn to if they have a question. Things are different in the "Real World." This transition from nursing student to registered nurse is referred to as **transition shock** or **reality shock.**

MAKING THE TRANSITION FROM STUDENT TO NURSE

At any point in their lives, most people fulfill several different roles simultaneously. For a nursing student, the biggest role conflict might be in the transition from student to registered nurse (Bradlby, 1990). The roots of the conflict may lie in integrating three distinct aspects of any given role: the ideal, the perceived, and the performed.

In the academic setting the student is generally presented with the **ideal** of what a nurse should be. The ideal role projects society's expectations. It clearly delineates obligations and responsibilities, as well as the rights and privileges, that those in the role can claim. Although the ideal role presents a clear image of what is expected, it often is static and somewhat unrealistic to believe that everyone in this role will follow the expected patterns of behaviors.

The ideal role of nurse might require someone with superhuman physical strength and ability and unlimited stamina, one who possesses superior intelligence and decision-making ability, yet remains kind, gentle, caring, and able to communicate with any client at any time. Ideal nurses function independently, know more than the physician, and are able to prevent the physician from making grievous errors in client care while continuing to be responsive to client requests and to carry out any physician's order with unerring accuracy and absolute obedience. Some perceptive students, early in their clinical experiences, may begin to suspect that this ideal role of nurse is not the way it actually is in the real world.

The **perceived role** is an individual's own definition of the role, which is often more realistic than the ideal role. When individuals define their own roles, they may reject or modify some of the norms and expectations of society in establishing the ideal role. Intellectually, though, the ideal role is often used as the yardstick against which the perceived role is measured.

After a minimal amount of clinical experience, the nursing student may realize that nurses do not possess extraordinary physical strength or intellectual ability but may continue to cling to the idea. Many students accept unconditionally, as part of their perceived role, that nurses must be kind, gentle, and understanding at all times with all clients. The perceived role is the role with which the nursing student usually graduates.

Reality shock occurs at the point where the ideal or perceived role comes into conflict with the performed role. The **performed role** is defined as what the practitioner of the role actually does. The reality soon recognized by many new graduate nurses is that carrying out role expectations depends on many factors besides their perceptions and beliefs about how it should be performed. Environment has a great deal to do with how the obligations of the role are met (Gardiner, 1992).

In nursing school, where students are assigned to care for one or two clients at a time, plenty of time remains to practice the therapeutic communication techniques taught in class and to provide completely for the physical, educational, and emotional needs of the client while developing an insightful care plan. The realities of the workplace may dictate that a nurse be assigned to care for six to eight clients at a time. In this situation, the perceived role of the nurse as expert communicator may have to be shelved for the more realistic performed role of the nurse as expert task organizer. Meeting all the client's physical and emotional needs becomes impossible, and the care plan may be forgotten.

Such situations can produce what is termed **cognitive dissonance** in many new graduate nurses; that is, they know what they should do and they know how they should do it, yet the circumstances do not allow them to carry it out. The end result is increased anxiety. High levels of anxiety, left unrecognized or unresolved, can lead to a variety of physical and emotional symptoms. When these symptoms become severe enough, a condition called **burnout** may result.

The reality shock that new graduates often experience can be lessened to some degree. Recently, some schools of nursing have instituted a **preceptor clinical experience** during the last semester of the senior year. The main goal of this type of clinical experience, just before graduation, is to produce a type of anticipatory socialization into the role of registered nurse, in which the student is allowed to fill the requirements of an employment situation before actually graduating.

In the preceptor clinical experience, the student is assigned to one registered nurse for supervision for most of the semester. The student works the same hours and on the same unit as the nurse he or she is assigned to, thus allowing the student to practice in the role of a graduate nurse. As the student becomes more competent in the skills being developed, the values and ideals learned in the classroom are modified to fit the workplace, but they are also reinforced by practice. As the role expectations of the workplace are absorbed by the student during the preceptor experience, the student's perceived role expectations also change, allowing movement from the student role to that of practicing professional with less anxiety and stress (Lindquist, 1989).

Finally, nursing students themselves can lessen the reality shock by becoming involved in the "internships" that many hospitals offer for nursing students between their junior and senior years. These internships allow the students to work in a hospital setting as nurse's aides, while permitting them to practice, with a few restrictions, at their level of nursing education. These experiences are invaluable for gaining practice in skills and for becoming socialized into the professional role.

BURNOUT

Although it has existed for many years, the burnout syndrome has only recently been recognized as a problem that can be reduced or even prevented. A widely accepted definition of **burnout** is a state of emotional exhaustion that results from the accumulative stress of an individual's life, including work, personal, and family responsibilities. Although the term is not often applied to students, many of the symptoms of burnout can be observed in these aspiring nurses.

Symptoms of Burnout

- Extreme fatigue
- Exhaustion
- Frequent illness
- Overeating
- Headaches
- Sleeping problems
- Physical complaints
- Alcohol abuse

- Mood swings
- Emotional displays
- Anxiety
- Poor-quality work
- Anger
- Guilt
- Depression

The people who are most likely to experience burnout tend to be more intelligent than average, hard-working, idealistic, and perfectionist. There are certain categories of jobs and careers that tend to produce a higher incidence of burnout: situations and positions in which there is a demand for consistently high quality performance, expectations are unclear or unrealistic, there is little control over the work situation, and the financial rewards are inadequate. These jobs or careers tend to be very demanding and stressful with little recognition or appreciation of what is being done. Also, jobs in which there is constant contact with people (customers, clients, students, or criminals) rank high on the burnout list (Kramer, 1979).

Even with the most superficial knowledge of nursing, it is easy to see that many of these elements are present in the nurse's work situation. It is possible to recognize nurses who are in the early stages of burnout by identifying some classic behaviors.

One of the earliest indications is the attitude that work is something to be tolerated, rather than eagerly anticipated. Nurses in the early stages of burnout often are irritable, impatient, cynical, pessimistic, whiny, or callous toward co-workers and clients. These preburnout nurses take frequent sick days, are chronically late for their shifts, drink too much, eat too much, and often are not able to sleep. Eventually, as their idealism erodes, their work suffers. They become careless in the performance of their duties, uncooperative with their colleagues, and unable to concentrate on what they are doing, and they display a general attitude of boredom and apathy. If allowed to continue, burnout may lead to feelings of helplessness, powerlessness, purposelessness, and guilt (Chenevert, 1993).

Dealing with Burnout

Despite this bleak picture, nurses do not have to fall victim to the burnout syndrome. There are many nurses who practice their profession for many years, manage to deal with the stress, and find great personal satisfaction in what they do. These satisfied and motivated nurses have developed ways to deal with the stress of their careers while maintaining their goals and purpose as nurses.

The first step in dealing with burnout is to be able to recognize its signs. Many nurses who are burning out use denial and rationalization to block recognition of burnout because it is just too painful for them to think that they put so much time, money, and effort into preparing for a career that they no longer want or enjoy. It is important to realize that it is not the career that is producing the burnout, but rather the difficulty in coping with the stresses the career is producing. Although it may not be possible to change the requirements of the profession significantly, it is possible to learn how to cope more effectively with stress.

Managing Stress and Time

Although there are many schools of thought about stress and time-management techniques, several common threads run through many of these theories. These include setting goals, identifying problems, and using relaxation techniques.

Setting Personal Goals

Goals and goal setting are an important part of client care. Nursing students, and by extension, practicing nurses are highly proficient in the *planning* stage of the nursing process, in which goal setting is the primary task. They know that a good set of goals should be client centered, time oriented, and measurable, and that they should write these goals with every care plan they prepare.

In their personal lives, however, these nurses may rush full-tilt into one erratic day after another, subordinating their own needs to the needs of others, working long, hard hours, but without accomplishing very much and feeling frustrated about it. What is the problem here? Very simply, they can prepare realistic, beneficial goals for their clients, but are not able to do the same for themselves.

Personal goals should include both long-term and short-term goals. Typically, personal long-term goals look into the future at least 10 years and include a statement about what the nurse wants to achieve during his or her lifetime. Some examples are going back to school to obtain an advanced degree, becoming a director of nursing, or even writing a book about nursing. Practicing nurses who are caught up in the whirlwind of everyday life find it difficult to formulate statements about the future. One other important characteristic of long-term goals is that they need to be flexible. As life circumstances change, modifications are required.

Short-term goals are those the nurse expects to accomplish in 6 months to 2 years. These should be aimed primarily at making the nurse's professional or personal life more satisfying and fulfilling. Like long-term goals, they do not need to be work related. Perhaps visiting a foreign country, a skiing trip in the mountains, even learning how to paint a picture or play the piano may be achievable in a relatively short time. In the professional realm, joining a professional organization, becoming a head nurse, or changing an outdated hospital policy are all achievable in a short time. The fact that everyone ages over time cannot be altered, but that time can also be used to achieve personal satisfaction in life and increase knowledge and accomplishments.

Although setting goals is an important first step in dealing with the stress that leads to burnout, any good nurse recognizes that a plan without implementation is useless. As difficult as goal setting may be for nurses, carrying it out may be even more difficult. Although goal achievement requires a degree of hard work and personal sacrifice, when people are working towards something they really want, the effort it takes to achieve the end actually becomes enjoyable. For example, planning a family vacation requires many activities, including mapping out the route, selecting specific sights to see, and deciding where to stay and where to eat. At first glance, this process may seem like a lot of work (and it is), but as the family gets caught up in the process, it actually becomes an exciting adventure in its own right.

Identifying Problems

Another important step in dealing with burnout is to identify the actual problems that are producing the stress. Again, nurses are taught as students that they need to identify client problems so that they can work toward solving them. Formulation of a nursing diagnosis is nothing more than precisely stating a client's problem. One thing nurses realize early in the learning process is that what may appear to be an obvious problem may in reality not be a problem at all. And, conversely, something that may only be mentioned in passing by a client may turn out to be the real source of the client's nursing needs. Perhaps nurses should look at their own lives and attempt to formulate nursing diagnoses that deal with their stress-related problems (setting the North American Nursing Diagnosis Association list aside).

For example, a new graduate has just completed a shift where he has been assigned to eight complete-care clients, has had to supervise two badly prepared nurses aides, and has put in 55 minutes of overtime, for which he will not be paid, to complete the charting. This nurse is feeling tired, frustrated, and even a little bit guilty because of an inability to provide the type of care that was taught in nursing school. What is the problem? A possible nursing diagnosis might be: Alterations in personal satisfaction related to excessive work load, evidenced by sore feet, headache, shaky hands, feelings of guilt, frustration, and small paycheck.

Now that the problem has been identified, goals and interventions can be introduced to solve the problem. The goals may range from organizing time better to refusing to care for so many complete-care clients. Interventions, depending on the goals, can include activities such as attending a time-management seminar, talking to the head nurse, or changing a policy in the policy and procedure book (Chenevert, 1993). Nurses already know the nursing process as a client problem-solving technique. Why not apply the same knowledge and skills to personal problems? Leaving problems unsolved only increases stress.

Strategies for Problem Solving

Although specific problems may require specific solutions, a number of widely accepted methods exist to deal with the general stresses produced by everyday work and personal life. Included in these methods are such activities as recognizing that nurses are only human, improving time-management skills, practicing what is preached, and decompression.

Improving Time-Management Skills

In modern life there is not enough time to do everything that needs doing. The key to time management is setting priorities. In the world of nursing and client care, some activities are essential to the safety and well-being of clients. These include getting the medications to the clients on time, meeting their comfort needs, and preventing accidental injuries. Beyond these actions, nurses really have a great deal of discretion in what they can do when providing care to clients.

Burnout largely results from personal and professional dissatisfaction. If nurses feel fulfilled in what they are doing, burnout is much less likely. Activities that may increase nurses' satisfaction include spending time talking with clients, learning new skills, and decreasing the anxiety of families through teaching and listening. After such activities have been identified, time should be set aside for them during the shift. The real secret in using time management to prevent burnout is for the nurse to use the time left for those nursing activities that bring the most professional and personal satisfaction.

Several skills need to be developed to be able to allow time during a shift for these preferred activities. First, the nurse must learn to delegate by letting the LPNs or aides do those tasks that they are supposed to be able to do. Many nurses graduate from nursing school with the attitude that if you want it done right, you need to do it yourself. After becoming familiar with the LPN and nurse's aide job descriptions, nurses need to give others a chance to prove themselves (Chenevert, 1993).

Another necessary skill is overcoming procrastination. Most people have a natural tendency toward procrastination, particularly when unpleasant or difficult tasks are involved. The primary reasons that people postpone or delay doing something is because they either do not want to begin or do not know where to begin. More time and energy are expended in inventing excuses for putting off tasks than would actually be taken in doing the task.

The best way to overcome procrastination is by starting the task, even if it is only a small step. An effective method is to select the most distasteful task to be done that day and to commit just 5 minutes to it. After 5 minutes are over, the task can be either set aside or continued. It is very likely that once the task is started and momentum builds, the task will be carried to completion.

Tasks can be prioritized by listing them in three categories. Category A tasks (e.g., passing out medications, treatments, and dressing changes) are those that need to be completed on time. Category B tasks (bath, linen change, lunch break, charting) can be postponed until later in the shift. Category C tasks (cleaning up the room, attending to personal grooming tasks other than those that are absolutely required) are tasks that can wait until the next day.

For daily tasks, both pleasant and unpleasant, the best time to do it is immediately. If achievement of the plan requires delegation, then it needs to be done at the beginning of the shift, not at the middle or end. Often nurses have a built-in fear of taking chances; as a result they avoid doing things where there is a chance for failure in the hopes that somehow the problem will resolve itself. Any time an important decision is made, there is a chance that someone will disagree, or that the decision will be incorrect. These types of situations need to be looked at as a challenge or an opportunity, rather than life-altering risk to be avoided. Although mistakes in health care do have the potential to be fatal, learning from mistakes is one of the most fundamental ways for increasing knowledge.

Time management, life other skills, requires some practice. Once a nurse masters this skill, life becomes a great deal more satisfying.

Practicing What Is Preached

Because nursing is oriented towards keeping people healthy as well as curing illness, nurses spend a large amount of their time teaching clients about eating right, getting enough sleep, going for regular dental, eye, and physical examinations, avoiding too much drinking and smoking, and exercising on a regular basis. It might make an interesting project for a student taking a nursing research course to have nurses rank themselves on how well they have incorporated these health maintenance activities in their own lives. The results would probably indicate a low overall score on the "practice what you preach" scale.

Nurses know all about the food pyramid, but they do not translate that knowledge into feeding themselves properly. In reality, there are going to be some busy days when it is impossible to eat right. But it should be possible, at least occasionally, to follow a diet that will promote health and reduce the build-up of fat-plaques in the arteries.

It is important to get enough sleep to avoid chronic fatigue. People can adjust to a state of fatigue, but it tends to decrease the enjoyment they find in life, as well as make them irritable, careless, and inefficient. Most people need between 5 and 8 hours of good-quality sleep each night. It also probably would not hurt for nurses to take short a nap during the afternoon on their day off.

Many nurses feel that they get enough exercise during their busy shifts. And, in truth, the average staff nurse will walk between 2 and 5 miles during each 8-hour shift. Unfortunately, this type of walking does not qualify as the type of aerobic exercise recommended for an improved cardiovascular condition. Exercise, in order to be beneficial, must be done consistently and must raise the heart rate above the normal range for an extended period. The short sprint-type walking involved in client care does not accomplish this goal (Kramer, 1979).

Walking 1 or 2 miles a day outside the hospital is a beneficial, simple exercise that will improve health. Nurses can also use a wide variety of exercise equipment for those days when walking outside is undesirable. The important requirement is that the exercise be done consistently and frequently. Regular exercise not only improves the cardiovascular system but also helps improve stamina, raise self-image, and promote a general sense of well-being.

Decompression

Nurses Need Time to Decompress. The profession of nursing is stressful, even under ideal circumstances. Nurses are required to deal with other people constantly and to carry out a large number of tasks that are potentially dangerous. At the end of any shift, even the most skilled and best-organized nurse has a sense of internal tension. This tension must be released or in time it will cause a major explosion or, if turned inward, produce anxiety.

Establish a Daily Decompression Routine. It may take a little time for an individual to discover, through trial and error, what works to reduce the tension built up during the shift. Some effective techniques include setting aside a half-hour or so of private, quiet time during which the nurse can dream and reflect about the day's activities. Perhaps relaxing in a tub of hot soapy water or sitting in a favorite reclining chair might meet the nurse's need for decompression. Relaxing activities, such as swimming, shopping, or even going for a drive, can help reduce tension and act as a time for decompression. Of course, stress-management techniques learned at seminars, such as self-hypnosis or meditation, can be used by those who have developed these skills. Finally, meeting with a nurse support group can help the nurse to vent feelings and make constructive plans for solving problems.

THE MYTH OF THE NURSING SHORTAGE

The lack of qualified nurses has been present in the health care system for so long that the term **nursing shortage** has become a truism. Even recent studies about employment opportunities project that there will be shortage of nurses well into the 21st century (Shugars, 1991). As a result, high school counselors, as well as employment agencies, are encouraging young people to enter nursing schools. Many nursing schools reflect this trend in their record numbers of applicants and high rates of enrollment and graduates. Unfortunately, the truth of the situation is that there is beginning to be an oversupply of nurses.

The first indicators that the nursing shortage may be over were seen in 1992. It was initially most evident in large city hospitals, although it has continued to spread to smaller facilities in rural areas. Probably the first sign was the decreasing number of hospitals that were actively recruiting senior students during career days or conventions. Although some hospitals were still actively seeking nurses, they were more interested in hiring nurses with 1 or 2 years of experience than inexperienced new graduate nurses (Anderson, 1992).

There are many reasons for the lack of nursing positions. Primary is the increasing concern for cost reduction in the health care system. Although no significant health care reform bills have passed at this time, the writing is on the wall. Health care is going to have to become more efficient and to reduce the cost of operations (Kirkwood, 1993). One of the most obvious places to cut costs is in personnel. Many hospitals are currently following the practice of not replacing nurses who retire or leave. A few hospitals who have found the attrition method of cutting staff to be too slow have initiated staff cuts during which large numbers of nurses are laid off. Although cutting nursing positions may markedly reduce the costs in the short run, the long-term effects to the health care system most likely will be devastating. Exchanging qualified nurses for lower-paid unlicensed technicians will eventually have an effect on the quality of client care (ANA, 1994). When quality of client care goes down, so does the number of those seeking care.

The picture is not completely bleak, however. Although the overall demand for nurses has taken a drastic turn for the worse during the past several years, certain groups of nurses are in higher demand than ever, such as nurses who can practice independently in several different settings, home care nurses, community nurses, and hospice nurses (Hegner, 1995). A major trend in health care today is to move the care out of the hospital and into the home. Providing nursing services in these settings often requires at least a bachelor's degree, however, and often education beyond the level of the bachelor's degree. Fewer than 50% of all new graduate nurses today are graduating from bachelor's degree programs (Shugars, 1991).

Another area of health care in which there is no oversupply of nurses is in the realm of the nurse practitioner. Nurse practitioners are advanced practice nurses who have completed at least 2 years' additional education beyond the bachelor's degree. Advanced practice nurses are able to provide a variety of services that were traditionally kept within the physician's scope of practice.

Although most nurse practitioners are currently based in community clinics, there is an ever-expanding opportunity for them to become involved in the care of hospitalized clients (Sabatino, 1991). A key element in many of the proposed health care reform plans is that clients would be required to be evaluated by a primary health care provider before they could be referred to secondary health care providers or specialists. The advanced-practice education of nurse practitioners would make them eminently qualified to fill this role of primary health care provider.

Certain specialty areas, such as intensive care units, neonatal units, and burn units, are still seeking nurses. Again, however, experienced nurses are preferred. And as with community nurses, nurses who provide care in specialty units must be able to work independently and to draw from a large base of theoretic knowledge.

Although the current oversupply of nurses may at first glance appear to be harmful to the profession, it can also be viewed as an opportunity to improve it.

During the long years of the nursing shortage, there was great impetus to turn out more nurses with less and less education, even though advances in technology and changes in society were demanding nurses with more and more education. The present oversupply may offer nursing a chance to regroup, reorganize, and regain the professional status it has long been seeking. The worsening situation that exists in the workplace may lead to expanded roles for nurses in the future.

Nursing education must pay attention to these trends and begin to prepare nurses for expanded roles in the community. Professional nurses who are not employed in the community will most likely find challenging and meaningful careers in the specialty units of large urban hospitals. The few nurses who are employed in community hospitals will likely be in positions in which they are supervising a number of unlicensed workers. Many of the other jobs currently filled by nurses will be taken over by lower-paid technicians.

FINDING A JOB IN A TIGHT JOB MARKET

In the past, nurses have not had to face a tight job market. Until recently, it was common for senior nursing students to have as many as half a dozen job offers even before they graduated. And nurses who were returning to the profession after taking several years off were often asked if they could start working on the same day they had their employment interview. The bleaker current employment picture, however, is likely to continue for many years.

Nevertheless, there are some strategies that can be used to increase the chances of being hired. Students should take advantage of preceptor and "extern" experiences in their senior year and attempt to meet their clinical obligations in the institution where they desire employment. That way the student can evaluate the hospital closely and observe its working conditions and the type of care provided to clients. The hospital, on its part, has the opportunity to examine the student's knowledge, skills, personality, and ability to relate with clients and staff closely. The hospital benefits by getting employees who are familiar with the hospital before employment starts, thus decreasing the overall time of paid adjustment (referred to as "orientation").

Resumes

In the days of multiple job offers before graduation, preparing a resume was a necessary but low priority, part of the hiring process. In today's tight job market, the resume is often the institution's first contact with the nurse seeking employment and it has a substantial effect on the whole hiring process. First impressions *are* important. Preparing a neat, thorough, and professional looking resume is worth the time and effort. If you have access to a computer, a good looking resume can be prepared at almost no cost. If a computer is not available, it is a good idea to spend a few dollars to have the resume professionally prepared and reproduced.

The general goal of a resume is to provide the hospital with a complete picture of the prospective employee in as little space as possible. It should be easy to read and visually appealing and have flawless grammar and spelling. Although various formats may be used for a resume, they should all contain the same information. This information includes, in the following order:

- Full name, current address (or address where the person can always be reached), with telephone number including area code.

- Educational background (all degrees), starting with the most recent first, naming institution, location, dates of attendance, and degrees awarded.

- Former employers, again starting with the most recent. Give dates of employment, title of position, name of immediate supervisor, supervisor's phone number, and a description of the job responsibilities.

- Describe any scholarships, achievements, awards, honors, or activities that have been received, starting with the most recent.

- List professional memberships, offices held, dates of the memberships.

- List any publications. If both books and journal articles were published, list the books separately, starting with the most recent.

- Include an "Other" category to describe any unpublished materials produced (e.g., an internal hospital booklet for use by clients), research projects, grants, and so forth.

- Provide professional license number and annual number for all states where licensed, along with date of license and expiration date.

Each area of information should have a separate heading. References should also be included on a separate sheet of paper. Most institutions require three references. After obtaining permission from the individuals listed as references, the nurse preparing the resume should make sure to have accurate titles, addresses, and phone numbers. In selecting individuals for references, it is important that the individual should know the applicant well, either in a professional or personal capacity, have something positive to say about the applicant, and be in some type of position of authority. Although the prestige of the reference is not an essential, listing the Dean of the Department of Nursing as a reference may carry more weight than listing the janitor. It is best not to list relatives, unless the hospital is asking for a specific personal reference (Fig. 7–1, p. 161).

A cover letter should be sent with every resume. Like the resume itself, it should be neatly typed without errors, short, and to the point. Although a friendly, rambling letter might provide insight into a prospective employee's underlying personality, most personnel directors or directors of nursing are too busy to read through the whole document. The letter should be written in a business letter format and include the name and title of the person who will receive the letter. Letters beginning "To Whom It May Concern" do not make a favorable impression. The primary purpose for writing this letter is to express interest in a position at the hospital where the letter is directed. The statement of interest and the name of the position should be the opening statement of the letter. Where the prospective employee heard about the position should be included in this first paragraph, as well as when the applicant will be able to begin working.

The second paragraph should give a brief summary of any work experience or education that would especially qualify the applicant for this position. Newly graduated nurses will have some difficulty with this part, but they should include their graduation date, the name of the school they graduated from, and the director of the program. This paragraph should also state which shifts the applicant is willing to work.

The third paragraph should be very short. It should express thanks for consideration of the nurse's resume and include a short list of times the applicant will be available for an interview, as well as a phone number. Both the letter and the resume should be sent by first class mail in a $9'' \times 12''$ envelope so that the resume will remain unfolded, thus making it easier to handle and read (Fig. 7–2, p. 162).

Waiting for a reply can be the most difficult part of the whole process. The applicant needs to avoid the urge to call the hospital too soon. Because most health care institutions recognize the high anxiety levels of new graduates, they return calls within 1 or 2 weeks after receipt of the application. If no response is made after 3 weeks, the nurse should call the hospital to see whether or not the application was received. Mail does get lost. If the application has been received, the applicant should make no further phone calls. Harassing the personnel director or director of nursing about a job is not usually an effective employment strategy.

Interviews

The next important step in the process is the interview. The interview allows the institution to obtain a first-hand look at the applicant, as well as an opportunity for the applicant to obtain important information about the institution and position requirements. The interview often produces high levels of anxiety in new graduates, who are interviewing for what might be their first real job.

Again, first impressions are important. The interview starts from the moment the applicant enters the office. Conservative business clothes that are clean, neat, and well pressed are recommended. Similarly, a conservative hair style and a limited amount of accessories, jewelry, and makeup produce the best impression. Smoking, chewing gum, biting finger nails, or pacing nervously do not make good first impressions. The interviewer recognizes that interviews are stress producing and will make allowances for certain stress-related behaviors.

Arriving a few minutes early allows time for last minute touch-ups of hair and clothes and gives the applicant a chance to calm down. Carrying a small briefcase with a copy of the resume, cover letter, references, and information about the hospital also makes a favorable impression.

Mental preparation is as important to a successful interview as physical preparation. Most interviewers start the interview by asking about the resume, so a quick review just before the interview is helpful. Expect questions about positions held for only a short time (less than a year), gaps in the employment record (longer than 6 months), employment outside the field of nursing (waitress, clerk), educational experiences outside the nursing program, or unusual activities outside the employment setting. Answer the questions honestly but briefly. Most personnel directors or directors of nursing are busy and do not appreciate long, detailed, chatty answers. Applicants can anticipate being asked why they want the position, why they have selected this particular hospital, why they think they are qualified for the position, and what unique qualifications they will bring to the job to make them more desirable than others.

Because of the emphasis placed on discrimination issues in recent lawsuits, there are a number of areas that prospective employers are not supposed to discuss, but sometimes do anyway. These include questions about sexual preferences or habits, age, race, plans for a family, personal living arrangements, and religion or political beliefs. If these questions are asked, the applicant needs to consider the implications of not answering them. Although there is no legal obligation for the applicant to answer, refusing to do so or pointing out that the question should not have been asked in the first place may be unwise.

At some point in the interview, usually towards the end, applications are asked if they have any questions. Although most do have questions, many applicants are afraid to ask. In fact, asking questions can be seen as a demonstration of independence, initiative, and intellectual curiosity, all traits highly valued by hospitals. It is important that the first questions are not about salary, vacations, and other benefits. Questions that indicate interest in the institution would inquire about:

- Responsibilities involved in the position
- Other staff or personnel involved in the area
- The client to staff ratios
- Requirements for rotating shifts, weekend obligations, and floating
- Opportunities for continuing education, advancement, or movement to other departments

After these questions have been answered, the applicant may want to ask, in passing, about salary, raises, vacations, and other benefits. The applicant should also ask for written material on the nurse's contract with the agency, including benefits and job descriptions. Often the interviewer will provide this information without being asked in the course of answering some of the other questions.

Mary P. Oak
100 Wood Lane
Nicetown, PA 22222
(333) 555-1234 (H)

Education:
Bachelor of Science—Nursing, 1995
Mountain University (1993–1995)
Nicetown, PA 22222

Associate in Science—Nursing, 1993
Hillside Community College (1991–1993)
Hilltown, PA 33333

Employment Experiences:
1993–Present
Supercare Hospital
Hilltown, PA 33333
Position: Registered Nurse, Staff 3-11 shift on a 28-bed surgical unit. Responsible for care of 8 to 10 postoperative clients at a time; including all aspects of physical care, monitoring for complications, and evaluating effectiveness of medications and care given. Supervised 1 to 2 unlicensed assistant personnel each shift.
Immediate Supervisor: Jane Smith, RN , Head Nurse, (333) 555-4321.

1990–1993
Kindcare Nursing Home
Ashtown, PA 23232
Position: Certified Nursing Assistant, 7-3 shift. Provided direct care of residents, including bathing, personal hygiene, therapeutic communication, and effective collaboration with nursing and non-nursing staff.
Immediate Supervisor: John Doe, RN, Director of Nursing, (333) 555-6789.

Awards:
1995–Student of the Year
Mountain University, Nicetown, PA

1993–Nightingale Society, New York, NY

1991–Presidential Scholarship
Hillside Community College, Hilltown, PA

Professional Memberships:
National Student Nurses Association
Secretary, 1993–1995
Mountain University, Nicetown, PA

National Honor Society
President, 1989–1990
Nicetown High School, Nicetown, PA

Professional Licenser:
Pennsylvania, 444-555-67890 Biannual Number, PA02468

Figure 7–1. Sample resume.

Mary P. Oak
100 Wood Lane
Nicetown, PA 22222

April 15, 1995

Mr. Robert L. Pine
Director of Personnel
Doctors Hospital
Gully City, PA 44444

Dear Mr. Pine:

I am interested in applying for the Staff Nurse position in the Intensive Care Unit as advertised in the April 1, 1995 issue of the Gully City News. I would be able to begin employment at your facility any time after May 10, 1995.

As you may have noted in the attached resume, I am already an RN from an associate degree program who has just completed a Baccalaureate degree in Nursing at Mountain University, Nicetown, PA. I have had several years, experience in providing care for seriously ill clients, and feel confident that I can meet the challenge of caring for clients in an intensive care unit. Although I prefer to work the 3-11 shift, I would be willing to accept any shift assignment at this time.

Thank you very much for considering my resume. I would be available between 9:00 and 11:00 AM on Mondays, Tuesdays, and Thursdays for an interview. Please feel free to call me at home (333) 555-1234.

Sincerely,

Mary P. Oak, RN

Figure 7–2. Sample cover leter.

It is appropriate to close the interview by asking for a tour of the facility. This allows first-hand evaluation of the workplace and a chance to observe the staff and clients in a real work setting. The interviewer may not be able to provide a tour at that time and so may ask another individual, like a secretary, to take the applicant on the tour. It would also be wise to inform the interviewer of the dates scheduled for the National Council Licensure Examination (NCLEX) so that arrangements can be made for time off.

As with the resume, making frequent calls about the results of the interview is not wise. It is, however, appropriate to send a letter within a week after the interview thanking the interviewer for his or her time, expressing how appreciative the applicant is to be considered for the position, and acknowledging how much it would mean to the applicant to become a member of the staff at

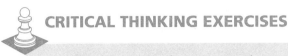

CRITICAL THINKING EXERCISES

1 Make a list of the characteristics that would be found in the "perfect nurse." Make a second list of characteristics found in nurses observed in actual practice. Discuss how and why these lists differ from each other.

2 Outline a plan for implementing a "Preceptor Clinical Experience" for the senior class of a nursing program. Make sure to include how many hours of practice are required, criteria for the selection of preceptors, student objectives from the experience, and methods of evaluation.

3 Write at least three long-term and five short-term personal or professional goals. Develop a realistic plan and time frame for achieving these goals. Make sure to include what is required to achieve these goals.

4 Complete this statement, using as many examples as possible. "I feel most satisfied when I am done with my shift in knowing that . . . . Analyze these answers and discuss how they can be implemented in everyday practice.

5 Think of at least three situations in which you were asked to do something that you really did not want to do. How did you handle these situations? How could they be handled in a more assertive manner?

such a fine hospital. If the position is offered, a formal letter of acceptance or refusal should be sent to the institution. Hospitals will not hold positions indefinitely, and failure to accept the position formally may cause the hospital to offer it to someone else. In today's health care system, many applicants are after a few positions.

SUMMARY

Although transition shock and burnout are realities of the nursing profession, they can be lessened or even avoided altogether. Recognizing the causes and early symptoms of transition shock and burnout make the nurse aware that a problem is developing or exists. Putting into practice the techniques to prevent these disorders prevents them from becoming insurmountable obstacles to nurses who want to practice their profession in a high-quality manner and gain the satisfaction that only nursing can provide.

ISSUES IN PRACTICE
Facing Cultural Diversity in Nursing

When dealing with clients from different cultural backgrounds, nurses can unwittingly impose their own values and standards.

A woman from a Middle Eastern culture had delivered a stillborn baby. After the delivery, she was transferred to the medical-surgical unit for post-partum care, a practice commonly followed after stillbirths. Becky, an experienced nurse, was assigned to care for this client. While reading through her chart, Becky noticed that the woman's husband refused to let his wife see the baby. The chart also contained a photograph of the dead baby, an ultrasound picture, and the foot and hand prints that had been taken after the delivery.

As expected, the woman was very depressed and Becky felt a great deal of sympathy for her. While caring for her, Becky mentioned to her client that there was a photograph and other mementos of the child and asked if she would like to see them. The woman's husband, who was visiting at the time, called Becky out of the room and indicated his displeasure at letting his wife know that these pictures existed without first asking him. He expressed his desire to see them but refused to let his wife see them. He also admonished Becky to stop talking with his wife and emphasized the fact that Becky really had no understanding at all of their culture.

Becky completed the shift without speaking to the woman, who was discharged before Becky returned the next day. Becky was plagued by a feeling that she had made a major error in providing care for her client by failing to meet her emotional needs.

As the immigrant population of the United States grows, nurses will have an increased likelihood of caring for culturally diverse clients. Understanding the requirements of transcultural nursing improves the care for these clients and prevents the nurse from committing major cultural blunders. It would be easy for some to dismiss the husband as a domineering male chauvinist who had no feelings for his wife's distress; but in his culture the woman's role is different from that of an American woman. But who is the client, the woman or her culture—or can the two be separated? Would your answer be different if the situation were the same, but the woman and her husband were American? Connecting nonjudgmentally with the family's culture and strengths increases the nurse's ability to communicate and help that family. The challenge nurses face is finding a means to increase their understanding and sensitivity to cultures to which they may never have been exposed.

A Closer Look

PRAYER: A POTENT FACTOR IN HEALING

Science and religion have come full circle. Many ancient cultures believed that disease and illness could be cured by prayer. As mankind took a more rational viewpoint, knowledge and science looked for a medical cure for disease and illness and came to view prayer as a meaningless ritual. In a new book, Larry Dossey, M.D., demonstrates that prayer is a potent force in producing healthy physiologic changes in patients.

Although many in the health care professions are hesitant about mixing prayer and medicine, evidence indicates that prayer can improve and sometimes even cure a client's condition. These positive results do not necessarily occur as a result of the client's own beliefs, faith, or hopes that healing will occur. In double-blind studies conducted by Dr. Dossey, clients receiving prayer who did not know they were being prayed for had higher rates of improvement. This evidence seems to eliminate the factors of positive thinking and placebo effects as elements in the clients' improved conditions.

Nurses seem to be particularly fascinated with the data about prayer and cure and view it as a way to enhance recovery in clients in critical care units and to increase the healing rates of wounds and other disease states.

Modified from Dossey, L: Healing Words: The Power of Prayer and Medicine, Harper, San Francisco, 1993 as printed in AACN News, February 1995, page 1.

ISSUES IN PRACTICE
It Isn't Always What It Seems to Be

My heart sank. The list of assignments for my clinical section was posted, and next to my name was "Room 234—Paulo Simonetti, 72—CHF." As the only male nursing student in a class of 58 students, I had become used to being assigned difficult, very large or highly hostile clients, or any combination thereof. My fellow students had been discussing Mr. Simonetti that morning before classes, and the general conclusion was that he was a demanding, "dirty old man" who liked to fondle the young female nurses. I tried to think back to where this topic was covered in my course work, but couldn't remember it ever being discussed.

I carefully went through his chart gathering the appropriate data for my care plan. Then I went to visit him to obtain some of the subjective assessment data that can only be gotten through a direct interview. The gods smiled on me that day. He

Continued on following page

was sound asleep, and his nurse admonished me not to wake him because of his weakened state. A reprieve.

The next day dawned clear and cold. I hardly noticed. That night had been one of the longest in my life—stretched by little sleep and lots of worry about what I was to face the next day. The little "call-in-sick" voice of my subconscious was starting to get very loud, but my instructor's admonition that the only excuse for not coming to clinical was death (mine) with a 48-hour prior notification outweighed that temptation.

Change-of-shift report that morning seemed much too short, and then I was out on the floors. Let's see, I need to check my medications, look through the chart for any changes in physician orders or lab results, make sure the care plan and cardex are current. . . .

My instructor wants to know why I've been out of report for 30 minutes and haven't checked on my patient yet. "I was just on my way" seemed like a good answer.

When I walked into his room, his bed was empty. Another reprieve? Hardly. His roommate said he was in the bathroom and should be out any time now. I wanted to run. I wanted to hide. I wanted . . . the door to the bathroom began to open. I took a deep breath and said: "Hi, Mr. Simonetti, my name is Don and I am going to be taking care of you today."

Without a word, he walked over to me, wrapped his ample arms around me and gave me a bear hug. Then he said in heavily accented English: "Thank you, I'm happy to meet you."

A bit surprised, I responded: "I thought you were only supposed to hug the girls?" He replied: "I hug everybody!"

At that point, it became clear to me where Mr. Simonetti's reputation had originated. In his Italian background, greeting people with hugs and the physical demonstration of affection were a natural part of his behavior. In our more aloof American culture, actions that would be a natural part of his behavior could be easily misinterpreted as sexual advances. Coupling that with the fact that his English-language skills were limited would only deepen the misunderstanding.

The nurses would respond to his behavior by avoiding him. His response to the nurse's avoidance was to put his call light on frequently. The call light often went unanswered for long periods of time. Mr. Simonetti's response to the unanswered call lights was to yell loudly for a nurse. Thus a reputation is born.

My day with Mr. Simonetti was very pleasant, hugs included. I never was able to get all the background data for the subjective portion of the care plan due to the language difference, but the communication was sufficient for the normal daily care activities. I even convinced one of my more adventurous female classmates to come in and get a hug.

Probably the most important lesson I learned that day was that you need to form your own opinion about clients based on your own observations. Client behavior, like all human behavior, is very complex and often defies simple explanations. Appreciation of a client's culture and their ways of expression is essential in providing high-quality nursing care.

BIBLIOGRAPHY

Al-Assaf, AF: Executive stress: An ounce of prevention. Nurs Management 23:69–72, 1992.
Anderson, H: Hospitals seek new ways to integrate health care. Hospitals 66:26–36, 1992.
Blegen, MA, Gardner, DL, and McCloskey, JC: Who helps you with your work? Am J Nurs 91:26–31, 1992.
Bradlby, M: Status passage into nursing: Another view of the process of socialization into nursing. J Adv Nurs 15:1220–1225, 1990.
Chenevert, M: Pro-Nurse Handbook. CV Mosby, St. Louis; 1993.
Gardiner, DL: Conflicts and retention of new graduate nurses. West J of Nurs Res 14:76–85, 1992.
Hegner, BR and Caldwell, E: Nursing Assistants: A Nursing Process Approach, Delmar, New York, 1995.
Jamieson, EM, Sewall, MF, and Suhrie, EB: Trends in Nursing History. WB Saunders, Philadelphia, 1968.
Kalish, PA and Kalish, BJ: The Advance of American Nursing, ed 3. JB Lippincott, Philadelphia, 1995.
Kirkwood, C: Your Services Are No Longer Required: The Complete Job Loss Recovery Book, Plume Books, New York, 1993.
Kramer, M: Reality Shock, CV Mosby, St. Louis, 1979.
Lindquist, KD: Finding the perfect match. Hlth Care Trends and Transition 1:6–8, 1989.
Morgan, A and McCann, JM: Problems in nurse-physician relationships. Nurs Admin Q 7:28–32, 1983.
Sabatino, F: Foundations funding priority shifts from acute to primary care. Hospitals 65:34–37, 1991.
Shugars, DA, O'Neill, EH, and Bader, JO: Health America: Practitioners for 2005, An Agenda for Action, PEW Health Professions Commission, Durham, N.C., 1991.

HISTORICAL PERSPECTIVES

Early Nursing Leaders: Florence Nightingale (1820–1910)

Although she has been immortalized as "the woman with a lamp" in Longfellow's famous poem of that name, it would be more appropriate, if less poetic, to call Florence Nightingale "the woman with a brain." She is universally credited with being the founder of modern nursing. Although English, she was born in Florence, Italy, while her parents were there on business. Contrary to the prevailing Victorian beliefs about the role and place of women, her father believed in educating his daughters. Nightingale was considered highly educated for her times.

Through her travels with her family, she became acutely aware of the substandard health care that existed in many countries, including England. She began to study health care throughout England and on the continent and was particularly interested in home care nursing. She also observed the substandard public hospitals and the higher-quality religious hospitals run by the nursing orders of the Roman Catholic Church in Italy, France, and Spain. She became particularly interested in the church-run hospital at Kaiserwerth, Germany and in

Continued on following page

1851 attended its 3-month nurses' training program. Although impressed with the organization and the dedication of the institution, she came to believe that a 3-month nursing education program was insufficient. She was forced to abandon her studies at the Sisters of Charity hospital in Paris because of illness, however.

She later assumed the charge position in a private nursing home for sick governesses and soon reorganized it so that it ran smoothly and provided first-rate care for the residents. Her interest centered on hospitals and on improving the educational standards for nurses. She was contacted by other health care reformers and a few visionary physicians about developing plans for a school of nursing in England. However, these plans were interrupted by a widespread cholera epidemic in England in 1854. Florence Nightingale volunteered her services to care for the sick and dying. From this experience, she learned a great deal about the spread of diseases and methods to contain that spread, such as hand washing, good personal hygiene, and disinfection of contaminated linens and equipment.

The year 1854 saw another major social upheaval in Europe, the Crimean war. As in the wars that preceded it, the health care provided to the wounded and sick soldiers was wretched (Woodham-Smith, 1951). This time, however, British correspondents at the front lines began sending reports back to England about the conditions found in the field hospitals. The public outcry forced the British politicians into action. By this time, Florence Nightingale had become recognized as a leader in health reform and was therefore a logical candidate to try to improve the health care being provided by the British army.

Nightingale's earlier request to take a group of 37 volunteer nurses to the battlefield was finally accepted by the Minister of War, Sir Sidney Herbert. Initially, the British medical officers running the hospital refused them admission to the wards. Nightingale waited patiently while correspondents' reports were published about the nurses' treatment and the increasing mortality rates among the wounded. Eventually, the physicians relented.

The conditions the nurses found were worse than they had imagined. As many as 3500 of the sick, wounded, dying, and dead lay crowded on stone floors in dark, damp, evil-smelling wards. Many wore the same bloody and dirty uniforms in which they had been wounded, now additionally fouled with excrement and urine. Medical supplies were not available, food was scarce, and inadequate water and sewage systems were additional problems. Hordes of rats roamed freely throughout the wards. Four of every 10 patients who entered the ward died there.

The first order of business for Nightingale and her nurses was to improve the sanitary conditions of the hospital and to separate soldiers with infectious diseases from those with wounds. The physicians strongly resisted her efforts, whereupon the nurses left, returning only after an agreement that there would be no more interference from the medical staff. Nightingale agreed to be under the supervision of the Chief Medical Officer, but she insisted on sole control over her own nurses. Over a 6-month period that saw the use of only these relatively simple nursing measures, the mortality rate fell from 42.7% to 2.2%.

Nightingale extended the reform of the British Military medical system to other areas. She established a consistent line of supply for such items as beds, medicines, and bandages and started a military post office so that soldiers could communicate with their families. She also expanded the health care system to include convalescent camps for long-term recovery and facilities where the families of soldiers could live. At the height of the war, she supervised 125 nurses in several large hospitals.

Once the hospitals in the rear were running smoothly under the supervision of her nurses, Nightingale began to improve the care at the front lines, helping to prevent many of the complications (for example, dehydration, hemorrhage, and infection) she observed in the wounded by the time they reached the hospital. She was at the front lines only a short time when she herself contracted Crimean fever (probably typhoid) and almost died. During her protracted recovery, she remained in the Crimea until all her nurses had left. Although she never completely recovered, Nightingale's accomplishments were later recognized by Queen Victoria of England. Nightingale was awarded the highest English award given to civilians, the Order of Merit.

Modified from Woodham-Smith, C: Florence Nightingale, McGraw-Hill, New York, 1951.

8

THE EVOLUTION OF LICENSURE, CERTIFICATION, AND ORGANIZATIONS

Learning Objectives

After completing this chapter, the reader will be able to:

1 Identify the purposes and needs for nurse licensure.
2 Distinguish between permissive and mandatory licensure.
3 Explain why institutional licensure is unacceptable in today's health care system.
4 Evaluate the importance of nurse practice acts.
5 Analyze the significance of professional certification.
6 Evaluate the importance of nursing organizations in the nursing profession.
7 Differentiate between specialty nursing organizations and national nursing organizations.

THE NEED FOR LICENSURE

Imagine what the quality of health care would be if any one could walk into a hospital, claim to know how to care for clients, and be given a job as a nurse based on that statement. This situation might sound impossible in today's health care system, but not too many years ago that type of situation was the norm rather than the exception.

Throughout the last half of the 19th century, and during the first half of the

20th, rapid growth in health care technology led to the increasing use of hospitals as the primary source of health care. Individuals who were qualified to provide this care, however, were in short supply. There were wide variations both in the abilities of those who claimed to be nurses and in the quality of the care that they provided. Paradoxically, nursing leaders who had always advocated some type of credentialing for nurses to ensure competency found their attempts to initiate registration or licensure met with strong opposition from physician groups, hospital administrators, and practicing nurses themselves (AAN, 1987).

EARLY ATTEMPTS AT LICENSURE

Although the idea of registering nurses had been in existence for some time, Florence Nightingale was the first to establish a formal "register" for graduates of her nursing school. In the United States and Canada, there was widespread recognition of the need for some type of credentialing of nurses as far back as the middle 1800s. The first organized attempt to establish a credentialing system was initiated by the Nurses Associated Alumnae of the United States and Canada (later to become the American Nurses Association) in 1896. As with other early attempts at licensure, it was met with resistance and eventual failure (Kelly, 1991).

The nursing leaders at this time recognized the existence of widespread misunderstanding about what licensure was and why it was needed. In 1901, after an extensive and lengthy campaign to educate the public, physicians, hospital administrators, and nurses themselves about the need for licensure, the International Council of Nurses passed a resolution that required each state to establish a licensure and examination procedure for nurses. It took 3 years before the state of New York, through the New York Nurses Association, developed a licensure bill that passed the legislature. Some of the key points in this bill:

- Establishing minimum educational standards
- Establishing the minimum length of basic nursing programs at 2 years
- Requiring all nursing schools to be registered with the state board of regents (who oversee all higher education)
- Establishing a state board of nursing (SBN) with five nurses as members
- Formulating rules for the examination of nurses
- Formulating regulations for nurses which, if violated, could lead to the revocation of licensure (Hirsh, 1988)

Other states that soon followed New York's lead were North Carolina, New Jersey, and the Commonwealth of Virginia. Although these states had bills that were weaker than New York's nurse practice act, passage of such legislation was considered a major accomplishment for several reasons. First, women did not even have the right to vote in general elections at the time these bills were passed. In addition, few requirements and regulations for licensure existed during this period in U.S. history, even for the medical profession.

IMPORTANCE OF LICENSURE EXAMINATIONS

The thought of having to take an examination that can determine whether or not one can practice nursing can make even the best students anxious. Adding to the tension is the fact that the examination is given outside of the academic setting and is created by individuals other than the students' teachers.

Some type of external means, however, to prove that the individual is qualified to practice nursing safely is necessary to protect the public from unqualified practitioners. Early attempts at creating licensure examinations for nurses were met with resistance. Although all states had some form of licensure examination by 1923, the format and length of the examination varied widely. Some states required both written and practical examinations to demonstrate safety of practice, whereas others added an oral examination.

Although licensure was and is a state-controlled activity, the major nursing organizations in the United States eventually realized that in order to have some consistency of quality across the country, a single examination that all nurses needed to pass should be devised. The American Nurses Association (ANA) Council of State Boards of Nursing was organized in 1945 to oversee development of a uniform examination for nurses that could be used by all state boards of nursing. The National League of Nursing Testing Division developed such a test, which was implemented in 1950. Originally the test was simply called the State Board Examination, but it was renamed the National Council Licensure Examination (NCLEX) in 1987. In 1994, the computerized version of the examination was implemented—the National Council Licensure Examination—Computerized Adaptive Testing, for Registered Nurses (NCLEX-CAT, RN).

REGISTRATION VERSUS LICENSURE

The terms **registration** and **licensure** are often used interchangeably, even though this is incorrect. Although they serve a similar purpose, some technical differences exist.

Registration is the listing, or registering, of names of individuals on an official roster when they have met certain pre-established criteria. Before universal licensure by the states, any health care institution that wanted to know whether a person applying for a position had met the standards for that position by graduating from a school of nursing or by passing an examination could call the school and see if the applicant's name appeared on the official roster or register, hence the origin of the term **registered nurse**. With the advent of state board examinations, an institution merely has to call the SBN to find out if the individual was registered.

Licensure is an activity conducted by the state through its enforcement powers to protect the public's health, safety, and welfare by establishing professional standards. Licensure for nurses, as for other professionals who deal with the public, is necessary to ensure that everyone who claims to be a nurse can function at a minimal level of competency and safety. There are several different types of licensure.

Permissive licensure allows individuals to practice nursing so long as they do not use the letters "RN" after their names. Basically, permissive licensure protects the "registered nurse" designation but not the practice of nursing itself. Most early licensure laws were permissive. Texas, the last state to continue with a permissive licensure law, today has mandatory licensure.

Mandatory licensure requires anyone who wishes to practice nursing to pass a licensure examination and become registered by the SBN. Because different levels of nursing exist, different levels of licensure also became necessary. At the technical level, the individual must take and pass the licensed practical nurse (LPN) examination; at the professional level, the individual must take and pass the RN examination.

Mandatory licensure forced SBNs to distinguish between the activities that nurses at different levels could legally carry out. This differentiation is referred to as the **scope of practice.** As more levels of nursing practice (e.g., the Associate Degree in Nursing, or ADN) have been added, however, lines dividing the different scopes of practice have become blurred. In today's health care system, it is not unusual to find LPNs carrying out activities that are generally considered professional and RNs performing chores that are clearly technical.

A particularly confusing element in today's health care system is the use of unlicensed individuals to provide health care. The advent of Certified Nurses Aides (CNAs) and Unlicensed Assistive Personnel (UAP) in recent years has led to widespread use of such individuals in all health care settings. Although they are to be supervised by an RN or LPN, these individuals can be assigned nursing tasks much more advanced than their levels of training. Despite the fact that permissive licensure is no longer legal, CNAs and UAPs appear to fall under an unofficial type of permissive licensure.

Although universally rejected by every major nursing organization, **institutional licensure** has become a reality for many other types of health care workers, such as respiratory therapists and physical therapists. In some state legislatures, bills have been introduced to allow nurses who are licensed in foreign countries to work in specific institutions without taking the U.S. licensure examination. Institutional licensure has been proposed periodically over the years as an alternative to governmental licensure.

The idea behind institutional licensure is that the individual health care institution will be permitted to determine which individuals are qualified to practice nursing within general guidelines established by some outside board. Although this type of licensure appeals to hospitals and nursing homes because it would allow them to hire individuals with less training at a reduced cost, it has some serious difficulties associated with it.

Probably the most critical problem is the lack of any external control to determine a minimal level of competency. The designations of RN and LPN would be virtually meaningless under institutional licensure. These nurses would not be under the control of the SBNs of the various states and so would not be held to the same standards of practice as other nurses who were licensed by the states. A second problem is that nurses who wished to move to a new place of employment would have to undergo whatever licensure procedure the new institution had established before being allowed to work there.

DEVELOPMENT OF NURSE PRACTICE ACTS

A nurse practice act is state legislation that regulates the practice of nurses to protect the public and make nurses accountable for their actions. Nurse practice acts establish SBNs and define specific SBN powers regarding the practice of nursing within the state. Rules and regulations written by the SBNs become statutory laws under the powers delegated by the state legislature (Moloney, 1992).

Although nurse practice acts differ from state to state, the SBNs have many powers in common. All SBNs have the power to grant licenses, to accredit nursing programs, to establish standards for nursing schools, and to write specific regulations for nurses and nursing in general in that state.

Particularly important is the SBN's power to deny or revoke nurse licenses. Some common reasons for this include:

- Conviction for a serious crime
- Demonstrating gross negligence or unethical conduct in the practice of nursing
- Failure to renew a nursing license while still continuing to practice nursing
- Use of illegal drugs or alcohol during the provision of care for clients
- Willful violation of the state's nurse practice act

Other functions of nurse practice acts include a definition of nursing and the scope of practice, ruling on who can use the titles RN and LPN, setting up an application procedure for licensure in the state, determining fees for licensure, establishing requirements for renewal of licensure, and determining responsibility for any regulations governing expanded practice for nurses in that particular state.

CERTIFICATION

At first glance, not much difference may be seen between certification and licensure. Strictly defined, **licensure** can actually be considered a type of legal certification. In the more widely accepted use of the term, however, **certification** is a granting of credentials to indicate that an individual has achieved a level of ability higher than the levels required for licensure (Fenton, 1992). In some states, certification also carries with it a legal status, like licensure, but in many cases certification merely indicates a specific professional status. One element that adds confusion to the understanding of the process of certification is that a large number of groups can offer certification. These are usually professional specialty groups like the National Association of Pediatric Nurse Associates and Practitioners (NAPNAP) and the American Association of Critical-Care Nurses (AACN) but they can also be governmental organizations or national organizations like the National League for Nursing (NLN).

The most common type of certification is called **individual certification.** When a nurse has demonstrated that he or she has attained a certain level of ability above and beyond the basic level required for licensure in a defined area of practice, that nurse can become certified. Usually some type of written and practical examination is required to demonstrate this advanced level of skill (Diers, 1985). The American Nurses Association (ANA) offers several certifications that are widely recognized.

Organizational certification is the certification of a group or health care institution by some external agency. It is usually referred to as accreditation and indicates that the institution has met standards established by either the government or by a nongovernmental agency. Often the ability of the institution to collect money from insurance companies or the federal government depends on whether or not the institution is certified by a recognized agency. Most hospitals are accredited by the Joint Commission on Accreditation of Healthcare Organizations (JCAHO) as a minimum level of accreditation.

In some states, the state government may either award or recognize certification granted to nurses in areas of advanced practice. In such cases, the certification then assumes the legal force of a license. Depending on the individual state's nurse practice act, nurses thus certified fall under regulations in the states practice act that control the type of activities nurses may legally carry out when they perform advanced roles. For example, many states recognize the position of nurse midwife as an advanced practice role for nurses. In these states, a nurse midwife is allowed to practice those skills allowed under the nurse practice act of that state after obtaining certification. Generally nurse midwives are allowed to conduct prenatal examinations, do prenatal teaching, and deliver babies vaginally in uncomplicated pregnancies (Porter-O'Grady, 1991). They are not usually allowed to perform cesarean sections.

Unfortunately, from state to state, no uniformity exists in the recognition of certification of advanced practice nurses. Some states recognize almost all certifications and have provisions in their nurse practice acts to help guide these practices. Other states have very little legal recognition of certification levels and thus few guidelines for practice. This confusion may result from so many different organizations offering certification in different areas. In some advanced practice areas, like nurse practitioners, two or more organizations may offer certification for the same title. The certification standards vary from organization to organization, and the method of determining certification may also be different.

An independent certification center was proposed in 1978 to establish uniform criteria and standards and to oversee all certification activities. Although it would eliminate much of the current confusion about certification and would help with the legal recognition of advanced practice nurses (Edmunds, 1992), this proposal has not yet been acted upon.

It is expected that advanced practice nurses will play a larger role in the rapidly evolving health care system of the future. What that role will be depends on how well governmental organizations and the public understand the contributions practitioners can make as primary care providers. Without a uniform definition of this specialty, such nurses will not be utilized to their full potential.

Licensure, registration, and certification are all methods of granting credentials to demonstrate that an individual is qualified to provide safe care to the public. Without proof of competency, the profession of nursing would become chaotic, disorganized, and even downright dangerous. It is important for nurses to keep a watchful eye on pending legislation and practices that health care institutions are initiating. Many of these proposals and practices mask, using legalistic language, the old nemeses of professional nursing: permissive licensure and institutional licensure.

NURSING ORGANIZATIONS AND THEIR IMPORTANCE

Establishment of a professional organization is one of the most important defining characteristics of a profession. Many professions have a single major professional organization to which most of its members belong and several specialized suborganizations that members may also join. Professions with just one major organization generally have a great deal of political power.

Nurses need and use power in every aspect of their professional lives, ranging from giving a bed bath to negotiating with the administration for increased independence of practice. Clearly, an individual nurse probably does not have much power, but for nurses as a group, the potential is increased exponentially by the organization. The dedication to high-quality nursing standards and improved methods of practice by the major nursing organizations have led to improved care and increased benefits to the public as a whole.

National nursing organizations need the participation and membership of all nurses in order to claim that they are truly representative of the profession. A large membership allows the organization to speak "with one voice" when making its beliefs about health care issues known to politicians.

THE NATIONAL LEAGUE FOR NURSING

Purposes

The National League for Nursing's (NLN) primary purpose is to maintain and improve the standards of nursing education. All levels of nursing education in all settings are now under the regulatory powers of one organization. The NLN is also a strong force in community health nursing, occupational health nursing, and nursing service activities. Its bylaws state that its purpose is to foster the de-

velopment and improvement of hospital, industrial, public health, and other organized nursing services and of nursing education through the coordinated action of nurses, allied professional groups, citizens, agencies, and schools so that
the nursing needs of the people will be met.

Membership

Although membership is open to individual nurses, the primary membership in
the NLN comes in the form of agency membership, usually through schools of
nursing. One of the major functions of this organization is to accredit schools of
nursing through a self-study process. The schools are given a set of criteria and
are then required to evaluate their programs against these criteria. After the
evaluation report is written and sent to the NLN, site representatives visit the
school to verify the information in the report. If the school meets the criteria, it
is accredited for up to 8 years. NLN accreditation of a school of nursing indicates that the school meets national standards. In some work settings, it is a requirement that a nurse be a graduate of an NLN-accredited school of nursing
before the nurse can be hired.

Other Services

Other services and activities that the NLN carries out include testing, evaluating new graduate nurses, supplying career information and continuing education
workshops and conferences for all levels of nursing, publishing a wide range of
literature and videotapes covering current issues in health care, and compiling
statistics about nursing, nurses, and nursing education.

THE AMERICAN NURSES ASSOCIATION (ANA)

Purposes

The ANA grew out of a concern with the quality of nursing practice and the care
that nurses were providing. The major purposes for the existence of the ANA,
as stated in its bylaws, include improvement of the standards of health and the
access to health care services for everyone, improvement and maintenance of
high standards for nursing practice, and promotion of the professional growth
and development of all nurses, including economic issues, working conditions,
and independence of practice (AAN, 1987).

Membership

Membership in the ANA is primarily individual. It is open to all nurses, including graduate nurses. Certain discounts in membership are offered for new mem-

bers and new graduate nurses. Various levels of membership are available for nurses who work part-time or those who are retired. The ANA makes every effort to encourage individual nurses to join the organization. Unfortunately, most nurses do not belong to this potentially powerful, politically active, and very influential organization.

Although dues are not inexpensive (they change from year to year, but are less than $200 per year), the ANA offers various plans for paying them. They can be paid in three equal payments over the course of a year or even through monthly payroll deductions. At least partly because of the efforts of the ANA, nurses' salaries have risen to a point where this sum is affordable.

Other Services

When nurses go on for advanced education and levels of practice, as many are doing today, the ANA is essential for testing and certification of these practice levels. Without the ANA, there would be even less standardization for advanced nursing practice and less recognition of these practice levels by the public, physicians, or lawmakers.

Another extremely important issue that the ANA has been involved in for years is the entry-level education requirement for professional nurses. The ANA has supported the baccalaureate degree as the minimum educational requirement for nurses for the last 25 years. This issue will continue to be hotly debated into the next century with the ANA at the helm.

Additional functions carried out by the ANA include the most important, that is, the establishment and continual updating of standards of nursing practice. These standards are the yardstick against which nurses are measured and held accountable by courts of law. The ANA also established the official code of ethics for nurses to measure these professionals. In the recent past, the ANA has become very concerned with supplying credentials for advanced practice nurses and has expanded this service greatly.

Many of the political and economic activities of the ANA are carried out behind the scenes in the halls of legislatures and offices of legislators. Such activities have a profound effect on the role nurses play and will continue to play in health care well into the next century. These activities require money (members' dues) and the influence of a large membership.

The political activities of the ANA seek to influence legislation about nurses, nursing, and health care in general. It has been and will be a strong voice in the formulation of current national health care reform. Another important function of the ANA is economic. In many states, the ANA is the official bargaining agent for nurses in the negotiation of contracts with hospitals, nursing homes, and other health care agencies that employ nurses. Professional organizations represent professional groups better than a labor union with little knowledge of what the professional does or needs.

NATIONAL STUDENT NURSES ASSOCIATION (NSNA)

Purposes

The NSNA is an independent legal corporation established in 1953 to represent the needs of nursing students. Working closely with the ANA, which offers services, an official publication, and close communication, the NSNA is composed of state chapters that represent student nurses in those particular states.

The main purpose of the NSNA is to help in maintaining high standards of education in schools of nursing with the ultimate goal of educating high-quality nurses who will provide excellent health care. Students' ideas, concerns, and needs are extremely important to nursing educators. Most nursing programs have committees in which students are asked to participate in curriculum development, evaluation techniques, and even selection of incoming students. It is important that students belong to these committees and actively participate in the committees' activities.

Membership

Membership is composed of all nursing students in registered nurse programs; like the ANA, the NSNA has several different membership levels. Dues are low with a discount for first year's membership.

Other Services

Additionally, the NSNA is concerned with developing and providing workshops, seminars, and conferences that deal with current issues in nursing and health care. These issues take on a wide range of subjects, from ethical and legal concerns to recent developments in pharmacology, test-taking skills, and professional growth. Student nurses who belong to the NSNA and who take an active part in its functions are much more likely to join the ANA after they graduate. Professional identity and professional behavior are learned. By beginning the process during the formal school years, student nurses develop professional attitudes and behaviors that they continue for the rest of their lives.

Many benefits exist for student nurses who belong to the NSNA. Many scholarships are available through this organization to members of the NSNA. Members receive the official publication of the organization, *Imprint*, as well as the *NSNA News*, which together keep the student nurse current on recent developments in health care and nursing. The student member also has political representation on issues that may affect the student now or in the future. Some of the issues include educational standards for practice, standards of professional practice, and health insurance. The NSNA is also concerned with the difficulty that many nursing students from minority groups experience in the educational process. Project Breakthrough is an attempt by the NSNA to help such students enter the profession of nursing.

Student nurses who join the NSNA experience first hand the operation, activities, and benefits of a professional organization. In schools with active memberships, the NSNA can be a very exciting and useful organization for students. Many NSNA chapters are involved in community activities that provide services at a local level and allow the student to practice "real" nursing. These services include providing community health screening programs for conditions such as hypertension, lead poisoning, and vision, hearing, and birth defects; setting up information and education programs; giving immunizations; and working with groups concerned with drug abuse, child abuse, drunk driving, and teen pregnancy. All nursing students should be encouraged to belong to this organization.

SPECIAL-INTEREST ORGANIZATIONS

The historical origins of special-interest organizations in nursing are even older than those of the main national organizations. The Red Cross, established in 1864, can be considered a special-interest organization for nurses. Like the Red Cross, most specialty organizations in nursing were founded when a group of nurses with similar concerns sought professional and individual support. These organizations usually start out small and informal, then increase in size, structure, and membership over a number of years. There were relatively few of these organizations until 1965, when an explosion in specialty organizations in nursing took place. During the next 20 years, almost 100 new organizations were formed, with the associated effect of diminishing membership levels in the ANA.

Specialty organizations are usually focused on one particular aspect of their membership. By far, the most common focal point is clinical practice area. Organizations exist for almost every clinical specialty and subspecialty known in nursing. These include such obvious areas as OB/GYN, critical care, operating room, emergency room, and occupational health, to less known areas such as flight nurses, urology, and cosmetic surgery. Another focal area for these organizations is education. Organizations such as American Association of Colleges of Nursing and the Western Interstate Commission for Higher Education fall into this category. Often organizations focus on the common ethnic, cultural, or religious backgrounds of nurses. The National Association of Hispanic Nurses and the National Black Nurses Association represent this type of specialty organization.

Although many of these organizations promote the personal and professional growth of their membership, they also carry out many other activities. Particularly important among these activities is establishing the standards of practice for the particular specialty area. Much as the ANA establishes overall standards of practice for nursing in general, the specialty organizations establish standards for their particular clinical areas. Providing educational services for their members is another important activity the specialty groups conduct. Conferences, workshops, and seminars in the clinical area represented are important venues for nurses to keep current on new developments and to maintain high standards of practice.

How many of these specialty nursing organizations are there? No one really knows. Many such organizations are informal and run by volunteers. A continual stream of organizations is being formed, while others are being disbanded. Should nurses belong to these organizations? The answer is yes, but only *after* they belong to the ANA. Many of the larger specialty organizations have recognized this fact and have established close ties with the ANA. The ANA, in its turn, is well aware of the membership bleed-off from the specialty organizations and has initiated efforts to become more involved in the specialty nursing areas.

Before nurses join a specialty organization (see Appendix D for a listing), they should determine if its purposes are at odds with those of the ANA. Many of the large specialty organizations have their own lobbyists in both state and national legislatures. Because the legislators really do not know the differences between the various nursing organizations, they can become easily confused over health care issues if they are receiving pressure from two nursing groups representing opposing sides of the same issue. At this point, legislators may simply surmise that nurses really do not know what they want and vote on an important issue without regard to nurses and nursing.

SUMMARY

Nursing, in its journey toward professionalism, has been propelled and shaped by its nursing organizations, which were the main vehicles for the development of educational and practice standards, initiation of licensure, promotion of advanced practice, and general improvement in the level of care nurses provided. From their beginnings, nursing organizations have served as channels of communication between nurses, consumers of health care, and other health care professionals. In many cases, the nursing organizations have served as focus of power for the profession to influence those important health policies that affect the whole nation. That continued unity is essential for the survival of nursing.

The tendency toward specialization has led to an ever-increasing number of nursing organizations, however, each focusing on a particular practice field within the profession. This trend has diluted the unity and ultimately lessened the power that nursing as a profession can exert in health care issues. Although

CRITICAL THINKING EXERCISES

1 Develop a strategy for increasing the membership in the ANA.

2 A labor union is attempting to organize the nurses at your hospital. Is it better for the professional nursing organization to represent the nurses? Why?

3 A new graduate nurse is working in the ICU of a large hospital. She wants to join a nursing organization, but only has a limited amount of money to spend. Her co-workers in the ICU want her to join the AACN, but she would also like to join the ANA. Basing her decision on economic and professional issues, which organization should she join?

4 Compare and contrast certification and licensure. Should certification be legally recognized? Justify your answer.

5 Current proposals for health care reform are likely to increase the demand for advanced-level nurse practitioners. Identify possible changes that may occur in the profession of nursing as a result of these changes.

it is important to recognize the complexity of today's health care system and the pluralism inherent in nursing, unity of opinion on major issues is essential if nursing is to have any influence on the future of the profession. The challenge for nurses in the future is to use the diversity in the profession as a positive force and to unite as a group on important issues. Awareness of earlier development of nursing organizations provides a perspective for the current situation and can act as a framework for planning the future.

BIBLIOGRAPHY

American Academy of Nursing: The Evolution of Nursing Professional Organizations: Alternatives for the Future. ACN, Kansas City, 1987.

American Nurses Association: Federation of Specialty Nursing Organizations and ANA–A History. ANA, Kansas City, 1980.

Billingsley, M and Harper, D: The extinction of the nurse practitioner: Threat or reality. Nurse Practitioner 7:22–30, 1982.

Bower, K: Case Management by Nurses. American Nurses Association, Washington, DC, 1992.

Christman, L: Opinion: Knowledge is power. Reflections 17:40, 1992.

Cristy, T: First fifty years. Am J Nurs 9:1778–1784, 1971.

Diers, D: Preparation of practitioners, clinical specialists, and clinicians. J Prof Nurs 1:41–47, 1985.

Durham, J and Hardin, J: Promoting advanced nursing practice. Nurse Practitioner 10:59–62, 1985.

Edmunds, MW: Council's pursuit of national standardization for advanced practice meets resistance. Nurse Practitioner 17:81–83, 1992.

CERTIFIED NURSE PRACTITIONERS—KEY TO FUTURE HEALTH CARE

With their additional education and advanced practice skills, nurse practitioners (NPs) are able to provide high-quality care and to serve a population that either avoids or is unable to afford the cost of physician-based health care. Many states, however, continue to place burdensome restrictions on nurse practitioners that severely restrict their practice.

In a recent study by the University of Buffalo School of Nursing, it was found that the states with the most restrictive laws for nurse practitioners (Illinois and Hawaii) not surprisingly have the fewest nurse practitioners per capita. The states with the least restrictive laws for nurse practitioners (Alaska, Arizona, Montana, New Mexico, and Wyoming) allow NPs full prescriptive authority and have the highest rate of nurse practitioners per capita.

The study also showed that most (85%) of the nurse practitioners practiced in urban areas, whereas only 15% practiced in rural areas. Those states with the most restrictive laws had fewer than 100 NPs for the whole state.

Advanced practice nurses are important to the future of health care in the United States as providers of health care services to a segment of the population that otherwise would not receive services. It is essential that all nurses support advanced practice legislation that allows the widest scope of practice for these dedicated practitioners.

Modified from Study finds NPs still face barriers. The American Nurse 27(1):7, 1995.

Elder, R and Bullough, B: Nurse practitioners and clinical nurse specialists: Are the roles merging? Clinical Nurse Specialist 4:78–84, 1990.

Fenton, MV: Education for advanced practice of clinical specialists. Oncol Nurs Forum 19:16–20, 1992.

Ford, LC: Nurse for all settings: The nurse practitioner. Nurs Outlook 27:516–521, 1979.

Hamric, AB and Spross, JA: The Clinical Nurse Specialist in Theory and Practice. WB Saunders, Philadelphia, 1989.

Hirsch, IL: Statement on nursing's scope describes how two levels of nurses practice. American Nurse 20:13, 1988.

Kelly, LY: Dimensions of Professional Nursing. Pergamon Press, Elmsford, NY, 1991.

Moloney, M: Professionalization of Nursing: Current Issues and Trends. JB Lippincott, Philadelphia, 1992.

Porter-O'Grady, T: Changing realities for nurses: New models, new roles for nursing care delivery. Nurs Admin Q 16:1–6, 1991.

HISTORICAL PERSPECTIVES

Florence Nightingale's Contributions

Florence Nightingale's experiences with her basic nurses' training, supervision of the nursing home, and her ordeal during the Crimean War only strengthened her conviction that nursing education required major reforms. She believed that nursing schools should be run by nurses, independent of control by hospitals and physicians. She advocated a program for nurses of at least a 1-year duration that included information about basic biologic sciences as well as techniques to improve nursing care and provide actual supervised practice. Nursing education should be a life-long endeavor, she believed, and the status of nurses should be raised above that of housemaids and servants. Educated nurses should not spend their time with menial jobs such as cleaning and cooking but rather in direct contact with the clients, providing nursing care.

Although she remained in a state of self-imposed semi-isolation for the rest of her life, Nightingale worked tirelessly for the reform of health care and nursing. She was appointed to a number of committees and commissions dealing with health care reform and improvement. She was a prolific writer and wrote extensively about improving hospital conditions, sanitation needs, health care in general, and nursing education. Her famous Nightingale Training School for Nurses opened in 1860 and soon her trained nurses were in great demand all over Europe and the United States.

Despite strong opposition from physicians who felt that her nurses were overtrained, The Nightingale School flourished. The main goal of her school was to educate nurses who could provide hospital and home care and who could also educate other nurses. Many of the early graduates from this school went on to become important nursing leaders in their own right. A Registry of Nurses who had graduated from the school was established. These listed nurses were certified as having achieved at least the minimal level of required education. She emphasized health maintenance and promotion in her school and advocated the philosophy that nursing was both an art and a science. She taught that each client should be treated as an individual and that nurses were to meet the needs of the clients, not the demands of the physicians.

Despite the many forward-looking and progressive ideas that she advocated, Nightingale was a product of her time and held some ideas that seem strange by today's standards. For example, she never completely accepted the theory that pathogens cause disease, even though she had extensive experience in caring for clients with all types of contagious diseases. She opposed establishing a national licensure procedure for nurses, perhaps because she thought the national licensure standards would be lower than her own registration standards. Her standards for admission to her school were strict—only unmarried women of good character were admitted to the school. Any indication of moral weakness was considered grounds for dismissal.

Florence Nightingale dedicated her long life to the improvement of health care and nursing. Through these efforts, she formed the foundation on which the practice of modern nursing is built. It is easy to see much of her underlying philosophy about health care and nursing reflected in the theories and models discussed in Chapter 2. This philosophy includes an emphasis on health maintenance and promotion, and not just care of the sick, treating each client as an individual and the center of nursing care, thus raising the status of nursing to a collegial level equal to that of medicine. She insisted on the requirement that nurses be educated in all sciences in formal schools of nursing. Although her ideas were diluted and lost to some degree during the first 50 years of the 20th century, they have since resurfaced and are now being evaluated in the light of a rapidly changing health care system (Christy, 1971).

9

NCLEX—WHAT YOU NEED TO KNOW

Learning Objectives

After completing this chapter, the reader will be able to:

1. Describe the NCLEX-RN, CAT test plan.
2. Discuss the NCLEX-RN, CAT test format.
3. Analyze and identify the different types of questions used on the NCLEX-RN, CAT.
4. Select the most appropriate means for preparing for the NCLEX-RN, CAT.
5. Apply key test-taking strategies to help improve examination grades.

THE NATIONAL COUNCIL LICENSURE EXAMINATION (NCLEX) TEST PLAN

The primary purpose of licensure examinations is to protect the public from unsafe or uneducated practitioners of the profession. When nurses pass the NCLEX, it indicates that they have attained the minimal level of competency deemed necessary by the state in order to practice nursing without injury to clients. Licensure is a legal requirement for all professions that deal with public health, welfare, or safety.

The NCLEX is a computerized test that is taken after the student graduates from a school of nursing. The examination measures nursing knowledge of a wide range of material. With computerized adaptive tests, such as the NCLEX, the computer selects questions in accordance with the examination plan and how well the graduate answered the previous question. There are three major components to the examination plan: Nursing Process, Client Health Needs, and Levels of Cognitive Ability.

NURSING PROCESS

The NCLEX-RN, Computerized Adaptive Testing (CAT) uses the five-step nursing process: assessment, analysis, planning, implementation, and evaluation. Each of the questions that the graduate answers will fall into one of these categories. It is important that the graduate keep in mind the steps of the nursing process when answering questions. Often questions that ask: "What should the nurse do first?" are looking for answers based on assessment because that is the first step in the nursing process. Questions on the nursing process are equally divided on the examination (i.e., 20% for each category).

1   The assessment phase primarily establishes the database on which the rest of the nursing process is built. Some components of the assessment phase include both subjective and objective data about the client, significant history, history of the present illness, signs and symptoms, environmental elements, laboratory values, and vital signs. Often the examination will ask the nurse to distinguish between appropriate and inappropriate assessment factors. An example of an assessment phase question is:
A client's respiratory status continues to worsen. Which of the following signs and symptoms would be most indicative of a deterioration of respiratory status?
a   Increased restlessness and changes in LOC.
b   Bradycardia and increases in blood pressure.
c   Complaints of chest pain and shortness of breath.
d   Rapidly dropping PCO_2 and pH.
The correct answer is **a**. The brain is one of the first organs to be affected by a decrease in oxygenation. Restlessness and changes in level of consciousness indicate this decrease. All the other choices are assessments for other conditions.

2   The analysis phase of the nursing process involves developing and using nursing diagnosis for the care of the client. The NCLEX uses the NANDA nursing diagnosis system. Questions concerning nursing diagnosis often ask the graduate to prioritize the diagnoses. An example of an analysis phase question is:
A client is admitted to the unit with a diagnosis of bronchitis, congestive heart failure, and fever. The nurse assesses him as having a temperature of 101°F, peripheral edema, dyspnea, and ronchi. The following nursing diagnoses are all appropriate, but which one has the highest priority?
a   Anxiety related to fear of hospitalization.
b   Ineffective airway clearance related to retained secretions.
c   Fluid volume excess related to third spacing of fluid (edema).
d   Ineffective thermoregulation related to fever.
The correct choice is **b**. Nursing diagnoses that deal with airway always have highest priority.

3   The planning phase of the nursing process primarily involves setting goals

for the client. Included in the planning phase are such factors as determining expected outcomes, setting priorities for goals, and anticipating client needs based on the assessment. An example of a planning phase question is: A client is determined to be in respiratory failure and is placed on oxygen. Which of the following goals would have the highest priority for this client?

a   Walk the length of the hall twice during a nurse's shift.
b   Complete his bath and morning care before breakfast.
c   Maintain an oxygen saturation of 90% throughout the nurse's shift.
d   Keep the head of the bed elevated to promote proper ventilation.

The correct answer is **c**. Choice **a** is unrealistic for this client. Choice **b** is not client-centered, and choice **d** is a nursing intervention, not a goal. Maintaining an oxygen saturation of 90% is realistic and within normal limits.

4   The intervention and implementation phase of the nursing process involves identifying those nursing actions that are required to meet the goals stated in the planning phase. Some of the material in the intervention and implementation phase includes provision of nursing care based on the client's goals, prevention of injury or spread of disease, therapy with medications and their administration, giving treatments, carrying out procedures, charting and record keeping, teaching about health care, and monitoring changes in condition. An example of an intervention/implementation phase question is:

When the nurse ambulates a client who has been on bed rest for 3 days, he suddenly becomes very restless, displays extreme dyspnea, and complains of chest pain. Which of the following would be most appropriate nursing action?

a   Call a code blue.
b   Continue to help the client walk, but at a slower pace.
c   Give the client an injection of his ordered pain medication.
d   Return the client to bed and evaluate his vital signs and lung sounds.

The correct answer to this question is **d**. These are symptoms of a pulmonary embolism, which is a common complication of prolonged bed rest.

5   The evaluation phase of the nursing process determines whether or not the goals stated in the planning phase have been met through the interventions. The evaluation phase also ties the nursing process together and makes it cyclic. If the goals were met, there is no problem. If they were not met, then the nurse has to go back and find the difficulty. Were the assessment data inadequate? Were the goals defective? Was there a deficiency in the implementation? Material in the evaluation phase includes comparison of actual outcomes to expected outcomes, verification of assessment data, evaluation of nursing actions and client responses, and evaluation of the client's level of knowledge and understanding. An example of an evaluation question is:

A client is being prepared for discharge. He is to take theophylline by mouth at home for his lung disease. The nurse will know that her teaching concerning theophylline medications has been effective if the patient states, a "I can stop taking this medication when I feel better."

b "If I have difficulty swallowing the time-released capsules, I can crush them or chew them."

c "If I have a lot of nausea and vomiting or become restless and can't sleep, I need to call my physician."

d "I need to drink more coffee and cola while I am on these medications."

The correct answer to this question is **c**. Choice **c** lists some side effects of theophylline medications that may indicate the onset of toxicity. The physician needs to know about these so that the theophylline level can be determined and the dosage adjusted accordingly. Other factors that the client could be taught about theophylline medications include: to avoid excessive amounts of caffeine, never to suddenly stop taking the medication, to take it with a full glass of water and a small amount of food, and to watch for interactions with over-the-counter (OTC) medications.

CLIENT HEALTH NEEDS

The NCLEX asks questions about four general groups of material called client health needs. These are Safe and Effective Care Environment, Physiologic Needs, Psychosocial Needs, and Health Promotion and Maintenance Needs.

Safe and Effective Care Environment questions make up approximately 20% of the questions on the NCLEX. These questions deal with overt safety issues in client care, such as use of restraints, medication administration, safety measures to prevent injuries like putting up side-rails, preventing infections, special measures for pediatric clients, and special safety needs of clients with psychiatric problems.

This needs category also includes questions about laboratory tests, their results and any special nursing measures associated with them, legal and ethical issues in nursing, a small amount of nursing management, and quality assurance issues. Questions on these issues are intermingled with other questions throughout the examination.

Physiologic Needs are concerned with adult medical and surgical nursing care as well as with pediatric clients. It comprises the largest groups of questions, with 50% of the total number of questions. It generally includes the more common health care problems that the nurse deals with on a daily basis, such as diabetes, cardiovascular disorders, neurologic disorders, and renal diseases. Questions about nursing care of the pediatric client, such as growth and development, congenital abnormalities, abuse, burn injury, and fractures, are a few of the many potential topics.

Psychosocial Needs are those health care issues that revolve around the client with psychiatric problems. This category comprises 15% of the examination and includes questions about the care of clients with anxiety disorders, depression, schizophrenia, and organic mental disease. Also included in the psychosocial needs section are questions about therapeutic communication, crisis intervention, and drug abuse.

Health Promotion and Maintenance Needs deals with pregnancy, labor, delivery, and care of the newborn infant. This section comprises 15% of the examination and evaluates the nurse's knowledge of the care of pregnant women. Teaching and counseling is an important part of the nurse's care during pregnancy, and knowledge of diet, signs and symptoms of complications, fetal development, and testing used during pregnancy is necessary.

LEVELS OF COGNITIVE ABILITY

The levels of cognitive ability is a component of the NCLEX that measures how knowledge has been learned and how it can be used by the nurse. For the NCLEX, knowledge is tested at three different levels.

1   Level 1 consists of knowledge and comprehension questions. Only about 15% of the questions are at this level. These questions involve recalling specific facts and the ability to understand those facts in relationship to a pathophysiologic condition. Examples of these types of questions would include: knowledge of specific anatomy and physiology, medication dosage and side effects, signs and symptoms of diseases, laboratory test results, and the elements of certain treatments and interventions. Being able to remember and understand information is the most basic way of learning. Although this type of knowledge is important and underlies the other levels of knowledge, it is not itself sufficient to ensure safe nursing care. An example of a Level 1 question is:
A client is admitted to the medical unit with respiratory failure. Which of the following is the normal range for the PO_2?
a   10–30 mmHg
b   35–55 mmHg
c   10–20 cm H_2O
d   70–100 mmHg
The correct answer is **d**. You either have or do not have the knowledge for this particular laboratory test.

2   Level 2 consists of questions that ask the nurse to analyze and apply the memorized information to specific client-care situations. Analysis and application questions are more difficult to answer because they require the nurse to take the learned information and do something with it. Analysis requires the ability to separate information into its basic parts and decide which of those parts are important. Application requires that the nurse be able to use that information in client-care decisions. Examples of this type of question may include questions about the interpretation of electrocardiographic (ECG) strips, interpretation of blood gas values, making a nursing diagnosis based on a set of symptoms, or deciding on a course of treatment. These types of questions provide a better indication of the nurse's ability to safely care for clients. An example of a Level 2 question is:

A client is becoming progressively short of breath. The results of his arterial blood gas (ABG) tests are: pH—7.13, PO_2—48, PCO_2—53, and HCO_3—26. These values indicate:

a Uncompensated metabolic acidosis with moderate hypoxia.
b Respiratory alkalosis with hyperoxia.
c Uncompensated respiratory acidosis with severe hypoxia.
d Compensated respiratory acidosis with normal oxygen.

The correct answer is **c**. Not only does the nurse have to *know* the normal values for each of the blood gas components given, he or she must also be able to use that information in determining the underlying condition.

3 Level 3, synthesis and evaluation, takes the process a step further. Approximately 85% of the questions are at either Level 2 or Level 3. Questions at the synthesis and evaluation level ask the nurse to make judgments about client care. One factor that adds to the difficulty of answering this type of question is that there is often more than one correct answer. The nurse is asked to choose the best answer from among several correct answers. Questions at this level often ask about the priority of care to be given, the priority of nursing diagnosis formulated, how to best evaluate the effectiveness of care that has been given, and the most appropriate nursing action to be taken. It is believed that the ability of the nurse to make decisions about nursing care at these higher levels is the best indication of the thought processes expected of a nurse demonstrating safe nursing care. An example of a Level 3 question is:

A client has become cyanotic and is having Cheyne-Stokes respirations. The best action for the nurse to take at this time is:

a Call a code blue and begin cardiopulmonary resuscitation.
b Call the physician and report the condition.
c Make sure the client's airway is open and begin supplemental oxygen.
d Give the ordered dose of 200 mg aminophylline intravenous piggyback (IVPB) now.

The best answer to this question is **c**. Choices **b** and **d** are also actions that should be carried out, but at this particular time opening the airway and oxygenating the client must receive highest priority. Not only does this question require that the nurse know some specific facts (definitions of "cyanotic" and "Cheyne-Stokes respirations"), but it also requires that a decision be made about the seriousness of the condition (analysis) and a selection of the type of care to be given from several correct options (judgment).

EXAMINATION FORMAT

Knowledge of the material covered by the NCLEX is evaluated by a multiple-choice test taken on a personal computer. The questions are all constructed similarly and usually include a client situation, a stem or stem question, and four answers or distractors. All the questions on the NCLEX stand alone, although a similar situation may be repeated. Occasionally a single question may be included without a case situation.

The graduate is asked to select the best answer from among the four possible choices. No partial credit is given for a "close" answer: there is only one correct answer for any particular question. The questions are totally integrated from the content areas already listed in the approximate percentages identified. Each question carries an equal weight or value toward the final score.

The graduate may take between 75 and 265 questions. There is a time limit of 5 hours for the entire examination, although there is no minimum time limit. The test is graded on a statistical model that compares the graduate's responses with a pre-established standard. If the graduate can demonstrate to the computer a knowledge level consistently above that standard, then the student will pass the examination.

Each question is assigned a difficulty value from 1 to 6. The first few questions are at the easier end of the scale of difficulty. As the graduate answers those questions correctly, the difficulty level is raised until the graduate begins to answer questions incorrectly. Then the computer lowers the difficulty level. The computer has a pool of about 20,000 questions from which to choose.

The NCLEX is given at Sylvan Learning Centers. After the graduates have completed the nursing program, they apply to the state board of nursing. Appointments at the examination sites are made on a first-come, first-served basis. The centers are required to schedule the examination within 30 days from the time the graduate applies. Each state establishes its own time interval for application after graduation, generally within 1 year. There are both morning and afternoon sessions of 5-hour duration. Depending on the size of the center, between eight and fifteen graduates may be accommodated at one time.

The computer skills required are minimal. After the graduate types in his or her name, address, and identification number, the only two keys that are used are the space bar and the enter key. All other keys are locked. The computer screen is split with the situation and stem question on the left side and the answers on the right (see example in Box 9–1). The space bar highlights a different answer each time it is pushed. When the graduate decides which answer is correct, he or she pushes the enter key. A message comes on the screen asking the graduate if that is the desired answer. If yes, the enter key is pushed again. The question is replaced with another question and answers. No question is ever repeated, nor is the graduate able to change the answer once it has been selected.

The NCLEX is graded on a pass/fail basis. If the student has failed the examination, the entire examination must be taken again. The National League for Nursing (NLN) recommends a 45-day waiting period for retaking the examination, although the majority of the states require 90 days. The results are sent to the graduate 7 to 10 days after the examination has been completed.

Box 9-1 EXAMPLE OF COMPUTER EXAMINATION	
A client is being prepared for discharge. He is to take theophylline by mouth at home for his lung disease. The nurse will know from her teaching that theophylline medications have been effective if the patient states:	**a** "I can stop taking this medication when I feel better." **b** "If I have difficulty swallowing the time-released capsules, I can crush them or chew them." **c** "If I have a lot of nausea and vomiting or become restless and can't sleep, I need to call my physician." **d** "I need to drink more coffee and cola while I am on these medications."

STUDY STRATEGIES

There are a number of ways to prepare for the NCLEX. To attempt to take the examination with an attitude of "if I don't know it by now, I never will" is to court failure. Carefully directed study and preparation will considerably increase the chances of passing the examination.

Review books. The material covered by review books is the key material found on the NCLEX. These books usually follow the NCLEX Test Plan very closely. A review book is, however, just that; it reviews the material that graduates should already know. Reviewing is important to reinforce learning and recall unused information.

Review books are not really designed to present any new information about key material. If a nurse is totally unfamiliar with the material in a particular section of the review book, then reading a more complete textbook on that particular subject area will be necessary.

Another important function that a review book serves is to point out areas of weakness. If the graduate finds sections that seem to contain "new" material, it is important to investigate that particular section in more detail. If graduates find most of the material familiar and easy to grasp, then they are probably prepared for the NCLEX examination.

Group study. Group study can be an effective method of preparation for an examination such as the NCLEX examination. To optimize the results of group-study sessions, there are several rules that should be followed.

Rule 1. Be very selective of the members of the study group. They should have a similar mind frame and orientation toward studying. They should be nurses who are also going to be taking the NCLEX. The ideal size for a study group is between four and six people. Groups larger than six become difficult to organize and handle. After the group has been formed and has begun its study sessions, it may be necessary to ask an individual to leave the group for not taking part, or if he or she is disruptive to the study process or is displaying negative attitudes about the examination.

Rule 2. Have each individual prepare a particular section for each group study session. Study groups generally meet once or twice a week. Have each individual assigned a particular section of the study topic. For example, if next week the group is going to study the endocrine system, assign group member #1 the anatomy and physiology of the system, #2 the pathologic conditions, #3 the medications used for treatment, and #4 the key elements of nursing care. When the group comes together, have each individual present his or her prepared section. This type of preparation prevents the "what are we going to study tonight?" syndrome that often plagues group-study sessions.

By following this process, the study group is organized and allows for more in-depth coverage of the topic. It also permits the members of the group to ask questions of the other members, thereby reinforcing the information being discussed.

Rule 3. Limit the length of the study session. No individual study session should be longer than between 90 and 120 minutes. Sessions that go for longer tend to get off the topic and foster a negative attitude about the examination. Try to avoid making group-study sessions into party time. A few snacks and refreshments may be helpful to maintain the energy level of the group, but a real party atmosphere will detract significantly from the effectiveness of the study session.

Individual study. No matter what other study and preparation methods are used, individual preparation for the NCLEX is a must. This preparation can take several forms.

As previously discussed, use of a review book is valuable to indicate areas of deficient knowledge. Reading and studying the appropriate textbooks and study guides can be helpful if it is approached correctly. It is important that the graduate mentally organize the information being read into a format similar to that found in the NCLEX. After reading each page of a textbook or study guide, the graduate should be able to ask three or four multiple-choice questions about that information. These questions can be asked silently or actually written out, and should answer the question "how might the NCLEX test my knowledge of this material?"

A second and extremely effective method of individual study is to practice answering questions similar to those found on the NCLEX itself. When practice questions are answered, several important mental processes occur. First, the graduate is becoming more familiar with and therefore more comfortable with the format of the examination. In research, this process is termed the **practice effect**; it must be accounted for when analyzing the results from "Pre-test/Post-test"–type research projects. Individuals will have better results after a test even without any type of intervention because of having practiced answering questions on the pre-test. Similarly, the score on the NCLEX may increase by as much as 10% through answering practice questions.

A second result of answering practice questions is that it reinforces the information already studied. Although it is unlikely that a question on the CCRN examination will be identical to a practice question, there are many similarities in the questions. Realistically, only a limited number of questions can be asked about any given subject. After a while, the questions will begin to sound very similar.

A third advantage of answering practice questions is that it reveals subject areas that will require more study. It is relatively easy to say, "I understand the renal system pretty well." It is quite another to answer correctly 10 or 15 questions about that system. If the questions are answered correctly, then the graduate can move on to the next topic. If the majority of the questions are missed however, then further review is required.

In order to obtain the optimal benefit from working practice questions, it is probably best to spend 30 to 45 minutes each day working 10 to 20 questions rather than trying to do 100 questions on 1 day during the week.

After the questions are answered, the student reviews them and compares them with the answers the study book provides. The student should also look at the rationales and the categories into which the questions fall.

Formal NCLEX reviews. The NLN does not endorse or sponsor any review courses for the NCLEX directly, but many companies offer reviews shortly after graduation. These review courses range from 2 to 5 days and basically cover the information found in review books. They are rather expensive, and the quality of NCLEX reviews varies. In general they are only as good as the people who are presenting the material.

TEST-TAKING STRATEGIES

The multiple-choice question test format is one of the most commonly used. Some individuals seem always to do well on multiple-choice question tests, whereas others seem to have problems with that test format. The individuals who always do well are not necessarily more intelligent; rather, they most likely have intuitively mastered some of the strategies or "tricks" necessary to do well on multiple-choice tests. Fortunately, once graduates become aware of these strategies and master them, they also will be able to score well on this type of examination format.

Knowing how to take a multiple-choice examination and optimizing the selection of the correct answers is a skill that can be mastered. When mastery of this skill is combined with knowledge of the key material, the probability of passing the NCLEX increases greatly. The following section lists and describes these important test-taking strategies.

1   Strategy 1: Read the client situation, stem question, and answers carefully. Many mistakes are made on this type of examination because the person taking the test did not read all parts of the question carefully. As you read the question and answers, try to understand what knowledge the question is ask-

ing for. As you did when reading the stem question, look for any key words, qualifiers, or statements that may help select the correct answer or eliminate the incorrect ones.

2   Strategy 2: Treat each question individually. Use only the information that is provided for that particular question in answering. Even though there may be client situations somewhere else in the examination that are similar to the one currently on the screen, avoid returning to these previous items for help. You should also be careful about reading into a question information that is not actually provided. There is a tendency to recall exceptions or unusual clients that the nurse may have encountered. By and large, questions on the NCLEX examination ask for "textbook" levels of knowledge of the material.

3   Strategy 3: Monitor the time. Although the examination is not strictly speaking timed, the graduate is never sure how many questions will need to be answered. If the graduate plans on taking all 265 questions in 5 hours, he or she will need approximately 70 seconds per question. Actually, most individuals who take this type of test average approximately 45 seconds per question, so it is likely that the student will be finished well before the time limit is reached. Take a watch along to the examination. If any question takes more than 2 minutes, put an answer down and move on. Theoretically, the graduate could sit in front of the computer screen for 5 hours with the same question.

4   Strategy 4: An educated guess is better than no answer at all. There is no penalty for guessing on the NCLEX. If the graduate is unable to make any decision at all about the correct answer, he or she should just select one and move on. There is at least a one-in-four chance to hit the correct answer. Statistically, answer **b** has about a 30% higher probability of being correct than any other. Wild guessing for large numbers of questions, of course, will have a negative effect on the total score.

5   Strategy 5: Use the process of elimination to select the correct answer. Usually there are one or more of the answers that can easily be identified as being incorrect. By eliminating these from the possible choices, the graduate will be better able to focus attention on the answers that have been identified as having some chance of being correct. Go back and read the stem question over again to try to determine exactly what type of information is being figured. If you are still unable to decide which of the remaining two answers are correct, select one and move on. Using this method increases the probability of choosing the correct answer to 1 in 2.

6   Strategy 6: Look for the answer that has the broader focus. Another method that may be used when the choices have been narrowed down to two is to examine the answers and try to determine if one answer may include the other. The answer that is broader, that is to say includes the other answer, is the correct one. An example of this type of question is:

A client has been diagnosed as having Wolf-Parkinson-White (WPW) syndrome, type A. In evaluating the ECG, the nurse would note which of the following characteristics for this condition.

a PR interval less than 0.12 second and wide QRS complex.

b PR interval greater than 0.20 second and normal QRS complex.

c Delta wave present in a positively deflected QRS complex in lead V_1 and PR interval less than 0.12 second.

d Delta wave present in a positively deflected QRS complex in lead V_6 and PR interval greater than 0.20 second.

The correct choice is **c**. Answer **a** may also be correct, but answer **c** includes the information in answer **a** and adds additional information. Again, reading all the answers carefully is essential before making a choice. Just reading answer **a** and selecting it without reading the rest of the answers would have led to an incorrect choice.

7 Strategy 7: Trust intuition. When a question and answers are read for the first time, an intuitive connection is made between the right and left lobes of the brain. The end result is that the first answer selected is usually the best choice. When a question is read too many times, the graduate may start to read into it elements that are really not there.

8 Strategy 8: Look for qualifying words in the question stem. There are some important words that can help determine what type of information is being elicited in the answer. Some of these words are:

FIRST

BEST

MOST

INITIAL

BETTER

HIGHEST PRIORITY

When words like these appear in the question stem, it is an indication that more than one of the choices are correct. The task then becomes to select the one answer that should be first or the answer that ought to receive the highest priority. An example of a "first" type of question is:

A 62-year-old client has a history of coronary heart disease. He is brought into the emergency room (ER) complaining of chest pain. The initial action taken by the nurse is to:

a Give the client nitroglycerine gr 1/150 sublingually now.

b Call the client's cardiologist about his admission.

c Place the client in an elevated Fowler's position after loosening his shirt collar.

d Check his blood pressure and note the location and degree of chest pain.

The correct choice is **d**. It is important to remember that when asked for an "initial" or "first" action to think of the nursing process. The first step in the nursing process is always assessment. If there was not an assessment-oriented choice, then look for a planning choice, and so forth. The other three answers provided for this question are also correct and should be done at some point, but in this particular situation, the first need is to assess his chest pain to determine if it is indeed cardiac. Many other conditions can also cause chest pain.

9   Strategy 9: Look for negatives in the question stem. Although there are very few negative questions on the NCLEX, negative words or prefixes in the question stem change how the correct answer is selected. Some common negatives include:

NOT
LEAST
UNLIKELY
INAPPROPRIATE
UNREALISTIC
LOWEST PRIORITY
CONTRAINDICATED
FALSE
EXCEPT
INCONSISTENT
UNTOWARD
ALL BUT
ATYPICAL
INCORRECT

In general, when a negative question is asked, it indicates that three of the choices are correct and one is incorrect. The incorrect choice is the answer. When a negative question appears, the test taker needs to ask: "What is it they don't want me to do in this situation?" An example of this type of question is: A client is admitted to the medical unit. He is still having some mild chest pain. Which of the following medications would be inappropriate for relief of chest pain?

a   Diltiazem (Cardizem)
b   Propranolol (Inderal)
c   Digoxin (Lanoxin)
d   Meperidine (Demerol)

The correct answer is **c.** Digoxin is a positive inotropic medication, which increases contractility and the oxygen demands of the heart. It is likely it would actually increase chest pain in this client. The other three medications all relieve chest pain by somewhat different mechanisms. But notice that if the question was not read carefully and the reader missed the *in-* prefix of *in*appropriate, then certainly **c** would not have been selected.

10   Strategy 10: Avoid selecting answers that have absolutes in them. Answers that have absolutes in them are almost always incorrect choices. Some absolute words to be aware of include:

ALWAYS
EVERY
ONLY
ALL

NEVER

NONE

Health care providers deal with very complex biochemical entities called human beings. Every person is different and almost every rule will have an exception. An example of this type of question is:

Which of the following is an accurate statement concerning cardiac chest pain in clients?

a This pain is always caused by constriction or blockage of the coronary arteries by fat plaques or blood clots.

b True cardiac pain is never relieved without treatment.

c This type of pain is only relieved by nitroglycerine.

d Clients often attribute the pain to indigestion.

The correct answer is **d.** The answers to this question very obviously demonstrate the "avoid the absolute" strategy. Coronary-type chest pain can also be caused by spasms of the coronary arteries as in variant angina **(a)**. Chest pain sometimes *can* go away by itself, although it will probably return later **(b)**. A number of medications will relieve chest pain besides NTG (e.g., morphine and narcotics, calcium-channel blockers, and beta blockers) **(c)**.

11 Strategy 11: The answer that seems different is usually incorrect. The NCLEX is difficult because the material itself is difficult, but the examination is not designed to be "tricky" or difficult for the sake of confusing the test taker. On the other hand, the test question writers are not going to make the correct answer completely obvious. Therefore, if one answer is much longer or shorter than the other three, it is probably not the correct choice. Be wary of answers that sound like they are trying to rationalize the correct choice by using a lot of explanation. Such answers are probably incorrect. You should also avoid answers that are different from the other three because of measurements or the way in which they are presented. An example of this type of question is:

A client has developed congestive heart failure. Which of the following would be the correct loading dose of digoxin (Lanoxin) for an adult client?

a 0.75 mg divided into three doses every 8 hours.

b 0.75 gm divided into four doses every 8 hours.

c 10 mg because the client is from a Native-American background and is a very large man, thus causing slow absorption of the medication.

d 0.25 mg.

The correct answer for this question is **a.** The loading dose for digoxin is usually three times the maintenance dose (0.25 mg) divided over 24 hours. Choice **b** is in a different measurement form (grams instead of milligrams); choice **c** should be avoided because it exemplifies the longer-than-average answer syndrome; and choice **d** is much shorter than any of the others. Look for one of the average-length answers to be the correct choice.

12 Strategy 12: Avoid selecting answers that refer the client to the physician. The NCLEX is for nurses and deals with conditions and problems that nurses should be able to resolve independently. The answer that refers a client to the physician is usually incorrect and can be eliminated from the choice selection.

13 Strategy 13: Avoid looking for a pattern in the selection of answers. The questions and answers on the NCLEX are arranged in a random fashion without any particular pattern. If something appears to be in a pattern, ignore it. Any pattern is just coincidental. For example, if question 6 had choice **a**, question 7 had choice **b**, question 8 had choice **c**, question 9 had choice **d**, question 10 had choice **a**, and question 11 had choice **b**, you might expect that question 12 would require choice **c**. This is probably not the case. Here is another example of a pattern-type situation that sometimes occurs with answers on this type of test. Questions 22 to 29 all have choice **c** as their correct answers. The answer to question 30 also seems to be choice **c**, but the tendency may be to not select it because of all the other choice **c** answers on the previous questions. The correct answer may very well be choice **c**, and if that is the best choice, go ahead and select it. It is important that each question be treated individually.

14 Strategy 14: **DO NOT PANIC** if a totally unfamiliar question is encountered. Examinations such as the NCLEX are designed so that it is very difficult, if not impossible, for anyone to answer all of the questions correctly. As a result, there are questions that are very complex, which deal with disease processes, medications, and laboratory tests that may be unfamiliar to the graduate. Questions like this may be encountered no matter how much review or study has been done.

Nobody knows everything! The important element to remember when encountering these types of questions is to avoid panic. It is just one question out of many. Use some of the strategies already discussed in this chapter to select the best answer. Remember that nursing care given is very similar in many situations even though the disease processes themselves may be quite different. Select the answer that seems logical and involves general nursing care. Common sense can go a long way on this type of examination. An example of this type of question is:

A 33-year-old African-American male client has been diagnosed as having a pheochromocytoma. Appropriate initial nursing care would involve:

a Administering large doses of xylometazoline to help control the symptoms of the disease.

b Monitoring his vital signs closely, particularly his blood pressure.

c Preparing the client and family for the client's imminent death.

d Having the family discuss the condition with the physician before informing the client about the disease, because of the protracted recovery period after treatment.

The correct answer is **b.** A pheochromocytoma is a tumor of the adrenal medulla that increases secretion of epinephrine and norepinephrine. One important result of having this type of tumor is that a hypertensive crisis may occur in some individuals. Monitoring the blood pressure would be an important nursing care measure. Assessment is also the first step of the nursing process and fits well with the qualifying word, *initial*, as used in the question stem.

15 Strategy 15: When answers are grouped by similar concepts, activities, or situations, select the one that is different. If three of the four choices have some common element that makes them similar, and the fourth answer lacks this element, the different answer is probably correct. An example of this type of question is:

A female client has been treated for severe chronic emphysema for several years using bronchodilators and relatively high doses of prednisone (Deltasone). Which of the following activities would pose the least risk for this client in relation to the side effects of prednisone therapy?

a Shopping at the mall on Saturday afternoon.
b Spring-cleaning her two-story house.
c Attending Sunday morning church services.
d Serving refreshments at her 6-year-old son's school play party.

The correct answer is **b.** In choices **a, c,** and **d,** there is the common element of groups of strangers. Because of suppression of the immune system, clients need to be protected from exposure to potential infections when they are taking steroid medications. Spring-cleaning her house, although strenuous, poses the least exposure to infection.

16 Strategy 16: Be positive about the examination! It is a generally accepted fact that people who have a positive attitude about an examination will score higher on the examination than people who are negative about it.

SUMMARY

Taking and passing the NCLEX-RN, CAT is a necessary step in the process of becoming a professional registered nurse. Like all licensure examinations, its purpose is to protect the public from undereducated or unsafe practitioners. The examination is comprehensive and includes material from all areas of the graduate's nursing education. Although most graduates have some anxiety about taking this examination, knowledge about its format and content and strategies for taking the examination can lower the anxiety levels to an acceptable level.

In addition, many of these test-taking strategies can be applied to the student's course examinations during the nursing program. Although nothing is as effective for passing an examination as paying attention in class, good note taking, and thorough study, awareness of these important test-taking strategies may improve the student's overall score.

A Closer Look

A NEW GRAD'S PERSPECTIVE

I remember sitting in my first nursing class, listening to the Director of Nursing describe to what we were committing for the next two years of our life. She stood so confident, almost intimidating, as she described an overview of what we were expected to learn as nursing students. I experienced absolutely horrifying fear. As a result, one question kept coming to mind. "What am I going to do"? I considered running to the advisor's office and changing my major to Spanish, but I remembered why I wanted to be a nurse.

One evening I had to take my roommate to the emergency room. While I thumbed through a magazine in the waiting room, a man with a gaping wound in his forehead sat down next to me. Over it he held a small gauze pad, which a nurse had given him. I became curious—couldn't that nurse have done something more for him? What other options were available? What would I have done in this situation? Sure that there was more to nursing than this, I enrolled myself in the Tulsa University nursing program.

Looking at the four demanding years of nursing school I have just completed. I have a better understanding of our director's confidence. After only three semesters of lectures and clinical practice, I felt very overwhelmed with the knowledge I was "supposed" to have. As a hands-on learner, I couldn't quite grasp the concepts our instructors tried to convey. I focused on practicing skills and learning techniques in clinical. I became a technician instead of a nurse until the day I had no choice but to become a nurse.

On that day, the reporting nurse stated that my patient had suffered a CVA with right-sided weakness but was able to communicate her needs. She was to have an assessment done as well as an enema performed. I mentally planned how I would efficiently perform my skills in four hours, and set out for her room. Aphasia! Why hadn't I considered this in my plan? She motioned for me to come closer and began pointing to the phone. "Beer, beer, beer, beer," she said, as she pointed to the phone, the window, and then the phone again. I asked her if someone was going to call her, and she shook her head "no." She began pointing again, and as we both started to get frustrated, I told her I would return shortly.

I went to my instructor with tears in my eyes. "I can't understand!" I cried. She patted me on the shoulder and encouraged me to try. I returned, and after an hour of pointing and guessing, we succeeded. My patient wanted to call her daughter and wish her a happy birthday! I was excited that I finally understood what she was communicating, and she seemed

Continued on following page

A NEW GRAD'S PERSPECTIVE (Continued)

grateful that I had tried. I confidently left clinical that day with a new understanding of what it meant to be a nurse.

As a new graduate, I realize that spending one hour communicating with a patient is an unrealistic goal for a nurse with ten to twelve patients to care for within eight hours. I have learned that balance is a key to safe, efficient, holistic nursing care. With the possibility of health care reform approaching rapidly, flexibility in nursing will be vital. I am excited to learn all I can about future changes and growth in the nursing field to expand my current knowledge. Utilizing this knowledge base and my experiences as a student, I plan to continue delivering holistic care with confidence.

From Deming, Stacia: A new grad's perspective. The Oklahoma Nurse, April–June 1995, page 16. Reprinted with permission.

CRITICAL THINKING EXERCISES

1 Obtain an NCLEX-RN, CAT review book. Analyze the questions in the practice examination for type, cognitive level, and level of difficulty.
2 Identify three to five other students in your class with whom you would feel comfortable working in a study group. Organize a study-group session before the next major course examination.
3 When you get the results of your next course examination, identify why you missed the questions you did and what strategies might have been employed to answer those questions correctly.

HISTORICAL PERSPECTIVES

Early Nursing Leaders: Isabel Adams Hampton Robb (1860–1910)

As a teacher in her home city in Ontario, Canada, Hampton felt unfulfilled, and in 1881, her restlessness and ambition led her to the Bellevue Hospital Training School in New York City to become a nurse. Her orientation centered on the academic rather than the clinical side of nursing. Shortly after graduation, she moved to Rome, in Italy, where she became the superintendent of a hospital that provided care for American and British travelers. During her one-and-a-half years as superintendent, her conviction that nurses needed a solid theoretical education as the foundation for their nursing practice grew.

From that point, Hampton dedicated her life to raising the standards of nursing education in the United States. She accepted the directorship of the Illinois Training School for Nurses and soon made major changes in its curriculum. This was a unique school for its time. Unlike most nursing schools that were hospital-based, this school was university-based and had academic learning as its primary focus. The curriculum was changed so that simpler concepts were presented first, and the more complex ideas were presented later in the program. She also arranged for students to gain clinical experiences in various hospitals so that the students could practice those skills learned in the classroom.

Word of Hampton's revolutionary ideas about nursing education quickly spread throughout the country and she was offered a succession of prestigious and important positions. In 1893, she accepted the directorship of the newly founded Johns Hopkins Training School for Nurses. She instituted her ideas about the need for theoretical nursing education and also proposed the novel idea of limiting the student-nurses' working days to 12 hours, which included 2 hours for recreational activities. She also eliminated the unpaid private-duty services that were provided by nursing students.

Her next position was the chairmanship of the nursing section of the Congress of Hospitals and Dispensaries in 1896, consisting of a group of nursing leaders who were attempting to form some type of national organization for nurses. Under Hampton's leadership, a group of superintendents of the key American nursing schools was brought together as the American Society of Superintendents of Training Schools for Nurses. Hampton was elected chairman of the group. In this organization are found the seeds of what was eventually to become the National League for Nursing, which was dedicated to improving the standards of nursing education.

Many of her contemporaries felt that her marriage to Dr. Hunter Robb in 1894 would be the end of her nursing career. Nursing at that time was not considered a suitable occupation for married women, particularly those with a relatively privileged social background. But Hampton Robb did not let these ideas interfere with her active pursuit of her goals for the future of nursing.

Shortly after her marriage, she organized a separate group for staff nurses in active practice. She became the first president of the group in 1896 and called it the Nurses Associated Alumnae of the United States and Canada. This group would later become the American Nurses Association (ANA), which is dedicated to the improvement of clinical practice. A few years later, she helped develop the American Journal of Nursing, the first periodical dedicated to the improvement of nursing. This became, and remains, the official journal of the ANA.

Unfortunately, her dedication and work to improve nursing were cut short by a fatal accident at age 50. Her contributions to nursing education, however, had an influence that lasts to this day. Her belief that nurses need both theoretical and practical education and her insistence on the separation of nursing education from medical education were not well accepted by the medical community of her times. Through her efforts, nursing made major strides in its attempt to emerge as an important, and separate, health care profession.

Early Nursing Leaders: Lillian Wald (1867–1940)

Born into middle class Ohio society, Wald was well educated and lived the early part of her life in relative comfort. She attended the New York Hospital School of Nursing between 1889 and 1901. After graduation, she worked for a short time as a hospital nurse. She became interested in medicine and entered medical school, but left after an experience on the New York docks that opened her eyes to the plight of sick poor people.

While Wald was teaching a series of classes in home nursing and bed making to a group of poor women on the Lower East Side, a dirty and frail little girl told Wald about her sick mother, who had just had a baby. Wald went with the girl through the filth, stench, and garbage of the slums to a filthy, crowded, dark, and damp apartment, where the girl's mother lay in a pool of blood and excrement. Wald came to understand that conditions such as these existed because of a lack of knowledge. She saw that nursing was the best way to teach people and improve living conditions.

Wald, with the help of Mary Brewester, opened the famous Henry Street Settlement, a storefront clinic on the Lower East Side in one of the poorest sections of New York City. It provided both clinic and home nursing care for the poor. Through this clinic, nurses were sent into the homes of the poor to visit the sick and to offer instructions in how to improve living conditions to stop the spread of disease. These early community nurses paid special attention to children and aimed many of their teaching and preventive efforts at helping children remain healthy.

From her experiences with the urban poor and her attempts to get funding for her clinic, Wald developed into a dedicated social reformer and an effective fund raiser. She became politically active and was recognized as an eloquent speaker, particularly when supporting candidates for public office who agreed with her health care reforms. Although women still did not have the right to vote, her political influence was felt nationwide.

Under her auspices New York's Columbia University developed courses to prepare nurses for careers in public health. From her community-health experiences, Wald also became a strong advocate of wellness education. Although the medical community did not seem to be interested in the wellness aspect of health care, she saw it as becoming one of the important functions of nurses and nursing. The Metropolitan Life Insurance Company saw the value of her belief in health maintenance and she was asked to organize the nursing service branch of that company. She is also credited with beginning the Town and Country Nursing Service of the American Red Cross, as well as developing the concept and practice of school nursing. In 1912, Wald founded, and was elected the first president of, the National Organization of Public Health Nursing.

As a pioneer in public-health nursing, Wald demonstrated how much influence one dedicated person could have on the health of a whole population. Over time, many of her farsighted ideas were adopted by the federal government. Many of the child-health and wellness programs in use today have their origins in her efforts. Many of the current proposals for health care revisions, particularly those that work under a capitation system (i.e., HMOs, public-health nursing, independent clinics, and health maintenance) derive their success from important elements in Wald's work.

10

HEALTH CARE
DELIVERY SYSTEM

LEARNING OBJECTIVES

After completing this chapter, the reader will be able to:

1 Analyze the evolution of the health care delivery system in the United States.
2 Discuss the current and future roles of nurses within the health care delivery system.
3 Evaluate the factors that are influencing the evolution of the health care delivery system.
4 Describe how health care is paid for.
5 Synthesize the concerns surrounding the uninsured in this country.
6 Analyze industry efforts to manage health care costs.
7 Compare and contrast HMOs, IPAs, and PPOs.
8 Discuss the benefits of group practice arrangements.
9 Evaluate the efforts being made to ensure quality cost-effective health care.
10 Compare and contrast profit and nonprofit health care agencies.
11 Describe governmental and nongovernmental health care agencies and the services they provide.
12 Analyze the challenges of delivering health care in rural settings and the mechanisms proposed for meeting these demands.

GENERAL SYSTEMS THEORY

General systems theory, as discussed in Chapter 2, is an excellent tool for analyzing health care delivery systems. The American health care system is affected by many sources of input—clients, health care providers, third-party reimbursers, and technologic advances, to name just a few. Output is readily identifiable and consists of longer life spans, increased incidence of long-term health problems, elimination of some chronic conditions, and acute problems that can be easily managed. Finally, feedback is composed of expectations that care will be accessible, of high quality, and affordable.

HISTORY

The health care system in the United States has been evolving since before the Declaration of Independence was signed. Health care was originally provided in the home. Remedies were passed down from generation to generation and combined with superstitious and spiritual rituals. As formal education for physicians became available, a need for centralized locations for clinical practice presented itself. In many cases, physicians constituted the vital force behind the construction of hospitals. With the development of schools of nursing modeled on Nightingale's ideas, the problem of staffing these facilities was solved.

Early on, knowledge of effective therapies was minimal. For this reason, hospitals were initially considered places where people only went to die. As technology evolved and the growing pharmaceutical industry began to offer lifesaving antibiotics and other drugs, however, hospitals started to be thought of as acute care facilities where people came to be treated, cared for, and helped to recover. Gradually, acute care of the sick (**secondary intervention**) was moved from the home setting to the hospital setting.

Another layer of care was formed when technology provided the resources necessary to perform unprecedented procedures, such as open-heart surgery and organ transplants. To meet the demand for these types of services (**tertiary intervention**), hospitals offering complicated services over large catchment areas were developed. Unfortunately, as tertiary and acute care facilities became more popular, less attention was devoted to health promotion, illness prevention, early diagnosis, and treatment of common health problems (**primary intervention**).

To a great degree, delivery of health care became centralized within hospitals where professionals were thought to hold the key to well-being through technology. Individual responsibility was minimized, and concerns about cost were diminished because third-party reimbursers were responsible for paying a large proportion of the bills. Health care was essentially removed from the hands of consumers, as clients became pawns in an expansive, expensive, and high-tech system.

Consumers, health care providers, and third-party reimbursers remained relatively satisfied with this system until it became obvious that health care costs

TABLE 10–1. **Health Care Delivery System Changes**	
From	**To**
Hospital-based care	Community-based care
Acute care	Illness prevention, health promotion, long-term and rehabilitative care
Incidental fragmented care	Comprehensive, continuous, coordinated care
Patients as passive participants	Patients assuming responsibility for self-care
Expensive high-tech care	Cost-effective care provided at an appropriate level
Health care delivery system monopoly	Competitive health care marketplace

were out of control and that millions of Americans had little or no access to care. It also became evident that failure to focus on promoting health and preventing illness was resulting in countless instances of unnecessary suffering and death. To solve these problems, the health care industry is gradually moving toward a decentralized system in which more and more care is being provided on an outpatient basis; emphasis is being placed on health promotion, illness prevention, and responsible self-care practices; and health care providers are implementing cost-containment measures (Table 10–1).

During this period of rapid change, provider roles and reimbursement practices may be greatly altered. For this reason, it is important for nurses to understand the health care delivery system (see Table 10–2 for a glossary of terms). Nurses need to ensure that their services are fully used and that their ability to function independently and autonomously is promoted. In addition, third-party reimbursers must be cognizant of the nurse's role and the importance of sound reimbursement practices.

MEMBERS OF THE HEALTH CARE DELIVERY TEAM

Within the health care delivery system, countless numbers of diagnosticians, technicians, direct care providers, and support staff are employed. It is estimated that there are more than 300 job titles used to describe health care workers (Birchenall, 1989). Among these are nurses, doctors, dentists, clinical psychologists, social workers, radiologists, physical therapists, music therapists, dietitians, pharmacists, housekeepers, biomedical engineers, secretaries, and others. All of these individuals provide services that are essential to the day-to-day operation of the health care delivery system in this country.

Of particular importance, among this array of health care workers, are a variety of types of nurses—registered nurses, licensed practical (vocational) nurses,

TABLE 10–2. Glossary of Health Care Delivery System Terms

Term	Definition
case management	Method of delivering care in which providers serve as client advocates in the provision and coordination of quality, cost-effective care.
Civilian Health and Medical Program of the Uniformed Services (CHAMPUS)	Federal program providing health care coverage to individuals associated with the military.
copayment	Percentage of the cost of a medical expense that is not covered by insurance and must be paid by the client.
customary, prevailing, and reasonable charges	The typical rate in a specific locale that Medicare traditionally reimburses physicians.
diagnosis-related groups (DRGs)	System of classifying inpatient stays for purposes of determining payment.
Employee Retirement Income Security Act (ERISA)	Federal law that grants incentives to employers to offer self-funded health insurance plans to their employees.
fee for service	Fee charged for each service rendered rather than paying a premium for all services provided over a designated period.
for-profit (proprietary) agencies	Health care agencies in which profits can be used to raise capital.
group practice	Three or more physicians in business together to provide health care.
health insurance purchasing cooperative (HIPC)	A proposed system in which groups of people or employers band together to buy health insurance at reduced rates.
health maintenance organization (HMO)	Organization that strives to provide cost-effective quality care to enrollees for a fixed fee.
horizontal integration	Cost-cutting strategy in which health care agencies share resources and collective buying power.
independent practice association (IPA)	Type of HMO usually organized by physicians that requires fee-for-service payment.
Joint Commission on Accreditation of Health-care Organizations (JCAHO)	Organization that performs accreditation reviews for health care agencies.
managed care	Business ventures that attempt to provide cost-effective quality health care services.
not-for-profit (nonprofit) agencies	Health care agencies in which all profits must be used in the operation of the organization.
out-of-pocket expenses	Amount the client is responsible for paying.
peer-review organization (PRO)	Organization that reviews the quality and cost of Medicare services.

TABLE 10–2. **Glossary of Health Care Delivery System Terms** *(Continued)*	
Term	**Definition**
preferred provider organizations (PPO)	Network of health care providers that offer services at negotiated or reduced rates.
premium	Amount paid on a periodic basis for health insurance or HMO membership.
primary intervention	Health promotion, illness prevention, early diagnosis, and treatment of common health problems.
prospective payment system (PPS)	Reimbursement system that pays for services based on a predetermined fixed rate.
secondary intervention	Acute care designed to prevent complications or resolve health problems. Until recently, these services were primarily provided in hospitals.
sliding-scale fee	Fee that is calculated based on a client's income.
tertiary intervention	Services involving complex and/or specialized care. May also refer to long-term and/or rehabilitative intervention.
total quality management (TQM)	Method of promoting cost-effective high-quality health care that encourages ongoing assessment and proactive strategies. Also known as continuous quality improvement (CQI).
universal health care coverage	Health care reimbursement benefits for all U.S. citizens.
Utilization guidelines	Guidelines that stipulate the amount of services that can be delivered by a health care provider.
vertical integration	Competitive strategy in which health care agencies attempt to offer a full array of services.

nurse practitioners, anesthetists, midwives, clinical specialists, and nursing assistants. Each of these titles requires a different type of educational background and clinical expertise. In general, all nurses make valuable contributions within the health care delivery system. Recently, however, there has been an increased demand for individuals who are prepared to deliver care in the community and in long-term health care settings rather than in the hospital. In response to this demand, some nurses are moving or have already moved to long-term care facilities and health care settings in the community. Professional nursing education programs are attempting to meet this need by preparing individuals who can practice independently and autonomously and also by offering more clinical experiences in rehabilitation, nursing home, and community settings. Many advanced practice nurses who graduate with master's level (or higher) degrees already meet this demand.

FACTORS INFLUENCING THE HEALTH CARE DELIVERY SYSTEM

Demographics

The settings in which nurses practice suggest something about recent demographic changes in the United States. One of the most important demographic trends is the graying of Americans. By the year 2000, it is estimated that the median age of U.S. citizens will be over 36 years. This compares with 29 years in 1975. In the year 2000, it is also projected that 13% of the population will be over 65, compared with 8% of U.S. citizens who were over that age in 1950. One of the most significant changes will be the number of Americans who have celebrated their 85th birthdays. By the year 2000, the number of Americans over 85 will have increased by around 30%, to about 4.6 million (U.S. Department of Health and Human Services, 1991).

Health Care Problems

Another factor that is influencing the climate of health care delivery in the United States is the mix of health problems that must be dealt with today. Although significant strides have been made in the treatment of acute infectious diseases, significant challenges still exist in the management of health concerns such as cancer, heart disease, diabetes, and infection with HIV. Additional concerns include environmental and occupational safety, drug abuse, and mother and child health care.

Health Care Priorities

In light of the health care problems being faced, the U. S. Department of Health and Human Services in 1991 outlined proactive strategies for the year 2000 in the areas of health promotion, protection, and prevention. Health-promotion priorities involve physical fitness, adequate nutrition, reduced use of tobacco and other harmful substances, family planning, preservation of mental health, avoidance of violence and abusive behavior, and community support services. Health-protection areas that are being emphasized include reduced numbers of accidents, occupational safety and health, improved oral health, improved environmental quality, and food and drug safety. In addition, mother and child health, heart disease, stroke, cancer, sexually transmitted diseases, infection with HIV, and other infectious diseases are targeted for new preventive strategies. Finally, emphasis is being placed on access to health care services and the importance of individual, family, employer, community, and government responsibility in improving the profile of the nation's health.

Rising Costs

Rising costs are also affecting health care delivery in this country. Health care costs have been increasing at an alarming rate for many years. According to

U. S. government data, American health care spending rose from 9% of the gross national product in 1980 to 14% in 1992 (Congressional Budget Office, 1993). This figure is expected to reach 15% by the year 2000 (Brockopp, 1992). Although hospital admissions significantly declined in the 1980s, the total spent on hospital services rose from $42.2 billion in 1961 (in 1991 dollars) to $288.6 billion in 1991. This represents a sevenfold increase (Congressional Budget Office, 1993).

Many factors account for this trend. Among them is the way in which third-party payers have customarily reimbursed health care services with little attention paid to cost-control measures. Other factors include the great cost of innovative technology, an increase in the need for long-term care, providers who have not always delivered care in a cost-conscious manner, and the limited ability and motivation of consumers to compare health care prices.

WHO PAYS FOR HEALTH CARE?

Who pays for health care is not a simple question to answer. The citizens of the United States have traditionally valued independence, individualism, competition, and entrepreneurship. They have also felt compelled to act based on humanitarian concerns and a commitment to reduce suffering. These values have led to the development of one of the most fiscally complex health care systems in the world. Paying for health care involves all levels of government, private enterprise, and innovative commercial financing structures.

It is important for nurses to be familiar with health care reimbursement practices for several reasons. First, judgments about whether or not to perform diagnostic tests or to use certain treatment strategies sometimes are based on third-party-payer guidelines. Second, decisions relating to how long a client is allowed to stay in a care facility frequently derive from restrictions on reimbursement. Third, plans of care based purely on financial incentives may raise legal and ethical questions of which the nurse must be aware. Fourth, the type of care individuals seek out depends largely on the health care benefits they have. For example, it is common for people who lack adequate coverage to seek care in an emergency department rather than using more economical primary care agencies such as community health centers or doctors' offices. Finally, as client advocates, nurses must understand reimbursement practices in order to offer clients appropriate advice and to make necessary referrals (see Table 10–2).

Private Health Care Insurance

Private insurance companies were the first third-party payers to reimburse for health care. Plans provided by these companies gained popularity after World War II when unions began to promote benefit packages in lieu of wage increases. Today, there are approximately 1500 private commercial insurance companies that offer health care policies; however, only 12 of them control about 60% of the business (Hawkins, 1993).

Private companies that offer health insurance function largely through group employee plans. The client is usually responsible for a small **copayment,** (i.e., the charge the insurer expects the client to pay) and the insurer reimburses either consumer or provider directly. Traditionally, companies have avoided introducing cost controls except in cases where there appears to have been excessive use or abuse of services. An attractive aspect of most private health insurance is that the consumer can choose any health care facility or physician and still receive the same insurance benefit.

Self-insurance Arrangements

In an attempt to reduce costs, approximately 75% of the larger employers in this country are choosing to become self-insured (Schultz, 1994). This means that businesses are taking on the financial risk of offering their own health care plans.

Employers perceive that there are several advantages to self-funded plans. First, under the **Employee Retirement Income Security Act (ERISA)** of 1974, outside regulators who supervise private insurance plans are eliminated. Second, employer self-funded plans are shielded from state regulations and produce some tax advantages. As a result of these exclusions, the cost of insuring employees is reduced.

In spite of the advantages of self-insured plans, authorities have expressed concern about the lack of consumer protection. For instance, employers have been criticized for rejecting potential employees based on existing health concerns or those with a family history of health problems. Employers have also been known to reject potential employees because they ride motorcycles or smoke. Although this practice of eliminating bad risks is common among private insurers, the question remains whether the nation's workforce should be determined by these criteria.

Blue Cross and Blue Shield

Blue Cross and Blue Shield plans evolved during the Great Depression. Financial hardships among the rich resulted in fewer philanthropic donations, and nonprofit hospitals were forced to seek out new sources of revenue. The Blue Cross plan was sponsored by hospitals, and subscribers received hospital services in exchange for their **premiums.** Physicians became involved when they saw an opportunity to guarantee payment for their services and to deter the national health-insurance movement. As a result, Blue Shield coverage became readily available (Hawkins, 1993).

From the beginning of the Blue Cross and Blue Shield programs, the physicians' role in managing these plans raised questions. Traditionally, Blue Cross was controlled by hospital boards, which were largely composed of physicians.

Likewise, physicians made up a large percentage of the Blue Shield governing bodies. Moreover, physicians on Blue Cross and Blue Shield boards frequently also administered federal Medicare and state Medicaid programs. In short, those receiving payments had significant control over establishing prices. In recent years, sensitivity to this conflict of interest has led to an increased number of community representatives on Blue Cross and Blue Shield Boards and in more private insurance companies administering these programs (Hawkins, 1993).

Another criticism of Blue Cross and Blue Shield plans is that they have traditionally been oriented toward treating illness with little emphasis placed on health promotion or illness prevention. Because of their size, Blue Cross and Blue Shield have had a significant impact on health care legislation, but unfortunately, they have not led the way toward a primary health care focus (Hawkins, 1993).

Medicare and Medicaid

Medicare

The creation of Blue Cross and Blue Shield in the 1930s only temporarily slowed the movement toward government involvement in health care financing. By the middle 1960s, it became clear that changes needed to be made to ensure adequate health care for the elderly and indigent. In 1965, legislation was passed that resulted in the establishment of the Medicare and Medicaid programs (Hawkins, 1993).

Medicare is a federally run program that is financed primarily through employee payroll taxes; it covers any individual who is 65 years of age or older as well as blind or disabled individuals of any age. Part A of Medicare is free in most instances and covers acute hospital, nursing home, and home-care services. Part B may be purchased for a monthly premium and 97% of the individuals participating in Part A are enrolled in the program (Lockhart, 1992). Participants are covered for physician services, outpatient hospital care, laboratory tests, durable medical equipment, and certain other selected services. Although Medicare was designed for older Americans, long-term care is not covered and health promotion and illness prevention benefits are limited.

Medicare was originally designed so that, with few exceptions, services were fully covered. This arrangement did not provide cost-containment incentives, nor was the cost-benefit ratio of services taken into consideration. For example, heroic and costly measures were used to extend life with little consideration given to the quality of that existence. A financial crisis peaked in the middle 1980s, and cost-control measures were implemented.

In 1983, a **prospective payment system (PPS)** was implemented in which hospitals are reimbursed based on a fixed rate and incentives are in place to reduce the length of hospital stays. At the core of this scheme is a classification system made up of 475 **diagnosis-related groups (DRGs).** Based on the particular diagnosis-related group in which a client is placed, hospitals are reimbursed for a standard, predetermined amount. In the event that a client is discharged early or costs are kept under the allotted amount, the hospital keeps the difference. In contrast, if a client's bill exceeds the maximum reimbursable amount, the hospital absorbs the cost.

From the outset, developers of the DRG classification system feared that quality of care might be compromised in favor of cost containment. To prevent misuse of the DRG prospective payment system, the **Medicare Utilization and Quality Peer Review Organization (PRO)** was instituted. The purpose of this group is to ensure quality care and prevent misuse of the system.

A common criticism of the DRG prospective payment system is that cost shifting has occurred. For example, to make up for lost revenues, clients with other forms of insurance have been charged inflated amounts for their services. Reports of paying $7 or more for an aspirin tablet are not uncommon (Wasley, 1992).

Under the DRG prospective payment system, physician reimbursement remained untouched. Physicians continued to be reimbursed based on **customary, prevailing, and reasonable charges.** In other words, what was normally charged by physicians in a given geographic area is what they received for their services. If a physician charged more than the customary, prevailing, and reasonable rate for a service, he or she could bill the client for the remaining amount that Medicare did not pay. Little attempt was made to control physician costs, and as a result, between 1961 and 1991 the price of their services increased more than sixfold (Congressional Budget Office, 1993).

In an attempt to contain physician costs, Congress passed legislation in 1989 to establish: (1) a standardized physician reimbursement schedule, (2) limits on **out-of-pocket** expenses for clients, (3) ceilings on the volume of services provided by physicians annually, and (4) federal practice guidelines to identify the most effective and efficient means of managing client care (Lockhart, 1992).

To date, it remains unclear how or if these cost-containment measures will influence reimbursement for nursing services. Nursing care has traditionally been grouped with the cost of other health care services, and third-party payers have resisted direct reimbursement of nurses because they have feared cost escalation. Physicians have also been reluctant to support direct compensation for nurses because they have worried about losing their broad control over the health care delivery system. With a standardized fee schedule in place, however, similar reimbursement costs can be justified for all health care professionals and barriers to direct third-party reimbursement for nurses may be diminished.

Medicaid

Medicaid is a state-administered entitlement program that is designed to serve the poor. Funds are generated at the federal, state, and local level; each state has the freedom to customize its program based on the needs of its residents. The financial status of each state is different; thus Medicaid eligibility and services vary from place to place. States with more money tend to offer better benefit packages or to cover more people than states that have limited resources. Services that are typically covered include hospitalization, diagnostic tests, physician visits, and rehabilitative, nursing home, and outpatient care. States can opt to offer services such as home care for which they receive federal matching funds. Although Medicare was originally designed to serve the needs of the elderly, it is Medicaid that often covers long-term nursing home care after personal funds have been exhausted.

Uninsured

Despite what may appear to be a plethora of reimbursement options, there are an estimated 37 million U.S. citizens at any given time who do not have health care insurance and 25 million more with inadequate coverage (United States, 1993). It is a common misconception that these individuals receive adequate care through charitable donations. In reality, the insured receive 54% more ambulatory care services and 90% more hospital care than the uninsured (Davis, 1990).

The uninsured tend to be from minority groups, poor, young adults, and rural residents. Employees of small businesses and agricultural workers tend to be less well insured. On the whole, white-collar workers have better health care benefits than blue-collar workers and workers in service industries. Those in manufacturing still have relatively good benefits (Davis, 1990). Pre-existing or long-term health problems also preclude some individuals from receiving coverage. One of the reasons that the movement toward substantial health care reform gained so much momentum during the last decade was because of the large number of uninsured or underinsured.

Health Care Reform

In an attempt to meet the health care needs of individuals in the United States, efforts have been made at the federal level to implement a system under which all Americans have adequate health-insurance coverage. The Clinton administration has favored a plan in which the financial responsibility of **universal health care coverage** is placed on employers. Many have been critical of this strategy because they fear government intervention into private enterprise and escalating costs of doing business. Others are skeptical that employer mandates would cover the cost of universal coverage and predict that tax increases would be inevitable.

Nurses have also taken an official position on health care reform. The American Nurses Association called for employer-mandated universal coverage in 1993. Within this plan, a **case-management approach** is being prescribed in which nurses act as client advocates to provide and coordinate cost-effective comprehensive care. A care-versus-cure philosophy is part of the plan, coupled with health-promotion and illness-prevention strategies.

INDUSTRY EFFORTS TO MANAGE HEALTH CARE COSTS

Managed Care

Managed care is a term used to describe health care subsystems in which services are administered in order to enhance their efficient and effective use. The primary purpose of these business ventures is to deliver, finance, buy, and sell health care services as economically as possible. In order to reduce costs, private insurance companies have played a major role in encouraging their development.

Managed-care systems, also known as alternative delivery systems, consist of administrators, providers, and the physical facilities in which health care is delivered. Many times hospitals are the focal point of managed-care organizations with ancillary services providing an array of complementary care. These delivery systems are of interest to nurses, particularly nurse practitioners, because of the autonomous practice opportunities they offer.

Several different administrative structures are characteristic of managed care arrangements. Some of the more common structures include **health maintenance organizations (HMOs), independent practice associations (IPAs)** and **preferred provider organizations (PPOs)** (see Table 10–3). Each of these managed-care systems is discussed further within the context in which they were originally designed. It should be noted, however, that these systems are in a state of flux and efforts are continually being made to refine them.

Health Maintenance Organizations

HMOs are usually organized in one of two ways. The first is the staff model in which HMO employees provide health-care services and also function as ad-

TABLE 10–3. **Comparison of Private Insurance and Managed Health Care Options**

	Private insurance	HMO	IPA (HMO)	PPO
Copayment requirement	Yes	No	No	Varies
Fee for service	Yes	No	Yes	Yes
Limited number of providers	No	Yes	Yes	Yes
Out-of-plan provider option	N/A	Emergencies only	Emergencies ony	Penalty applies
Utilization guidelines	No	Yes	Yes	Yes

ministrative personnel. The second, the group model, consists of a medical group that accepts a contract from an HMO to provide health care services for its participants.

Regardless of their structures, the primary purpose of HMOs is to limit costs by decreasing referrals to specialists, restricting diagnostic studies, and decreasing client hospitalization. Reducing the number of hospitalizations is accomplished, in part, through the provision of health-promotion and illness-prevention services.

HMOs are attractive for several reasons. First, after premiums are paid, care is free or requires only a small copayment if a designated HMO provider is used. Second, cost-containment incentives are in place to keep expenses down, and third, paperwork is kept to a minimum.

Less attractive aspects of HMOs also exist. An important disadvantage is that a limited number of providers are under contract at any one time, thus, client options may be restricted. If individuals choose to use providers who are not employed by their HMO, they are held personally responsible for the cost of those services. The only exception is in emergency situations.

Independent Practice Associations

A variation of the traditional HMO is the IPA, which is usually organized by physicians. Within this structure, HMOs contract with physicians and hospitals to provide care for their members. Physicians are paid on a **fee-for-service** basis at rates that are usually predetermined and attractive to insurers. Fee-for-service means that IPA members are charged for each service at the time care is provided. This is unlike most HMO plans, in which members pay premiums and are not charged for each service individually. Similar to traditional HMOs, IPAs do not reimburse for payments to nonmember providers. Finally, hospitals and physicians must adhere to **utilization guidelines** in order to contain costs. This means that the number of services they can provide is limited.

Preferred Provider Organizations

PPOs are another type of managed-care organization that can be sponsored by providers, insurance companies, or employers. Contracts are established with a limited number of health care facilities and professionals, and lower-than-customary rates are sometimes negotiated. In an attempt to contain costs, providers may be required to adhere to PPO utilization guidelines. In return for these concessions, provider services are used by greater numbers of clients.

Within PPO systems, physicians are reimbursed on a fee-for-service basis and members are charged each time care is provided. In addition to the fee-for-service arrangement, some PPO plans demand participant copayments in which individuals pay a percentage of the cost of services. The copayment requirement is thought to decrease client use and thus reduce costs.

A critical difference between HMO and PPO plans is that use of the PPO providers is encouraged through preferential rates. Benefits extend beyond the use of their services, however. Penalties apply if providers outside of the PPO are used, but their use is not prohibited. Americans have traditionally valued the freedom to choose their health care providers and this is perceived as a notable advantage over HMO plans.

Group Practice Arrangements

An outgrowth of managed-care systems has been an increase in the number of **group practices.** As many as a third of all non–governmentally employed physicians are in a group practice and this number is expected to increase to 50% by 1995. A group practice usually consists of three or more physicians who are formally organized to provide medical care. They distribute income according to a prearranged plan and use equipment, records, and personnel jointly (Schryver, 1991).

Group arrangements are thought to be advantageous for a number of reasons. First, they preserve the ideal of private entrepreneurship while cutting overhead. Second, they are attractive to providers who prefer to hire professional managers. This arrangement enables practitioners to spend more time caring for clients and less time worrying about the mechanics of running a business. Group practice arrangements are also appealing because they offer providers more time off, better client coverage, and professional camaraderie. Finally, group practices frequently employ an array of specialists and clients are offered convenient, centralized, and comprehensive services.

QUALITY ASSURANCE

Over time, the delivery of health care has moved further and further away from its charitable origins and more toward a business orientation. As this transformation occured, considerable attention was given to delivering quality client care in a cost-effective, competitive, and profitable manner. In order to achieve these goals, the health care industry borrowed the philosophy of **total quality management (TQM)** from the business world. **The Joint Commission on Accreditation of Healthcare Organizations (JCAHO)** has been so impressed with TQM's potential to improve health care delivery that in 1994 it began requiring hospitals to implement TQM strategies.

TQM, also referred to as **continuous quality improvement (CQI),** is based on the notion that organizations that produce higher-quality services than their competitors will capture a greater share of the market. Emphasis is placed not only on meeting the expectations of the customer (in this case, the health care client) but in exceeding those expectations. Within the TQM philosophy, there are internal customers and external customers. The external customers are clients and their families, whereas internal customers are individuals working within the health care setting. Quality is valued above all else and every constitutent must be satisfied with the services provided.

TQM requires that the process used to deliver services receive close and constant scrutiny. Everyone is encouraged to generate ideas for improving quality. Although change based on systematically documented evidence is encouraged, standardization of the process is also valued to maximize efficiency. Because TQM is proactively oriented, emphasis is placed on preventing problems rather than reacting to them after the fact (Whetsell, 1991).

Nurses are in an excellent position to implement TQM strategies. On a daily basis, they can assess how the health care delivery system is functioning and can measure the effectiveness of specific treatment approaches. For example, based on evidence that inexpensive saline solution is as effective as heparin in keeping intermittent intravenous catheters working, nurses at one hospital implemented a new protocol and saved $70,000 within 1 year (Buterbough, 1992).

FINANCIAL STRUCTURE OF HEALTH CARE AGENCIES

Profit Versus Nonprofit

Health care in the United States is largely provided within agencies in the private sector. These nongovernment health care facilities are generally classified as **for-profit** (proprietary) or **not-for-profit** (nonprofit) institutions.

To qualify as nonprofit, an institution must be organized and operated exclusively for one or more specified purposes. For example, a health care facility might be run for charitable or educational reasons. Agencies operated in this manner must reinvest all profits into the operation of the institution. In turn, they can take advantage of significant tax benefits. In contrast to common belief, nonprofit hospitals do not have to provide free or low-cost care to be classified as not-for-profit; however, use of emergency department services must be unrestricted.

A majority of hospitals are classified as nonprofit (69%) (Theisen, 1993). During the 1970s and 1980s, however, there was a significant increase in the number of for-profit hospitals. Struggling nonprofit agencies were purchased by corporations and new proprietary care facilities were built.

Unlike nonprofit agencies, proprietary organizations do not have to reinvest their profits solely into the operation of the health care facility. Rather, they have the option of raising capital through the sale of stock. They tend to charge customers considerably more than cost for services, and they are also likely to use expensive support systems such as laboratory and pharmacy services.

For-profit hospitals are most common in the southern U.S.; many are owned by Humana Incorporated or the Hospital Corporation of America. A growing number of nursing homes are also part of for-profit chains. Regardless of their for-profit or nonprofit status, health care agencies are feeling increasing pressure to balance humanitarian objectives with the need to operate in a fiscally motivated manner.

HEALTH CARE AGENCIES

Integrated Hospital Systems

Hospitals date back to the Middle Ages, when they were traditionally affiliated with a church or monastery. Early in U.S. history, physicians were often clergy; untrained women served them as nurses. Over time, many hospitals evolved independently to serve small local populations, and little thought was given to collaborative efforts. Because of recent changes in health care, hospitals are feeling pressure to function cooperatively and to be more sensitive to the needs of the region they serve.

For years, hospitals were at the center of the health care delivery system. They were centralized facilities with physicians, nurses, equipment, and other resources necessary to provide high-quality care. Physicians in independent practice provided primary care, made diagnoses, and referred clients to hospitals.

Several factors have affected this centralized system of care since the early 1980s. First, the health care market has become more competitive. New providers such as HMOs and ambulatory care centers have emerged to threaten the independent hospital's client base. Second, technologic advances have made it possible for freestanding ambulatory care facilities to provide services that were traditionally available only in hospitals. Third, demographic changes have forced hospitals to change the types of services they offer. For example, some hospitals are now focusing on long-term rehabilitative care rather than only short-term acute services.

As a result of these influences and economic pressures, client census has fallen to about 65% in most hospitals (Vidaver, 1993) and a decentralized system is emerging. In this model, several providers offer services that, in the past, were offered only at a hospital. For example, there are multiple-care facilities consisting of home health care agencies, minor emergency clinics, ambulatory care centers, outpatient surgery facilities, and small speciality hospitals that are geographically removed from the hospital setting. Because of this plethora of new providers, hospitals are experiencing considerable competition and are making significant efforts to remain competitive.

One way hospitals are managing to compete is through **horizontal and vertical integration.** Horizontal integration simply involves several health care agencies working together to cut costs by sharing resources or by using their collective buying power. For example, several agencies may use the same high-quality computer system or they may organize purchasing groups to reduce the cost of buying supplies (Herzlinger, 1994).

Vertical integration is another cost-cutting, competitive strategy that hospitals are using. In a vertically integrated system, hospitals provide the entire scope of health care services. These services may include home, acute, long-term, and ambulatory care. In this way, clients receive whatever type of assistance they need without having to be referred outside the system (Herzlinger, 1994).

Public Hospitals

Special note should be made of the public hospital system in this country. Public hospitals are owned by federal, state, or local governments and were originally patterned after almshouses in England that serviced the poor. The almshouse tradition was transferred to this country and eventually evolved into public hospitals. Philadelphia General Hospital, established in 1731, was the first of these facilities in the United States (Allison, 1993).

Public hospitals have traditionally played a valuable role in caring for the underserved and underprivileged as well as in offering training opportunities for health care professionals. In 1976, there were 1905 public hospitals in the United States. Since that time, their numbers have been declining because of budget cutbacks, the availability of Medicare and Medicaid benefits, and the high percentage of unoccupied beds in private facilities. Because of the need to fill beds in private hospitals and the potential profit that can be made by servicing Medicare and Medicaid clients, referrals to public hospitals have fallen off in recent years. As methods of health care reimbursement continue to change, the mission of public hospitals may have to be re-evaluated (Allison, 1993).

Outpatient Care

In recent years, several factors have led to greater demand for outpatient services, also known as alternative ambulatory services. First, implementation of the Medicare prospective payment system has resulted in shorter hospital stays. Second, private insurers perceived that ambulatory services were less expensive. Third, new technology made procedures that were formerly considered complicated or dangerous available on an outpatient basis. Finally, clients demanded less expensive and more accessible health care services.

It is estimated that in 1995 and beyond a significant number of hospitals will generate over 30% of their client revenue from outpatient care (Lutz, 1990), and that, over time, ambulatory services will determine their overall financial success (Eubanks, 1990).

Some hospitals are embedding themselves within a cluster of outpatient services. Others are establishing satellite clinics in surrounding suburbs and rural communities. Outpatient facilities are also cropping up in renovated stores in retail shopping malls where families can shop or eat lunch while loved ones are having surgery or tests.

Nursing Homes and Other Long-Term Care Facilities

Today, more senior citizens need long-term care. In addition, individuals of all ages are managing their lives with AIDS or traumatic head injuries. Such clients require extended care and rehabilitation services. Hospitals and nursing homes are attempting to meet these demands by developing units to accommodate the long-term needs of these clients.

Hospitals are starting to provide care in a more homelike atmosphere. Skilled nursing facilities, subacute care facilities, and assisted living facilities are sometimes physically located in the hospital setting but operated independently from the acute care hospital. Large client rooms, comfortable dining areas, and space for activities are important in order to meet the psychosocial needs of clients who stay for extended periods. Emphasis is also being placed on interacting with family members and involving them in the client's care. Because the restorative process may be slow, priority is placed on long-term goals and adjusting to ongoing health concerns (Eubanks, 1990).

Nursing homes also provide long-term health care. Although clients in these settings experience complex health problems, acute care is usually not necessary. Nursing homes generally provide care for two types of clients. Some individuals are admitted to recuperate after being hospitalized and generally stay fewer than 90 days. They may be recovering from surgery and require assistance until they are able to manage independently. Other clients need care for lengthier periods because they are more disabled or do not have people who can assist them at home (Mezey, 1992). Such clients may require services ranging from personal assistance to skilled nursing care.

The nursing home industry has experienced considerable growth in recent years; there are now more beds in these facilities than in acute care hospitals. Traditionally, nursing homes were nonprofit agencies sponsored by organizations such as churches. Today, approximately 75% of all nursing homes are for-profit institutions (Mezey, 1992) that rely heavily on Medicaid and Medicare reimbursement. Medicare benefits may be limited, and private insurance frequently pays the balance charged.

Community Health Centers

Community health centers provide services primarily for medically underserved and disadvantaged individuals. They are supported by federal funds, and their focus is on health promotion and disease prevention. Based on their philosophic origins, community health centers make a special effort to tailor services to meet local needs. For this reason, community members are intimately involved with their operation, development, and governance.

Community health centers use a team approach, and nurses, along with physicians and physician assistants, play key roles in providing care. The variety of ambulatory services offered tends to vary with fluctuating government funding; Medicare, Medicaid, and **sliding-scale fees** are relied on more heavily. Along with disease-prevention and health-promotion activities, some centers offer emergency assistance, home care, mental health counseling, and rehabilitative support. Diagnostic, laboratory, and pharmaceutical services may also be available.

School-Based Health Care

Nurses provide a variety of services within local school systems. These services include screenings, health-promotion and illness-prevention strategies, and treatment of minor problems. Emphasis is placed on physical as well as social and psychologic well-being. Concerns relating to self-esteem, stress, drug abuse, and adolescent pregnancy are frequently addressed by the school nurse. In addition, children and adolescents with long-term health problems often attend school, and it is not uncommon for the school nurse to be consulted about colostomy care or nasogastric tube feedings.

Students who have health concerns are frequently referred to providers within the community; an important role of the school nurse is that of community liaison. For this reason, the nurse must be knowledgeable about community resources and adept at getting clients into the health care system in a timely and efficient manner.

Nurse-Run Clinics

Similar to community health centers, nurse-run clinics tend to focus on health promotion and disease prevention. Nurses who are interested in autonomous practice often work in these settings.

Several types of nurse-run clinics have been identified. Among these are free-standing agencies that rely on a variety of funding sources and provide a range of services to the medically underserved. Second are nurse-run outreach programs that are sponsored by medical centers. These clinics typically serve targeted populations and those who have specific health problems; care is usually based on a nursing model. Nurses in these settings are employees of the medical center and are expected to generate funds necessary to run the clinic (Riesch, 1992).

Third, nursing centers are organized around a wellness and health promotion model. Specific populations, such as the elderly who tend to gather at community centers, are frequently targeted. These clinics may be associated with academic institutions and offer opportunities for student and faculty practice and research (Riesch, 1992).

Finally, some nurses who practice independently are not affiliated with an institution. They provide counseling, consultation, direct care, and home services. These practitioners are primarily found in urban areas and rely on direct fees and insurance. Most nurses in independent practice supplement their income with teaching positions or other types of employment (Riesch, 1992).

Public Health Departments

Epidemics in the 18th and 19th centuries forced community leaders to take measures to prevent and control communicable diseases in their geographic area. Along with this mission came an emphasis on public education and home care.

Today, public health departments are administered by state, county, or city governments; there has been a shift away from home care. More emphasis is now being placed on the management of acute and chronic conditions in outpatient clinics. A large percentage of clients seen in these settings are indigent, members of minorities, uninsured, or on Medicaid and Medicare.

Home-Care Agencies

Nurses employed by home-care agencies have assumed almost total responsibility for care provided in private residences. These nurses may work for hospital-based or local independent agencies, regional and national chains, or private duty registries. They provide acute and long-term services but may also be specialists in areas such as hospice care. Home-care clients vary widely in age and their needs may be simple or complex. Unlike public health departments, about half of all home-care providers are for-profit agencies and receive payment from a number of sources (Bowman, 1992).

Adult Day Health Care Centers

In an attempt to meet the health care needs of the rapidly increasing number of elderly individuals in the community, adult day health care centers are becoming more common. These centers provide services for a large number of elderly clients who have physical problems, organic brain dysfunction, or mobility problems that make them liable to social isolation. Care is provided for clients during the day and they return to their homes or families at night.

Some adult day health care centers are associated with hospitals and provide sophisticated medical and nursing care to individuals recovering from acute illness. Others are extensions of psychiatric facilities and focus on management of psychosocial problems. A third type is freestanding or incorporated into a senior citizen complex. Clients who participate in these programs usually have long-term health concerns and benefit from social and restorative therapy and supervision. Finally, individuals may benefit from day health care centers that primarily provide social interaction. Often these programs are associated with senior citizen organizations or religious groups (Osterman, 1986).

Adult day health care centers are funded by governmental agencies, philanthropic organizations, and private payments. Third-party payers do not consistently reimburse charges for these services despite studies that suggest that these agencies provide an economical way to meet the needs of many elderly individuals (Osterman, 1986).

Parish Nurses

Working in conjunction with community-based programs are parish nurses, otherwise known as ministers of health. Churches are engaging nurses to: (1)

serve as health educators and counselors; (2) do assessments and make referrals; (3) organize support groups; (4) make visits to the sick and elderly; and (5) serve as client advocates. It is estimated that approximately 1500 parish nurses throughout the country are attempting to meet the needs of individuals who are without adequate primary care and experiencing escalating health care costs. Many of these nurses work part-time or are volunteers (King, 1993).

Voluntary Health Agencies

Since the inception of voluntary health agencies in 1892, their number has grown to more than 100,000. The first voluntary health agency was the Anti-Tuberculosis Society established in Philadelphia around 1839. Some of the better-known agencies that exist today include the American Cancer Society, the National Foundation for the March of Dimes, and The National Easter Seal Society for Crippled Adults and Children. In 1989, all volunteer agencies combined raised about $1 billion. These organizations play an important role in promoting the general welfare of individuals and in educating the public (Hawkins, 1993).

RURAL HEALTH CARE

Delivery of health care in rural areas presents unique challenges. These challenges result from: (1) an inadequate number of physicians, nurses, and allied health care professionals who are willing to live and practice in remote areas; (2) decreased access to advanced medical technology; and (3) the fact that rural hospitals often have higher expenses than revenues. In recent years, many rural hospitals have been forced to close or severely curtail their services.

Rural health care delivery problems are being overcome through integrated community health care systems that provide primary and secondary care to residents in the region. These systems are composed of a network of primary care physicians, nurse practitioners, nurses, physician assistants, and other ancillary health care personnel. Some acute care hospitals are merging, whereas others are being transformed into ambulatory health care centers. Physicians and nurse practitioners are employees of multistructured networks, in which constituents work under the aegis of the same administrative staff.

Paying for health care services is another concern for rural residents. Many of these individuals are farmers or employees of small businesses that do not offer health benefits. To overcome this problem, the use of **health insurance purchasing cooperatives (HIPCs)** has been proposed. These are large groups of people or employers who band together to buy insurance at reduced costs. HIPCs may be organized by private groups or by the government. So far, these organizations remain untested and may or may not be successful.

FEDERALLY FUNDED HEALTH CARE AGENCIES

The federal government has been involved in the development of health care institutions since 1798. At that time, the Marine Hospital Service for the Relief of Sick and Disabled Seamen was established. Today, the federal government administers several health care programs in order to meet the needs of select groups. Among these are military personnel, veterans, and Native Americans.

Military

The federal government provides health care for military personnel on active duty and retirees, their dependents and survivors. Services are available in conventional on-base hospitals as well as in less traditional settings such as field facilities.

Military dependents, survivors, retirees and dependents can also use nonmilitary health care providers. This option is made possible through the **Civilian Health and Medical Program for the Uniformed Services (CHAMPUS)**. CHAMPUS provides funding for nonmilitary health care services when care through the armed forces is not available (Hawkins, 1993).

Veterans' Administration

The Veterans' Administration (VA) was established in 1930 to meet the health care needs of individuals who had served in the military. Today the VA provides care for approximately 27 million veterans. The VA consists of medical centers, outpatient clinics, rehabilitation services, facilities for the chronically ill, nursing homes, and other services. The VA hospital system is the largest health care system in the United States (Hawkins, 1993).

Any veteran who developed a disability related to military service and received an honorable or general discharge is eligible to receive care in the VA system. In keeping with current health care trends, VA providers encourage self-care and expect clients to take responsibility for their personal well-being (Hawkins, 1993).

Public Health Service

Through the Public Health Service, the federal government provides health care in areas where there are critical shortages of providers. The National Health Service Corps has placed more than 16,000 professionals in hundreds of sites throughout the United States. Health care providers are encouraged to join the Corps through scholarships and stipends. In return, members are assigned to underserved areas and are encouraged to continue practicing in those settings (Hawkins, 1993).

Native Americans and Native Alaskans also receive health care through the federal government. Under the aegis of the Public Health Service, The Indian Health Service provides assistance for more than 1 million individuals. Health care is available in hundreds of facilities ranging from hospitals and large health centers to local clinics. Most of these facilities are located in remote or rural areas where problems such as malnutrition are common (Hawkins, 1993).

SUMMARY

The health care delivery system in the United States offers a variety of facilities, payment plans, and providers. The nurse has traditionally played a key role as a direct health care provider. As the delivery system changes, however, that role will be expanded and transformed. It is anticipated that nurses will take on additional responsibilities in primary care, case management, and the community. Nurses must understand the workings of this system so that they can provide cost-effective quality services and so they can help shape the health care delivery system of the future.

CRITICAL THINKING EXERCISES

1   Select three clients you are familiar with who have different health care needs. Describe these clients' medical histories, current problems, and future health care needs, then determine which health care setting and which health care practitioners would be most appropriate for them. Identify any difficulties that might be encountered during their entry into the health care system. How can the nurse facilitate the process?

2   Skilled nursing facilities, subacute care facilities, and assisted living facilities are all forms of long-term or extended health care. Identify five specific problems that nurses working in such facilities encounter. What is the best way to resolve these problems?

3   Identify cost-cutting measures used at a health care facility with which you are familiar. Have these measures affected the quality of client care? What other measures to cut costs can be implemented? How have changes within the health care delivery system altered nursing practice?

4   Identify four health care priorities that may be initiated by the year 2000. How are these likely to affect the profession of nursing?

5   Describe the advantages and disadvantages of various health care reimbursement plans. Which ones will produce the highest quality care? Which ones are best for the profession of nursing? Are there any payment plans that do both?

6   Identify those elements in health care reform that are most necessary. Should nurses support these changes and why?

HOME HEALTH CARE IS FRAUGHT WITH DANGER

All across the nation, the insurance company and HMO executives who are busily ejecting acutely ill patients from their hospital beds are singing the praises of home health care. Taking care of sick patients at home, they proclaim, saves money; reduces the risk of hospital-born infections, and spares the sick the experience of an often cold and impersonal hospital setting. Visions of mom serving up hot tea and chicken soup to a child with a bad case of the flu immediately come to mind.

But there's a major obstacle to the realization of this glowing scenario of a hospital-less future. Taking care of acutely ill patients in the home demands much more than a shift in the *locus* of the delivery of health care. It demands the presence of family caregivers or friends who are available to replace the 24-hour monitoring, intervention and assistance acutely ill patients receive in the hospital. That's because home care nurses, aides and other technical support staff are meant to supplement—not replace—family caregiving.

But today—as more and more patients are discharged from the hospital writhing in pain, suffering from infections, with tubes and draining wounds, on ventilators, IV medication or toxic chemotherapy regimens—there is often no one at home or no one who is allowed to stay at home to give them the 24-hour attention they require.

The issue is quite simple and yet seems to be utterly ignored as we embark on this bold new experiment. To shift the burden of health care from hospital to home and ensure that care is safe and effective, the country will have to undergo a major social transformation that includes changes in family policy as well as changes in health-care policy.

Consider the facts: In order to be safe, cautions home care expert Chris Kovner, professor of nursing at New York University, home care arrangements must combine four successful ingredients: Patients must return to a reasonably comfortable and clean setting; expert nurses must be available to provide teaching and support to help patients and family caregivers manage the medical and technical tasks they confront; patients must have access to on-going medical care at a clinic or physician's office; and a family caregiver or friend, plus home health aides, must be available to provide the kind of continuous care many patients need.

Although they have constructed an alluring fantasy of home care, the health-care entrepreneurs and employers who are now running America's health care system have consistently acted to prevent its realization. Home care is a highly fragmented industry with few quality controls; most insurance plans do not provide the level and intensity of services sick people

HOME HEALTH CARE IS FRAUGHT WITH DANGER
(Continued)

really need; physician care is still inaccessible to many, and the biggest problem of all is having caregivers in the home. The very businesses who won't pay for patients to stay in hospitals nonetheless refuse to allow their employees time off work to care for acutely, chronically or terminally ill family members.

In the United States today, women still provide most domestic services. But today most women work outside the home. The majority of these working women would be penalized—with lost promotions, docked pay, or a pink slip—if they left their posts to care for the sick.

This is because the Family and Medical Leave Act that was finally signed under President Clinton provides only unpaid leave. The act exempts from its provisions the majority of American workers. The minority who are covered by the act are unable to take time off work to care for a newborn or adopted child or sick relative because they cannot afford to take unpaid leave. Even those who are eligible for medical leave and could afford to take it are prohibited from so doing because top wage earners in firms with over 50 employees are also exempt from the bill.

If these working women—and men—thought they had trouble caring for a healthy child, or an elderly parent, imagine the kind of dilemmas they will face when the find they have to provide nursing care for an acutely ill family member. And what about those who have no family caregivers, or whose family members are as sick and frail as they are?

Ironically, in the 19th century, it was urban America's inability to care for the sick in the home that led to the development of hospitals with their professional caregiving staffs. Now, as the need for surrogate family caregivers increases, we are eliminating their expertise and, simultaneously acquiescing to a corporate culture that wants workers to have fewer opportunities for caregiving, not more.

Many changes in insurance benefits will have to be implemented if home care is to work. But the biggest challenge we face will be to make it possible for people to take paid time off from work so they can shoulder this new burden. And, in an age when women rightly refuse to bear this burden alone,we will have to make sure that men share it equally.

If America is ready to do all this, then home care can indeed be embraced as one of the solutions to our health care crisis. If it is not, home care will simply become a dumping ground for sick patients; the burden of professional care will be shifted from professional caregivers to unskilled, ill-equipped family members—mostly working or frail elderly women. Those who have no family will suffer even more.

Reprinted with permission from Baer, E. and Gordon, S.: Home health care is fraught with danger. Philadelphia Inquirer, April 10, 1995, page 9.

A Closer Look

CQI-NEW STRATEGY FOR BETTER NURSING CARE

Providing patient care of the highest quality has always been a concern of nurses. In the atmosphere of today's health care system, this concern has been amplified and enlarged to include all members of the health care team as equal members in the collaborative effort to give clients and families the best care possible.

One innovative approach is **Continuous Quality Improvement** (CQI). The key element in CQI is that the traditional authoritarian command and control hierarchical structure that has dominated the health care system for so long will be changed to a structure in which all members have equal input. No longer does the top (physician) think while the bottom (e.g., nurses, physical therapists, social services workers) merely reacts. In CQI, every health care provider at all levels thinks and acts to provide the best care possible at all times, recognizing that quality health care extends far beyond just one individual. High-quality health care results only when all individual providers work together, regardless of their roles in the organization.

In a well-organized and functional CQI system, the client's needs, *not* the providers' needs, are at the heart of the care being given. Client input is essential in the CQI approach to health care. Although the clients may not know all the details of what is being done, it is certainly possible to tell whether or not the care is meeting their needs.

Problems can be solved quickly and well and the quality improvement climate fosters an atmosphere wherein mistakes are prevented and client comfort is maximized. CQI stretches the use of the care-providers' knowledge and skills. Continually striving for improvement focuses the nurse's attention on client care delivery systems and creates a climate in which high-quality nursing services match client needs and family needs in the most cost-effective way.

Modified from AACN News February 1995, page 2.

A Closer Look

NURSING CENTERS FILL HEALTH-CARE VOID
The clinics are turning up in long-underserved areas

Sheri Pitts sat flopped over the table, her head cradled in her arms, when the woman wearing a lab coat and carrying a stethoscope walked into the examining room at the health center.

Five months pregnant with her third child, Pitts was feeling lousy. Vomiting, diarrhea, cramping.

Cheryl MacDonald was writing it all down in her patient's file.

MacDonald, a nurse practitioner at the Schuylkill Falls Health Center, helped her onto the examining table.

"Where are you living?" she inquired, checking her blood pressure and pulse. "Still with your mother?"

Pitts, who cringed from the cramps, nodded. "My sister moved out."

MacDonald helped the patient lie back on the table, and pulled up the teen's red Garfield the Cat T-shirt to expose her basketball of a stomach.

"Is anyone helping you with the kids during the day?" MacDonald asked, running a portable ultrasound machine over the stomach.

Pitts snapped her head to look at the nurse. "That was a joke, right?"

It was a typical scene at the center, one of a growing number of full-service clinics managed by nurse practitioners that are starting to dot the urban landscape in Philadelphia and nationwide.

This center at the Schuylkill Falls public housing project, on Ridge Avenue in East Falls, opened in September.

And what was a dank maintenance office is now a brightly lit wing of pastel-painted offices and examining rooms.

There are toys in the waiting area. Phones ring off the hook from people seeking appointments with nurses and advice from community outreach workers. Similar health centers will open soon at a housing project in North Philadelphia and at a recreation center in Southwest Philadelphia.

Nurse practitioners say it's about filling a void. They are working in rural and urban areas suffering a dearth of primary care physicians. Anything a family doctor can do, they can do—and cheaper, the nurses say.

Nursing centers take different forms, from full-service health clinics to others dedicated to a single population, like the elderly or pregnant women.

Just how many centers there are nationwide is unknown. Marjorie Buchanan, a consultant for the National League of Nursing who is doing research on the subject, estimates there are about 200.

Continued on following page

NURSING CENTERS FILL HEALTH-CARE VOID (Continued)

With pressures to bring down health costs, that number is sure to grow. There are 2,000 licensed nurse practitioners in Pennsylvania, more than 1,200 in New Jersey and 100,000 nationwide. They are registered nurses with special advanced training.

And while they are serving primarily the underserved, their turf is extending far beyond, Buchanan said.

Philadelphia is viewed as a leader in the movement, Buchanan said, with centers like the one Thomas Jefferson University Hospital geared to women's health and the University of Pennsylvania's nursing center for the elderly.

But the challenge for many is redefining the public's perception of nurses, and the role they play in the medical community.

"The nursing approach is not the same as the medical model," said Jane Pond, director of ambulatory services at Temple University's Neighborhood Nursing Center, which plans to open a nurse-run clinic in the fall at Norris Homes, a public housing project in North Philadelphia.

"We tend to look at things more in the vein of health promotion and disease prevention, and looking at the person in perhaps a more holistic way," said Pond.

Pond related a recent case of a doctor who prescribed painkillers and X-rays for a woman complaining that she couldn't sleep and was having pain in her neck and arm.

It was the nurse practitioner who asked what kind of bed she was using, and found out the woman was sleeping in the bathtub because she was so afraid of stray bullets.

"I tend to look at their environments much more, what's going on in the family and what's going on in their homes," Pond said, while doctors often don't have the time for those kinds of dialogues.

Carolyn Lewis-Spruill, who runs the first nurse-managed health center to open in New Jersey, does not feel in competition with doctors because she practices in an area long ignored by physicians.

Her clinic is in a renovated row-house in a rundown part of Trenton. Most of her patients are uninsured.

"Probably no one would come out here to do anything like this, but there is a great need," said Lewis-Spruill, director of St. Martins Center, which opened in August and serves about 300 adults and children.

"We do have a special commitment to the underserved," said Margaret Cotroneo, an associate professor of nursing at the University of Pennsylvania. "But we belong every place."

NURSING CENTERS FILL HEALTH-CARE VOID (Continued)

Rules determining how nurses can practice are set by both the state Board of Nursing and the Board of Medicine. They define a nurse's role as "diagnosing and treating . . . actual or potential health problems," by offering such services as counseling, teaching, patient support and following the medical regimens prescribed by licensed doctors.

The law goes on to say that nurses cannot diagnose any medical conditions or prescribe therapeutic or corrective measures unless such care is authorized by both boards. The two groups, however, differ on what this means.

In Pennsylvania, nurse practitioners can only prescribe medication for standard treatments, and those prescriptions must be signed by doctors.

What generally happens is that physicians, working as consultants for the nurse-run clinics, will sign their names to blank prescriptions that a nurse uses as needed.

Cotroneo said nurse practitioners are trained to recognize more serious conditions and make the appropriate referrals. She points to the states where nurse practitioners can prescribe medicine. "Can they all be encouraging nurses to practice medicine without a license? I hardly think so."

Whether nurse practitioner programs survive may depend more on medical reimbursement policies. Health care must start recognizing the nurse as a provider without tying the services to a physician, said Christine Fillpovich, an administrator for the Pennsylvania Nurses Association.

For instance, the state Department of Public Welfare reimburses nurse practitioners under Medicaid for low-income people, she said. But Medicare, for those over 65, will only pay for the services in rural areas, or if they are working for a physician.

Cheryl MacDonald's interest in health was aroused during the four years she served as a Peace Corps volunteer in Senegal. Though she was there to help in rural development, the natives went to her for everything from stokes to colds.

When MacDonald returned home, she received master's degrees in both nursing and public health at Yale University. She now teaches at Penn's nursing school and works two days at the Schuylkill Falls clinic.

"I knew it would be a holistic approach," said MacDonald, 37. "As nurses, we're trained to focus on health education and the psychosocial aspect of what's going on in a person's life, and how that impacts her wellness or illness."

Continued on following page

NURSING CENTERS FILL HEALTH-CARE VOID (Continued)

That's why she asks the pregnant Pitts not only about her health, but also about where she's living and whether she has help with her two children. There are outreach workers at the center educated about housing opportunities and child care.

"It's not just about that pregnancy," MacDonald said. "It's about all these other stressors."

For her part, Pitts said she notices no difference in the care she received at her former obstetrician's office on City Line Avenue and how she's treated at the nurse-managed health center a short walk from her public housing apartment.

"It's easier to get to, and less of a wait."

Reprinted with permission from Santiago, D.M.: Nursing centers fill health-care void. Philadelphia Inquirer, April 3, 1995, pages B1–B3.

BIBLIOGRAPHY

Allison, F: Public hospitals—past, present, and future. Perspect Biol Med 36:596–610, 1993.

American Nurses Association: Nursing's Agenda for Health Care Reform. American Nurses' Publishing, Washington, D.C., 1993.

Birchenall, JM and Streight, ME: Health Occupations: Exploration and Career Planning. CV Mosby, St. Louis, 1989.

Bowman, RA: Nursing returns to the home health frontier: Markets and trends in home health care. In Aiken, L and Fagin, C (eds.): Charting Nursing's Future: Agenda for the 1990s. JB Lippincott, Philadelphia, 1992, pp 235–254.

Brockopp, DY, Porter, M, Kinnaird, S, and Silberman, S: Fiscal and clinical evaluation of patient care: A case management model for the future. J Nurs Admin 22(9):23–24, 1992.

Buterbough, L: TQM: The quality-care revolution. Med World News 33:17–21, 1992.

Congressional Budget Office: Trends in Health Spending: An Update. U.S. Government Printing Office, Washington, D.C., 1993.

Davis, K and Rowland, D: Uninsured and underserved: Inequities in health care in the United States. In Lee, PR and Estes, CL (eds): The Nation's Health, Jones and Bartlett, Boston, 1990, p 298–308.

Eubanks, P: Outpatient care: A nationwide revolution. Hospitals, 64:28–35, 1990.

Hawkins, JW and Higgins, LP: Nursing and the American Health Care System. Tiresias Press, New York, 1993.

Herzlinger, R: The quiet health care revolution. Public Interest 115:72–90, Spring 1994.

King, JM, Lakin, JA and Striepe, J: Coalition building between public health nurses and parish nurses. J Nurs Admin 23:27–31, 1993.

Lockhart, CA: Physician payment reform: Implications for nursing. In Aiken, L and Fagin, C (eds): Charting Nursing's Future: Agenda for the 1990s. JB Lippincott, Philadelphia, 1992, pp 448–461.

Lutz, S: Ambulatory care of the 1990s stretches the imagination. Modern Healthcare, 20:24–26; 33–34, 1990.

Mezey, M: Nursing homes: Residents' needs; nursing's response. In Aiken, L and Fagin, C (eds): Charting Nursing's Future: Agenda for the 1990s. JB Lippincott, Philadelphia, 1992, pp 198–215.

Osterman, HM: In nursing's future: Establishing adult day health care centers. Nurs Management 17:50–52, 54, 1986.

Riesch, SK: Nursing centers: An analysis of the anecdotal literature. J Prof Nurs, 8:16–25, 1992.

Schryver, DL: Responding to managed care proposals. Med Group Management J 38:32–34, 1991.

Schultz, EE: Advantages of employer health plans are disappearing. Wall Street Journal June 17, 1994, pp. C1, C15.

Theisen, BA and Palfrey, S: The advantages and risks of being a tax-exempt, nonprofit organization. J Nurs Admin, 23:36–41, 1993.

United States Executive Office of the President, Health Security Act of 1993. U.S. Government Printing Office, Washington, D.C., 1993.

United States Department of Health and Human Services Public Health Service: Healthy People 2000: National Health Promotion and Disease Prevention Objectives. U.S. Government Printing Office, Washington, D.C., 1991.

Vidaver, VS: A position for home care. Caring 12:5, 7–8, 1993.

Wasley, TP: What Has Government Done to Our Health Care? Cato Institute, Washington, D.C., 1992.

Whetsell, GW: Total quality management. Topics in Health Care Finance, 18:12–20, 1991.

HISTORICAL PERSPECTIVES

Lavinia Lloyd Dock (1858–1956)

Much like Florence Nightingale, Lavinia Dock was born into an upper-middle-class family in which education was highly valued. As with Nightingale's family, Dock's family was surprised when she selected nursing as her life's calling. In 1885, when she left her home in Pennsylvania and entered the Bellevue Training School for Nurses in New York City, nursing was not considered an acceptable occupation for well-born, well-educated women. She did not find nursing school particularly difficult, because of the high-quality primary and secondary education she had received as a child, but she observed that many of her fellow nursing students had a great deal of difficulty learning about the many medications that were becoming available at that time. She later wrote a medication textbook for nurses, the first one ever published, called *Materia Medica for Nurses.* It sold about 100,000 copies.

Like many of the nursing leaders of this time period, Dock quickly became aware that the terrible social conditions of large segments of the population had a direct effect on their generally poor health. From this observation, she drew the conclusion that the poverty and squalor in which much of the population lived would have to be improved before their health could. She became a dedicated social reformer and tried to improve the conditions in the New York City slums by confronting legislators. Dock soon became disillusioned. Without the right to vote, and with the prevailing attitude that they were second-class citizens, women had little power and almost no influence over legislators' opinions.

Although Dock worked for a short time in the Henry Street Settlement with Lillian Wald and was Isabel Hampton Robb's assistant supervisor at the Johns Hopkins Hospital, she spent most of her nursing career in the pursuit of equal rights and equal social standing for women. Over 20 years of her life, she cajoled, berated, and lobbied legislators at all levels about the need for women to have the right to vote. Her belief was that only through the right to vote would women ever gain the power they needed to influence social reforms and health care. She was also an avowed pacifist and argued against America's entrance into World War I.

Dock provides an excellent example of what nurses are capable of doing in achieving higher-quality care, even if they are not at the bedside. Through a life dedicated to the improvement of society, women, and nursing, she is considered one of the most influential leaders in early 20th century U.S. history.

Early Nursing Leaders: Annie W. Goodrich (1876–1955)

As a contemporary of Lillian Wald and Adelaide Nutting, Goodrich also was involved in the Henry Street Settlement in New York City after having received her nursing education from the New York Hospital Training School for Nurses. She too was known as an outstanding nurse educator and taught in, or was superintendent of, several nursing schools in New York City. In 1910, she was appointed as a state inspector of nurse training schools, a position that ony physicians had held before that time.

She became interested in military nursing, and in 1918 Goodrich was asked by the U.S. Army to make a survey of their hospitals with nursing departments. After observing the many difficulties and shortages in the Army nurse corps, she proposed that the U.S. Army organize its own nursing school. Later that year, when the school was opened, Goodrich was appointed Dean. Other Army nursing schools, based on the one designed by Goodrich, were established at army hospitals during World War I.

After America's reluctant entrance into World War I, the demand for trained nurses increased dramatically. The many hospital-based nursing schools of the period could not keep up with the demand. To respond to this need, Goodrich established the Vassar Training Program at Vassar College to produce highly trained nurses after a 12-week classroom summer session of science and theory, followed by 2 years of clinical practice in a hospital. The response was tremendous, and after the war other colleges and universities became interested in developing their own nursing programs.

Goodrich returned to home care nursing, where the majority of nursing care was still being provided, through the Henry Street Settlement after the war. She eventually moved on to nursing education in the university setting and was dean of the Yale University School of Nursing until she retired in 1934. Her many writings about nursing education and her experiences with military nursing have made a great contribution to nursing education. Through the Vassar Training School, the viability of nursing education in a college setting was demonstrated, much to the dismay of the hospital-based schools of nursing. Physicians and the medical community still believed that nurses were overtrained and questioned the need for university-based education. Although university-based schools of nursing were slow to develop, Goodrich had demonstrated that classroom theory was just as important as clinical practice in the education of highly skilled nurses.

There are other nurses who lived during this period who made substantial contributions to the profession of nursing. This small group was selected for presentation because they are representative of the great drive and dedication of individuals who produced changes and influenced the course and development of professional nursing even to this day. There are many extensive, well-written biographies of these early nursing leaders, and it is recommended that nurses at all levels read about these dedicated women's lives.

11

THE POLITICALLY ACTIVE NURSE

Learning Objectives

After completing this chapter, the reader will be able to:

1 Explain why it is important for nurses to understand and become involved in the political process.
2 List four levels of political involvement.
3 Describe the basic structure of government.
4 Discuss how a bill becomes a law.
5 Identify the major committees at the federal level that influence health policy.
6 Identify four points at which nurses can influence a bill.
7 Give examples of how nurses may become politically involved.
8 List and describe four methods of lobbying.
9 Discuss the role of professional associations, nursing networks, and coalitions in influencing health-policy decisions.
10 Define terms relevant to legislative and political process.

WHY NURSES NEED TO BE POLITICALLY INVOLVED

"If nursing is to take its rightful place in setting health policy, nurses must know about the issues, understand the political system, and participate in it" (Goldwater, 1990).

Although the term **politics** holds negative connotations for many, it is actually a neutral term that means *influencing*—specifically, influencing the allocation of scarce resources (Mason, 1993). Nurses have become increasingly interested in public policy realizing that both their personal lives and professional activities are significantly influenced by government policy and programs. "Many nurses have become aware that health policy directly affects how they are educated, where they practice, and how they are reimbursed" (Goldwater, 1990).

The beginning of health care reform in our country has shown the impact that even "proposed" legislative action can have. For example, when President Clinton placed health care reform on the national agenda, it was expected that a comprehensive national health care law would be passed. Many even believed that the U.S. Congress might consider a national health insurance program (single-payer plan) similar to that in operation in Canada. This caused many special interest groups to mobilize and to oppose such sweeping changes in the system. Hospitals and health care agencies also reacted to the anticipated legislation. The result has been downsizing or "rightsizing" of hospitals, with subsequent layoffs of nurses or hiring freezes, done before the actual passage of any laws or regulations. In Philadelphia, a news article reported a "merger mania which fused one-time rival hospitals with each other and insurers with hospitals" and the attendant layoff of more than 4000 workers (Uhlman, 1994). As a result of the dramatic changes and retrenchment within the hospital industry, Maria Talamo, a nurse administrator with 17 years of experience and a master's degree, became so disheartened that she moved to Texas. A physician affected by the merger, Dr. David Nickin, sold his practice to the University of Pennsylvania. Dr. Nickin stated that he never thought the medical market would transform itself so quickly in the absence of a national plan for health reform (Uhlman, 1994). These dramatic changes all resulted simply from the agenda-setting phase of the health policy process.

Consider the impact of laws that have been passed and their effect on nursing. The establishment of diagnosis-related groups (DRGs) with Medicare reimbursement legislation led to the discharge of patients from hospitals in a manner described as "sicker and quicker." The implications of this single act for the nursing profession were profound. Although this law applied only to Medicare clients, after the Federal Government had set a precedent, other insurance carriers began to impose similar restrictions. The effect of this law can be seen in the case of Mrs. J.

Mrs. J, aged 86, was admitted to the hospital with paralysis of the esophageal musculature and aspiration pneumonia, having had a cerebrovascular accident and requiring insertion of a gastrostomy tube. The family expected that she would be hospitalized for an extended period. They were shocked when they learned of her early discharge and upset when informed that they would be responsible for required dressing changes and tube feedings, tasks with which they were clearly uncomfortable. It was the nursing staff who had to explain that hospital stays were reduced because of this prospective payment initiative, they are often the ones who must deal with the client's and with the family's frustration.

With earlier discharge of mothers and newborns from the hospital (within 24 hours after a normal delivery, 3 days after cesarean section) becoming a common practice, groups are mobilizing to educate the public on the effects of this "cost-saving measure." Not only is the client sent home before the nurse has adequate time to provide teaching, but certain potentially life-threatening conditions like jaundice and circulatory problems cannot be detected in newborns until 2 to 3 days after birth.

A number of state laws affect both nursing practice and education. Many states have passed laws providing third-party reimbursement for nurses. These laws allow certain categories of specialty nurses to be directly reimbursed by clients or insurance carriers, rather than through doctors. Legislation varies from state to state, but the types of nurses most frequently covered by such laws are nurse anesthetists, nurse practitioners, and nurse midwives. Such laws have helped to increase the autonomy of nurses and have set the stage for more nurses to enter into advanced practice. With legislation, insurance carriers have recognized the contributions of advanced practice nurses, particularly in the primary-care setting. At present more than 100,000 advanced practice nurses—nurses with education and clinical experience beyond the 2 to 4 years of basic nursing education—are providing essential primary care services as certified nurse midwives, nurse practitioners, and clinical nurse specialists (ANA, 1994).

State laws or regulations may also impact nursing education. In North Dakota, for example, the baccalaureate degree has been designated as the minimal requirement for entry into professional nursing practice. This requirement was the result of passage of a law; however, regulations promulgated by a state board of nursing may also affect both education and practice and, if passed, also hold the force of law.

NEEDS MAY PRECIPITATE ACTION

In some states, laws allow registered nurses to pronounce death. The need that precipitated a law that permits pronouncement of death by nurses in one state is illustrated in the example provided by a home care nurse who worked in rural area.

Mrs. Smith, an elderly woman who had a terminal illness, died peacefully at home surrounded by her family. When the family was unable to reach the physician or funeral director, however, they had no choice but to call the paramedic unit serving their area. When the paramedics arrived, approximately 3 hours after Mrs. Smith's death, they were required by law to initiate cardiopulmonary resuscitation (CPR) and to transport her to the nearest emergency department several miles from the family home.

Needless to say, this was emotionally disturbing to the family. It was also costly in terms of the paramedics' time, charges for the ambulance, and emergency room fees. Such situations can serve as a springboard to action prompting a nurse or a nursing group to approach a legislator to ask for support to introduce a bill to rectify the problem. In Pennsylvania, the case mentioned renewed the fervor of nurses, particularly those working in home care, hospice, and long-term care, to push for legislation that would permit the timely release of deceased persons to funeral directors in order to prevent unnecessary and unanticipated resuscitative measures at that time required by law. A bill had been introduced 10 years earlier by Mary Ann Arty, a nurse member of the legislature, but had failed. When the measure was reintroduced in 1991, nurses worked diligently to assure passage of the law, which was signed in 1992. (PNA, 1991)

Nurses can play a significant role in helping to get legislation that benefits their patients and families passed. But nurses also must remember that the nurse practice acts in their respective states are based in law and might be revised or completely eliminated through a single legislative action. The nurse practice act in each state provides nurses with the right to practice and delimits the parameters of professional practice. Most state practice acts contain basically the same major components including reason for the law, definition of nursing, requirements for licensure, grounds for revocation of a license, provisions for persons licensed in other states, creation of a board for nurse examiners, responsibilities of the board, and penalties for practicing without a license (Kelly, 1991). Unfortunately, the requirements in these categories vary from state to state. Because each state law differs, it is important for nurses to know about the law regulating their practice. Copies of the law can be obtained from one's state nurses' association or from the state agency responsible for distribution of laws.

Appointments to a state board of nursing are frequently political appointments. Therefore, nurses need to be aware of the composition of their respective state boards and to have a voice in the selection of candidates to serve on the board. Because regulatory changes made by a state board have the same force as law, it is important to remain aware of the activities of the state board of nursing that regulates nursing practice within each state. Nurses are often unaware that changes are even being proposed until it is too late to influence them.

Levels of Political Involvement

Mason and coworkers in 1993 identified four spheres of political influence in which nurses can influence change. These are the workplace, government, professional organizations, and community (the encompassing sphere). Nurses must recognize the workplace as a significant political arena, both in terms of creating optimal working conditions and in promoting decision making that ensures high-quality patient care.

In the workplace, as in other political situations, those in power must hear nurses' opinions and those opinions must be substantiated with facts. Nurses are also more likely to be heard, and to be listened to, if they are involved and are known to the people they are trying to influence. What does this mean in practical terms? First, nurses must take an active role in institutional decision making. This may be done at the unit level or by volunteering to serve on various hospital or agency committees. Second, nurses must remain current with the trends and issues in health care and with the latest research related to the work of patient care; this assists nurses to present factual data and to contribute to policy decisions. Hospitals in recent years have also begun to establish committees dealing with legislative issues. Some of these were set up by groups of nurses and others resulted from hospital-wide involvement. Serving as members of such committees offers nurses opportunities to learn about the legislative process and to contribute to this process. Finally, nurses must be a positive force for change and be assertive in making their opinions known. This is most easily done through fostering good interpersonal relationships and by learning as much as possible about the views of co-workers and those in positions of higher authority.

These principles of institutional politics are relevant at all levels of political involvement. The late Speaker of the U.S. House of Representatives, Thomas P. (Tip) O'Neill, Jr., is frequently quoted as saying "all politics is local." Sharp (1994) points out that Mr. O'Neill looked like the "man next door" in the working-class neighborhood where he lived and worked and that much of his power was based on personal relationships.

Considering this perspective, it makes sense for nurses to become involved in issues directly affecting their work, their profession, and their personal lives. An oncology nurse, for example, may choose to lobby for a bill that provides increased funding for cancer research at the state or federal level. In the workplace, nurses may become involved on committees or task forces seeking to institute alternate delivery patterns such as patient-focused care or may become members of a management team, to investigate a shared governance model.

At the local level, nurses' involvement again can be directed toward something that has meaning for them personally. Nurse activist Terri Swearingen has become nationally known for her work, which literally began in her backyard. Terri has been a key leader of a grassroots effort against the construction and operation of a hazardous waste incinerator which is only 2 miles from her home in Chester, West Virginia, and more importantly for her, only 1100 feet from an elementary school. Her passion about this issue stemmed from her concern for the children of the community and was based on her nursing knowledge of potential health hazards. Her commitment began when she read about the amount of lead the planned incinerator would be permitted to emit. Her efforts, and years of work, have led her from being an average citizen to being recognized nationwide, with appearances on television on *Nightline* and *60 Minutes*, among other programs. Although she has often been arrested, she was able to persuade the U.S. Congress to hold its first public hearing regarding the Environmental Protection Agency's favorable treatment of industries it was supposed to regulate. This resulted in an admission that the EPA was uncertain about the safety of hazardous waste incineration and led to an 18-month moratorium on construction (Hopey, 1994). Clearly, not every nurse can devote as many years to a cause as Terri Swearingen has done, but there are many ways for nurses to become involved on the local level.

Nurses who have children in school may choose to run for elected positions on the school board in order to influence decisions affecting their children. Others may simply become involved by attending meetings to voice their concerns. Nurses can have a powerful influence in their communities. Something as simple as recognizing the hazards of a dangerous traffic intersection and working with a borough or township to install a stop sign there may save lives.

The experience of one nurse called to the home of a neighbor who had suffered cardiac arrest demonstrates how nurses can spark changes that protect the health of the community. After she had arrived at the victim's home and had begun initiating CPR, the nurse learned that it was necessary for the local police to certify that an emergency actually existed before 911 emergency medical system calls were activated. When two police officers arrived, only one, who had been trained to provide CPR, was able to relieve the nurse.

This episode raised two issues, which the nurse brought to the attention of the mayor and borough council. First, precious time was lost in treating this individual (over 20 minutes elapsed between the time the police arrived and paramedics reached the scene). Second, the local borough had not provided appropriate emergency response training for their police force. By raising this important issue and working with local officials, the nurse was subsequently able to influence the decision to allow emergency calls to go directly into the 911 system. The borough also began to provide more extensive emergency preparedness training for their police officers in case the police were the first to respond at the scene of an accident or illness.

Nurses are often most active at the state level. For example, states where third-party reimbursement laws were passed to enable nurses to bill insurance carriers directly clearly had a cadre of organized nurses working very hard to advance this important issue. At the state level, individual nurses or a nursing organization can introduce a piece of legislation and seek a sponsor and co-sponsors for the proposed law. Once the legislation is introduced, they must lobby other legislators to support their initiative by providing facts about its benefits, particularly how it will benefit the legislator's constituents. Again, as in the workplace or organizations, establishing a personal relationship with a legislator is a vital part of the political process. Legislators recognize that nurses have expertise about the unique needs of clients (who are also constituents of their district) and of health care delivery. Nothing is more powerful than an anecdotal "human interest" story about a particular client or family in the legislator's district to help the legislator understand the importance of a piece of legislation or the need for increased funding for a certain program. The input of nurses is vital to legislators because few of them have a health care background. In fact, the only experience they may have is the personal knowledge of having been a client, or the views which they may have gained from a relative or friend who is a health professional. If these views are negative, the interests of nursing may not be served.

During 1995, approximately 45 nurses served in state legislatures and one nurse served at the federal level. Although it is rare to find other health care professionals serving in elected positions, things are beginning to change. There has, for example, been a dramatic increase in the number of physicians running for public office since President Clinton introduced health care reform to the national agenda. It is becoming more common to see more nurses elected to leadership positions and appointed to serve on boards at the state government level, but there is a great need to increase the numbers who are willing and prepared to serve in these roles. Often it is through involvement at the local level, such as working the polls on election day or serving in a position at the district or ward level, that nurses gain experience to move on to state level positions.

At the federal level, nurses' influence can help promote or defeat legislation or to help maintain funding for particular purposes, such as nursing education. At this level of government, it is especially important for nursing organizations to speak with a unified voice in presenting their nursing concerns. Although specialty groups may have their own particular needs, it can be detrimental to the cause for legislators to sense dissension among groups within the same profession because it diminishes the groups' power and credibility. Nurses should remain knowledgeable about the positions set forth by the professional organizations on issues that are likely to come before the Congress, should learn who the key legislators and their assistants are, and should communicate regularly about matters of concern.

THE STRUCTURE AND FUNCTION OF GOVERNMENT

In order to participate most effectively in the political process, it is essential to understand the structure of government at each level. Because government structures may vary with location throughout the country, each nurse should become familiar with the particular local governing body.

County government generally takes one of the following forms: board of supervisors, elected board of commissioners, county executive or county manager, or mixed county board (Majewski, 1993). City government forms include: mayor-council, council-manager, mayor-manager, or commissioner(s). Towns, boroughs, or villages also have a variety of elected officials similar to those of county government. School districts may also be regarded as governmental units, if their budgets are not tied to a longer municipal budget (Majewski, 1993). It is probably easiest for nurses to exert influence at this level because the issues addressed are those which that most directly affect their lives. They are also more likely to know the elected officials at this level. They may even be neighbors, members of the same club or religious organization, or colleagues of those serving in political office. Nurses should learn the names of elected officials and current officeholders in order to track their positions on various matters, especially those that pertain to the health of the community. This information can usually be obtained by calling one's city or town clerk, a county elections bureau, or the League of Women Voters.

Each branch of government plays a significant role in the development and implementation of health policy. The federal government and most state governments have three branches; the legislative, executive, and judicial. At the federal level, the executive branch includes the President, the cabinet governmental departments, and regulatory agencies. The executive branch is responsible for the administration of government and its laws. Additionally, the president sets the legislative agenda for Congress and a budget for the nation. The legislative branch includes the two houses of Congress and is responsible for lawmaking, representation, and administrative oversight (i.e., overseeing the agencies of the executive branch and providing their funding). The judicial branch includes the Supreme Court, which interprets the law.

Although nurses are most often involved with the legislative branch of government, the executive branch can also be of great importance to nursing and health care. The President's budget influences the monies available for health care and for nursing education, and the agenda set by the President determines what programs have a high priority for the administration. The President can also recommend legislation and can approve or veto legislation passed by Congress. It is also in the executive branch where appointments to government departments, volunteer boards, or committees are made.

The Congress of the United States receives its mandate from the U.S. Constitution. The Congress is bicameral, meaning that it is composed of two bodies. These are the Senate and the House of Representatives. In the smaller chamber (Senate), each state is equally represented; there are 100 Senators, two from each state. Senators are elected for 6-year terms. In order to provide stability, Senate terms are staggered so that every 2 years a third of the Senate is up for re-election. Members of the House of Representatives, called Congressmen or Congresswomen, are selected according to the population of each state as determined by the U.S. Census. Thus, more heavily populated states have a greater number of representatives, which may change with population growth or decline. There are 435 congressional representatives, with each one representing approximately 517,000 constituents. Terms of office are for 2 years, and every congressional representative must seek re-election every 2 years. The qualifications of those running for the House and Senate include age, U.S. citizenship, and place of residency. A summary of facts about the U.S. Congress is presented in Figure 11–1.

State government structures are similar to those described at the federal level, and also derive their powers from the U.S. Constitution. Most states have bicameral legislatures. State senators are generally elected to 4-year terms, and lower chamber legislators are elected for 2-year terms. As at the federal level, it is important for nurses to learn who the legislators are for their districts and to communicate with them regularly.

It is also important to understand the powers of the governor of each particular state. In some states, members of the state board of nursing, or other important health commissions, are appointed by the governor. As with the President, the governor can sign legislation into law and use the power of the veto.

	SENATE	HOUSE OF REPRESENTATIVES
NUMBER	100 Senators (2 from each state) Equal representation	Congress persons (435 members)* Representation based on population of each state
TERMS	Elected for term of 6 years	Elected for term of 2 years
RE-ELECTION	Every 2 years, one third of senators face re-election	Entire membership is up for re-election every 2 years
QUALIFICATIONS	30 years of age Citizen of U.S. for 9 years Resident of the state represented when elected	25 years of age Citizen of U.S. for 7 years Resident of the state represented when elected

* The House also includes delegates from the District of Columbia, Guam, the Virgin Islands, and American Samoa, and the resident commissioner from Puerto Rico.

FIGURE 11–1. U.S. Congress.

HOW LAWS ARE MADE

The idea for a law may originate with an individual concerned citizen, with a professional group such as the American Nurses Association (ANA) or the National League for Nursing (NLN), with a legislator, or with the executive branch (the President or governor). The bill is authored or sponsored by either a representative or a senator, who introduces it after it is written in suitable legislative language by the legislative counsel of either the House or the Senate. At the federal level, bills are referred to full committee and, generally, because of the enormous number of bills being introduced, to a subcommittee. It is within the committee structures that most of the work of Congress takes place. Committee action is perhaps the most important phase of the Congressional process, for this is where the most intensive consideration is given to proposed measures and where people are provided with an opportunity to be heard. The subcommittee studies the issue carefully, holds hearings, and reports the bill back to the full committee with recommendations. There are numerous standing committees in the House and Senate. In addition, there are several select committees and several standing joint committees. Each committee has jurisdiction over certain subjects, and often has two or more subcommittees. In the U.S. Congress, the committees with greatest jurisdiction over health matters and their subcommittees are:

1 *House Ways and Means Committee*: Social Security and Medicare (health subcommittees).
2 *House Commerce Committee*: Health legislation including Medicaid (Subcommittee on Health and the Environment).

3 *Senate Finance Committee*: Medicare and Medicaid (health subcommittees).

4 *Senate Labor and Human Resources Committee*: Health legislation in general; it also works cooperatively with Senate Finance Committee in considering issues involving Medicare and Medicaid.

5 *House and Senate Appropriations Committee*: Authorizes all money necessary to implement action proposed in a bill (Subcommittees for Labor, Education, and Health and Human Services).

As a result of full committee hearings, several things may happen to a bill:

- It may be reported out of committee favorably and be scheduled for debate by the full House or Senate.
- It may be reported out favorably, but with amendments.
- The bill may be reported out unfavorably, or killed outright.

After a bill has been reported out of a House committee (with the exception of Ways and Means or Appropriations Committees) it goes to the Rules Committee, which schedules bills and determines how much time will be spent on debate and whether or not amendments will be allowed. In the Senate, bills go on the Senate calendar, after which the majority leadership determines when a bill will be debated. After a bill is debated, possibly amended, and passed by one chamber, it is sent to the other chamber, where it goes through the same procedure. If the bill passes both the House and the Senate without any changes, it is sent to the President for his signature.

If the House and Senate pass different versions of a bill, however, the two bills are sent to a Conference Committee, composed of members appointed by both the House and the Senate. This committee seeks to resolve differences between the two bills; if the differences cannot be resolved, the bill dies in committee. After the Conference Committee reaches agreement on a bill, it goes back to the House and Senate for passage. At this juncture, the bill must be voted up or down, because no further amendments are accepted. If the bill is approved in both houses, it then goes to the President. If the President signs the bill, it becomes a law. If vetoed, it is sent back to the House and Senate. In order to override the veto, a two-thirds vote by both chambers is required.

Clearly, the passage of a law can be a long and difficult process. This is often quite frustrating for "action-oriented" nurses who are used to seeing immediate outcomes, forming plans, and making things happen. Nevertheless, nurses can and do play a significant role at several points in the legislative process (Fig. 11–2).

Nurses can influence the introduction of a bill as private citizens or as members of a professional organization. They can provide information to assist in drafting the bill and work to gather support from members of Congress on the proposed legislation. During committee or subcommittee hearings, nurses may provide testimony to inform committee members about their position. Nurses may also actively work to influence (lobby) the views of congressional members, both when they are in their home district or in Washington,

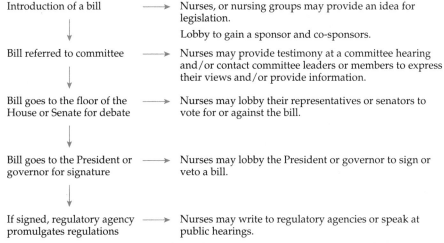

Introduction of a bill   ⟶   Nurses, or nursing groups may provide an idea for legislation.

Lobby to gain a sponsor and co-sponsors.

Bill referred to committee   ⟶   Nurses may provide testimony at a committee hearing and/or contact committee leaders or members to express their views and/or provide information.

Bill goes to the floor of the   ⟶   Nurses may lobby their representatives or senators to
House or Senate for debate   vote for or against the bill.

Bill goes to the President or   ⟶   Nurses may lobby the President or governor to sign or
governor for signature   veto a bill.

If signed, regulatory agency   ⟶   Nurses may write to regulatory agencies or speak at
promulgates regulations   public hearings.

FIGURE 11–2. How nurses may make an impact on the legislative process (at both the state and federal levels).

D.C. (or the state capitol). Finally, they may attempt to influence the President or governor, using telegrams, letters, and phone calls to either sign or veto the legislation.

After a law is passed, it is assigned to the appropriate department of the executive branch of government, which begins the process of regulation. The regulation-writing process includes study of the law and drafting and publishing regulations for implementation. Again, nurses can influence these regulations by writing letters to the regulatory agency or by speaking at public hearings. Clearly, nurses can do a great deal to help shape public health policy. If we as nurses fail to become involved in this process, however, others will simply determine policy for us.

GAINING SKILL IN POLITICS

In order to become politically astute, it is necessary to understand the political process and become convinced that although you may not always be satisfied with the way the system works, you can work to make significant changes (Winter, 1991). Figure 11–3 lists actions for becoming more involved.

Chalich and Smith in 1992 offered a model for individual political development that encourages grassroots involvement in local issues. As a nurse-activist herself, Chalich contends that whereas some involvement in partisan politics may be desirable, grassroots efforts may be more fulfilling and should certainly not be discounted. This model is an activity-oriented ladder, including activities at four distinct levels:

1. Register to vote, or if registered, encourage others to become registered. (It has been said that our nation is second only to the tiny African nation of Botswana in voter apathy.)
2. Learn who your legislators and other elected or appointed officials are at local, state, and national levels.
   (A phone call to the League of Women Voters or your county elections office will provide this much-needed information. For listings of local officials call your city or town clerk.) Be aware of the composition of your State Board of Nursing, and its influence on policy decisions affecting the profession.
3. Meet your legislators in their home district even if only to pick up information and become acquainted with the staff.
   (Legislators want to hear the concerns of their nurse constituents, and most will regard you as the credible professional that you are. Establishing personal relationships is an important step in building rapport.)
4. Call or write to elected officials or legislators on issues important to nursing and health.
   (Remember you are the expert when it comes to nursing and patient care, and legislators need to know what is actually happening in the practice area in order to make sound decisions in casting votes.)
5. Be informed about legislation and policy decisions that have important consequences for nursing or those for whom we care.
   (For national issues be certain to read the Political Nurse column in The American Nurse, the news section of the American Journal of Nursing, or the legislative commentaries in Nursing and Health Care.) State nurse's associations often publish a legislative bulletin or summary of bills in their publications, and many specialty groups also have government relations committees publishing information of current nursing issues.
6. Join and become involved in the professional nursing organizations. (Every nurse should consider belonging to one of the major nursing organizations and one specialty group. It is our profession and we must support it with our money and our efforts.)

FIGURE 11–3. How nurses can become more politically involved.

Rung 1—CIVIC INVOLVEMENT: Children's sports, PTA, neighborhood improvement group

Rung 2—ADVOCACY: Writing letters to public officials and newspapers and making organized visits to officials on local issues

Rung 3—ORGANIZING: Independent organizing on local issues, incorporation of single-issue citizens' groups, and networking with similarly situated citizen's groups

Rung 4—LONG-TERM POWER WIELDING: Campaigning for oneself or another, local government planning, and agenda setting

In order to be involved in the political process, nurses must know and understand the issues. At times an issue may be readily apparent in the nurses' community, for example an increased number of homeless people. Other issues are easily identified by reading newspapers. Issues are generally presented in the editorial section; most newspapers also have a political watch section, which reports the results of any significant votes at the State and Federal level.

The ANA newspaper, *The American Nurse*, is an excellent source of information on issues of concern to the profession. In addition, the *American Journal of Nursing* "Newsline" feature and *Nursing and Health Care's* "Washington Focus" serve as excellent, easily readable sources of information in journals. *Capitol Update*, the ANA legislative newsletter for nurses, reports on the activities of its nurse lobbyists and on significant issues in the congress and regulatory agencies. This publication requires a subscription but is available in most nursing school and hospital libraries.

State nurses' associations and many speciality nursing groups also publish newsletters or legislative bulletins. Many of these are free to members but may be sent only when requested. When one is a member of a nursing organization, *Action Alerts* may also be sent to inform members of vital issues and the action needed by nurses.

COMMUNICATING WITH LEGISLATORS

Nurses must establish a personal relationship with legislators and their legislative aides whenever possible. Although nurses may initially be hesitant or even a little fearful about approaching politicians, it is important to remember that these officials are elected to serve. Many elected officials have little, if any, background in health care matters. Therefore, a nurse's offer to serve as a personal resource is frequently welcomed by the legislator and the legislator's staff. This is particularly true at the local and state levels, where legislators may not have extensive staff to serve as legislative aides for legislation involving health care concerns. Writing a letter or stopping by a legislator's office to introduce oneself as a constituent and as a nurse and asking to be notified as matters related to health care arise (or volunteering to serve as a resource to secure information when needed) is a good way to become known and to increase nursing's visibility. Legislators *do* want to hear from nurses.

Lobbying

Sometimes communications with legislators take the form of lobbying. **Lobbying** may be defined as attempting to persuade someone (usually a legislator or legislative aide) of the rightness of one's cause or as an attempt to influence legislation. Lobbying methods include: letter writing, face-to-face communication or telephone calls, mailgrams, telegrams, or E-mail, letters to the editor, and providing testimony (verbal or written).

Guidelines for letter writing are presented in Figure 11–4. In order to lobby effectively, one should be both persuasive and able to negotiate. Lobbying is truly an art of communication, an area in which nurses are highly skilled. Before beginning any lobbying effort, it is vital to gather all pertinent facts. In politics, getting the facts and laying the groundwork are analogous to developing a nursing care plan. Before visiting or writing a legislator to gather facts, delineate a problem or concern you wish to discuss, and develop a plan to articulate your concerns. Determine a method for evaluating your effectiveness.

1. Write on your personal stationery if expressing your own views.
2. A handwritten letter is acceptable, and often preferred provided that it is legible.
3. Be certain that your name and address are on both the letter and envelope.
4. Identify yourself as a nurse or nursing student.
5. A legislator is referred to as "The Honorable" on the envelope and inside address (The Honorable Jane Doe) and in the salutation as "Dear Senator" or "Dear Representative."
6. Limit your letter to one subject.
7. Identify the specific issue or request. Include the bill number (e.g., H.R. 19) or Senate Bill 25 (S. 25), if known, or the intent of the bill.
8. Be brief. Limit your letter to one page, if possible; two at the most.
9. Be specific. Provide facts and figures to support your views or give anecdotal data on how your clients or families have been or may be affected. (Let them know what you want—vote for or against—oppose or support certain amendments.)
10. Emphasize needs or the positive or negative impact of proposed legislation and what the proposed legislation will mean to the legislator's constituents in terms of health care.
11. Be polite and reasonable. A positive-sounding letter is usually an effective tool even when asking your legislator to oppose a piece of legislation.
12. Write to thank legislators who supported your wishes or who have supported nurses in some manner.

Letters will reach legislators if addressed as follows:

FEDERAL LEVEL
The Honorable ————————————
United States Senate
Washington, DC 20510

The Honorable ————————————
House of Representatives
Washington, DC 20510

If you know the room number and building, the correspondence will arrive faster. You can call the official's local office to obtain this information.
To write to the President of the United States:

The Honorable ————————————
President of the United States
Washington, DC 20500

FIGURE 11–4. Guidelines for letter writing.

If the plan is to visit the legislator's office, an appointment should be set up in advance. Often the meeting may actually be with the legislative aide, particularly at the federal level. This should not be discouraging because this is the individual who is often responsible for assisting in the development of position statements and offering committee amendments for the legislator.

To ensure that legislators listen to your concerns, it is important not only to be well prepared but to show that others support your position. When one person speaks, legislators *may* listen, but when many people voice the same concern, legislators are much more likely to pay attention. This is one very important reason to join professional nursing organizations. Only through unified efforts will nurses be seen as a powerful group and only then will nursing's voice be recognized in the policy arena.

Increasing Your Power Through Professional Organizations

Although nurses are the largest group of health care providers in the United States (approximately 2 million practitioners), they have not historically been seen as powerful. Thus, they have not played a role proportionate to their size in shaping health care policy even though that policy profoundly affects them both as providers and consumers.

Nurses have always had a great deal of potential power (by virtue of numbers) but have only begun to actualize this power. One example of the exercise of this power was illustrated by the significant influence of organized nursing in advancing the concepts of the publication *Nursing's Agenda for Health Care Reform* with the Clinton Administration. This agenda, developed by the two major nursing organizations (ANA and NLN) and supported by approximately 58 specialty-nursing organizations, contained many of the provisions ultimately included in the Clinton proposal. According to ANA President Virginia Trotter Betts, this was perhaps the first time in history that nursing was included at the health care policy table along with corporate heads and other key leaders. Other major victories for nursing have been gained through the lobbying efforts and unified positions of nursing. Examples of nursing's ability to make a difference include the defeat of the Registered Care Technologist (RCT) proposal advanced by the American Medical Association (AMA) and the cancellation of the television program *The Nightingales*. The latter portrayed nurses in a negative light, and the RCT proposal suggested that physicians educate and supervise technicians to help nurses.

The AMA's announcement of their RCT proposal to establish a new level of health care worker, intended to help nurses and to alleviate a nursing shortage, prompted a prompt and unified response from the nursing community. The major nursing organizations opposed the plan as unnecessary, duplicative, and potentially unsafe. Concerns were also raised about legal liability as related to use of RCTs. Nursing summit meetings were convened by the Tri-Council for Nursing to develop strategies to address the nursing shortage by providing nursing solutions.

In 1994, through the efforts of the ANA Strategic Action Team (N-STAT), nurses scored a major legislative success, turning a potentially close vote on direct Medicare reimbursement in the Senate Finance Committee into a unanimous victory. This was accomplished by the grassroots lobbying efforts of nurses, which generated thousands of phone calls and fax messages to committee members (N-STAT, 1994). This is the type of lobbying effort that legislators understand and respond to. These examples show how powerful nurses can be when they join, support, and really become involved in their professional associations. All nurses should join one of the major professional organizations, as well as a specialty organization. This is vital because we need information about our chosen speciality and the opportunity to lobby for its specific issues but we must also invest our money, time, and efforts to advance and protect our profession. Too much time has been wasted with nurses fighting one another. This not only diminishes credibility in the policy area but also shifts the power to others.

Through the efforts of nursing organizations, professional nurse lobbyists have increased visibility on Capitol Hill and in state legislatures in recent years (Goldwater, 1990). The ANA has several nurse lobbyists working at the federal level and a significant number of their constituent state organizations (SNAs) also hire professional lobbyists. Money from dues-paying members allows such services to be offered to the profession.

Although ANA has the largest governmental affairs office, many other national nursing organizations also have professional lobbyists, and some nurses lobby for businesses that have health care interests (Goldwater, 1990). The legislative or political arm of the ANA is known as the Department of Governmental Affairs. In addition to its lobbying activities, it promulgates legislative and regulatory initiatives for each session of Congress. This department also contains the Political Action Unit, which is made up of the grassroots lobbying network, which functions through the activities of Congressional District Coordinators and Senate Coordinators, and the ANA Political Action Committee (ANA-PAC).

Political Action Committees (PACs)

It is a political reality that legislators are more likely to see and to hear from a group of people who have contributed to their campaign through political action committees. The American Nurses Association formed a political action committee in order to create power and influence for the nursing profession. Nurses who contribute to ANA-PAC donate because they want access to the policy makers who will work on advancing nursing practice and on promoting quality client care in the legislative arena. The PAC raises money from voluntary contributions (dues money may not be used for this purpose) to support candidates and officeholders who are concerned about nursing issues. As Curtis and Lumpkin pointed out in 1993:

> PACs and lobbyists serve different functions. Lobbyists persuade public officials to work for legislation that nurses consider important. Primarily they try to convince those already serving in public office. PACs work to influence the outcome of elections. By endorsing candidates and contributing time and money, nurses can help elect to office and keep in place public officials who support their point of view (Curtis, 1993).

A distinction must be made between "special interest" and "monied interest" PACs. The latter type has received adverse publicity because of the large sums of money given to legislators by groups who influence an issue by wielding lobby power through donating money. A recent example of this inflated PAC spending was the millions of dollars that the insurance companies gave members of Congress during debate on reform of the health care industry. Their lobbying goal was to further the financial needs of the companies, in comparison with the American Nurses Association, which was lobbying Congress for a universal health care program that would benefit all citizens. Large PAC donations cannot be comprehended by the average voter whose wages have not kept pace with the rising cost of living. There is a belief that money will buy a legislator's vote—this is where confusion arises over the value of PACs.

Special-interest PACs are organized according to conservative or liberal ideologies or according to trade associations (e.g., labor, teachers', environmental, and women's groups). These groups are representatives of an egalitarian society participating in the most current democratic process: contributing to political action committees. Voluntary financial donations to political campaigns require rigid reporting and disclosure requirements and cannot be taken out of the members' dues or the association's treasury. The money given to PACs is legally required to be kept in a separate account.

Political Nursing Networks and Coalitions

Various nursing and other grassroots networks have been established to provide for lobbying efforts to support the legislative goals and objectives of the state nurses' associations. In Pennsylvania, for example, the Pennsylvania Political Nursing Network (PPNN), as a part of the Government Relations Committee of the Pennsylvania Nursing Association (PNA) encourages nurses throughout the state to participate in the political process by serving as key contacts for their own legislators. These nurses have an opportunity to practice lobbying skills and to educate legislators about nursing issues. The membership of the network is depicted in Figure 11–5, which shows the channels of communication to be used when nurses need to respond to a key issue. One of the challenges with such a network is the effort needed to recruit and maintain contacts for each legislator or legislative district. Other nursing networks may include nursing groups from a variety of settings as well as clinical specialty groups.

The Arizona Nursing Network, established in 1978, is an example of such a network. Bagwell (1984), who was responsible for its design, stated its basic

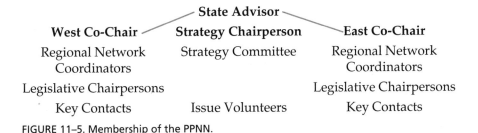

POLITICAL NURSING NETWORK

State Advisor
West Co-Chair   Strategy Chairperson   East Co-Chair
Regional Network   Strategy Committee   Regional Network
Coordinators   Coordinators
Legislative Chairpersons   Legislative Chairpersons
Key Contacts   Issue Volunteers   Key Contacts

FIGURE 11–5. Membership of the PPNN.

functions as follows: (1) to disseminate information and educate nurses about health legislation, (2) to increase the political awareness of nurses, (3) to encourage nurses to participate in the legislative process, and (4) to promote and support the advancement of nursing through the legislative process. These functions are still applicable today. As nurses (and nursing organizations) have become more sophisticated and have moved into a new age of technology, however, networks are also changing. The N-STAT, for example, was formed as ANA's grassroots rapid action network to send a strong message to Congress about health care reform. In addition to traditional methods of lobbying, faxed information and E-mail have been added to the nurse's repertoire.

Coalitions often result from networking. When one organization or group does not have sufficient power to make its voice heard, it may join with others who subscribe to similar goals. A coalition may be described as a temporary alliance of distinct groups or factions who act together in support of a common goal. An example of an effective coalition is provided by the example of nurse and community activist Theresa Chalich, founder and director of the Rainbow Clinic, a free primary-care clinic located in Homestead, Pennsylvania. Chalich mobilized seniors and other groups around a significant Medicare issue.

Coalition Building: In Numbers There Is Strength

A coalition that is united on a common issue increases the effectiveness of the group's work. In many cases, economic, environmental, and political restraints have brought together individuals and groups into collaborative formation: a pooling together of personal, organizational, and financial resources. An example of effective coalition building was the alliance formed for the passage of the Medicare Overcharge Measure in the Pennsylvania General Assembly in 1990. Senior citizens, as Medicare recipients, would benefit directly from the legislation. If passed, the legislation would mandate that a doctor would have to accept the assigned Medicare payment and could not require the senior citizen to pay out-of-pocket expenses toward the balance of the bill. The coalition was composed of grassroots senior-citizen groups and AARP chapters, labor unions, nurses, public interest groups, and elected public officials.

Each organization brought to this state-wide coalition its own particular assets and in the course of the work developed its own distinctive role. The senior-citizen groups were the backbone of this coalition because they provided the large numbers of people needed to influence Pennsylvania lawmakers. They organized their members to lobby their legislators through letter writing, phone calls, and bus trips. They also gave personal testimony about their inflated medical costs that resulted from Medicare overcharge payments. The senior groups were able to fill the buses for the many lobbying trips made to the state capital in Harrisburg.

The planning meetings were conducted in the offices of the various public-interest groups throughout the state. These groups offered their leadership and organizations as well as office equipment, such as telephones and photocopying machines. In these offices press releases and public service announcements (PSAs) were written and public hearings were organized.

The labor unions contributed by providing to the coalition their union halls for the public hearings. They also were the financial backers of these hearings and the lobbying bus trips. The politicians who represented areas heavily populated with senior citizens were able to present official testimony at public hearings and during the state lobbying sessions. Several of the elected officials also financed the bus trips. The nurses who worked in the coalition offered organizational, as well as leadership, skills to this movement. Because nurses are perceived to have moral authority, senior citizens appreciated their concern for this health care issue. Nurses believe that lack of finances directly affects client-care outcomes; they felt the involvement of this coalition was an extension of providing comprehensive care. They also viewed Medicare Overcharge Measure legislation as an effective strategy for health care cost containment.

In addition to supporting this particular legislation, each collaborating organization also worked on advancing its own agenda. Labor unions were concerned about economic issues for their retired members. The nurses joined because they wanted a constituency group, such as senior citizens, to understand that nurses have an interest in the lives of the elderly outside a hospital. The politicians assumed a political liability with groups opposed to this proposed legislation but also appreciated the possibility of losing a large percentage of senior citizen votes in their respective districts.

The Medicare Overcharge Measure coalition is an example of sustained, organized effort of approximately 10 years. Coalition work can last for any length of time depending on the group's activity and outcomes.

NURSES IN ELECTED OR APPOINTED POSITIONS

In order to increase the power base of nursing, it is essential that more nurses enter the political arena in positions that permit them to participate directly in health care policy decision making. Aburdene and Naisbitt in *Megatrends for Women* question what benefits women might reap by taking on the added burdens of responsibility and leadership. They conclude, "The answer is simple: the power to create, not just influence, the world in which they live." Much of nursing's lack of power is ascribed to its history as a profession predominantly composed of women. As they assume more power, they become part of the megatrend moving from liberation to leadership.

Nurses' grassroots involvement in community affairs (the local PTA, school boards, city or township planning commission, League of Women Voters, or a political party) often provides the skills necessary to run for elected office. Barbara Hafer, a registered nurse *and* Auditor General of the state of Pennsylvania, began her involvement in government when, working for a county rape crisis

ISSUES IN PRACTICE
How Do Politics Affect You and Your Family?

Why should nurses be involved in politics? Does it really make a difference who is elected and who makes the laws? Take a minute to go through the questions below and check the items that you think may be affected by politics.

Between the time you wake up and the time you leave the house several things usually happen to you. Do you think any of the following subjects are affected by politics?

☐ The water with which you wash your face and brush your teeth.
☐ The electricity that lights the room.
☐ The price and quality of food you have for breakfast.
☐ The safety of the products you buy.

As the average person's lifespan grows longer and the retirement age is lowered, these latter years become more meaningful. Are any of the following decisions affected by our political systems?

☐ The age at which you can retire.
☐ The income you get during retirement.
☐ The quality and cost of health care.
☐ The life expectancy of each of us.

We value our leisure time and the chance to get away from it all. Are any of the following areas affected by politics?

☐ The parks and lakes where vacationers fish and swim.
☐ The air you breathe.
☐ The radio and television programs that entertain you.

---

center, she became involved in a commission to study home rule for Allegheny County. She subsequently made a successful bid for County Commissioner of Allegheny County and served in that capacity for 6 years before being elected Auditor General. Hafer also ran for Governor of Pennsylvania during her political career. She frequently speaks of the fact that her nursing skills and knowledge have served her well during her political career. By virtue of their education, nurses do possess the necessary interpersonal and problem-solving skills to participate in the health care policy arena. Nurses are also generally well thought of by the public. In Auditor General Hafer's case, an uncomplimentary comment by a physician opponent actually helped her to win her first election by rallying the voters to support her.

Marilyn Goldwater, in recounting her success in being elected to the Maryland state legislature, recalls that her activity began with an active role in the PTA, which led to increasing community involvement. This was followed by her joining the League of Women Voters and active involvement in her local Democratic Party Organization (Goldwater, 1990).

A Closer Look

RUSHED HOME FROM THE HOSPITAL, A NEWBORN GETS OFF TO A BUMPY START

A few weeks ago, my sister had a baby. That's the good news. The bad news is that the baby was sent home with an undetected infection the day after she was born.

Within days, the baby was rushed back to the hospital and placed in intensive care, where a tube pumped antibiotics into a vein in her head.

Doctors diagnosed her condition and prescribed 10 days in the hospital. However, she was discharged after five because she was getting better.

So my sister took her baby home with an IV tube still pumping medicine into her head—and with the job of scheduling nurses to visit four times a day.

Enter the insurance company. They balked at paying the bill for visiting nurses and told my exhausted sister that she should care for the baby herself: that a nurse would teach her how to drip exact amounts of antibiotics into the IV, to flush and clean the tube, to check the baby for signs of dehydration, jaundice and weight loss.

No, my sister said frantically. I'm an English professor, not a nurse.

The insurance company persisted, arguing that these procedures were simple. My sister wouldn't give in.

Finally she won—if you can call it that. Nurses came to the house four times a day. The baby's IV tube dripped and leaked, jammed and had to be replaced. Nurses drew blood from the baby's head to dissolve air bubbles in the new tube.

So much for simple procedures.

Fortunately, the baby recovered and is doing well. Unfortunately, my sister's horror tale is not unique.

Everywhere, patients are increasingly being jeopardized as insurance companies decide how much and what kind of health care to reimburse.

These days the bottom line is the dollar sign—not the patient's well-being. And so, new mothers and fragile newborns are sent home 24 hours after delivery.

I know of one woman who gave birth five minutes before midnight and was ordered home the next day by her insurance company even though anesthesia had made her violently ill. Her doctor prescribed an additional night's stay, but the insurance company refused.

Increasingly, such stories are commonplace. In fact, my sister's tale was topped by those of friends who told of being sent home hours after surgery. Sore and groggy, they were discharged with raw stitches and oozing wounds—and with no one at home to provide trained care.

Continued on following page

RUSHED HOME FROM THE HOSPITAL, A NEWBORN GETS OFF TO A BUMPY START (Continued)

Matters are getting worse. As hospitals try to save money, they are replacing registered nurses with nursing aides, which means a serious decline in the quality of care.

And as insurance companies go about lowering costs, they are ejecting patients from hospitals far too soon. In some cases, they are even rationing care.

For instance, if you need cataract surgery, most insurance companies will pay for the removal of only one cataract unless you're young or need both eyes for work.

Those opposed to health-care reform warn about the dangers of rationed care. Well, I've got news for them. We already have rationed care in this country.

Insurance companies decide whether you qualify for surgery and how long you stay in the hospital. They determine if you're eligible for certain medical treatments—not your doctor.

We're in a crisis. Insurance company and health-care executives must start putting patients' well-being above profits.

Ironically, such a shift makes economic sense.

If my sister had stayed in the hospital a few more days, her baby's illness would likely have been diagnosed. If the hospital had not reduced registered nurses the week she gave birth, one of them might've noticed something wrong.

But no one did—so the insurance company ended up paying for five days in intensive care and five days of home health care.

Even worse, my sister and her new baby got off to an unnecessarily bumpy start.

Reprinted with permission from Steenland, S.: Rushed home from the hospital, a newborn gets off to a bumpy start. Philadelphia Inquirer, April 10, 1995, page B30.

There is nothing magical about political involvement. It is simply a matter of hard work and use of the critical thinking skills possessed by nurses. It is clear, however, that nurses can and do make a difference in the political arena. Nurses must ask how and where they can make a difference and how they can become involved in the process. Not every nurse may choose to run for political office, but each nurse can make a contribution. It is vitally important that nurses use their voices and individual power to empower nurse and nursing.

AS JOB LOSSES MOUNT, MASSACHUSETTS RNS KICK OFF CAMPAIGN FOR "SAFE CARE"

Boston, MA—What would happen if nurses got mad enough to say they wouldn't put up with it anymore?

Massachusetts hospitals may be about to find out. The Massachusetts Nurses Association is launching a "Safe Care Campaign" with town meetings across the state to alert the public to the dangers of understaffing.

MNA's board acted after a town hall-style meeting in Boston. More than 200 nurses turned out to testify about short-staffing, new moves to shorten length of stay, and the proliferation of unlicensed personnel.

The same concerns are spelled out in a new study of how the state's nurses are feeling the impact of work redesign.

Responding to a survey by Boston College Prof. Judith Shindul-Rothschild, an overwhelming majority of 858 randomly selected nurses said their hospitals had undergone significant changes in structure and organization. Bed closures were reported by 82%, mergers by 54%, and acquisitions by 74%. Nearly half were seeing declines in the volume of patients.

RN positions were frozen, said 79% of the nurses. RN layoffs were common (56%) as were cuts in RN positions (75%) and cross-training programs (69%). When the study team compared the responses with a similar survey of 928 RNs in 1989, they found striking changes in the way nurses view their workplaces.

More filings of unsafe staffing forms were reported this year by 43% of the nurses, primarily those working in state, city, and county hospitals where staffing was well below the private-sector norm. Asked about quality of care in the 1989 survey, only two of 928 said they were having trouble delivering safe care.

Nearly three-quarters said this year that they were working with unlicensed assistive personnel, compared with less than a quarter who said in 1989 that their hospitals were employing UAPs. Use of per diem and agency nurses was also on the increase.

In answer to a question about patient outcomes, 15 RNs described the circumstances of a patient's death that they attributed to inadequate staffing.

When staffing was analyzed at the hospitals where the deaths occurred, it turned out they typically assigned three RNs, one LPN, two nursing assistants, and one UAP to a 17-bed unit. Average staff levels, by contrast, were five RNs one LPN, one nursing assistant, and one UAP for a 19-bed unit.

Continued on following page

AS JOB LOSSES MOUNT, MASSACHUSETTS RNS KICK OFF CAMPAIGN FOR "SAFE CARE" (Continued)

(Coincidentally, the Massachusetts Board of Medicine has released documents pointing to 497 unexplained hospital death last year.)

Some survey findings were revealed on an NBC news broadcast in September. The Massachusetts Hospital Association reacted sharply, announcing that its own data don't support the nurses' "perceptions." Despite persistent reports of hospitals restructuring with techs taking over nursing work, MHA contended there's no overall trend to replace RNs with unlicensed workers.

The hospital association conceded that a record total of more than 2,000 RN positions were eliminated last year. But the association stressed that the years from 1989 to 1993 saw declines in hospital usage across the board: 10% in their numbers, 15% in licensed beds, and 19% in patient days. Given those losses, MHA estimated that RN FTEs per 100 patients had actually grown from 135.6 in 1989 to 165.2 this year.

"That's been warranted by the increase in case mix complexity and severity," MHA spokesperson Therese Smaha told *AJN*.

Preparing last month to present her study to the American Academy of Nursing, Shindul-Rothschild stressed that all its major findings were backed by secondary data. She was "standing by" the nurses in her survey, who said they were seeing no significant differences in RN-to-patient ratios.

With all their worries, the survey group believed the quality of care had been maintained on the whole; only 3% rated it "poor." But they saw themselves coping with a continued rise in acuity linked to longer delays in admissions. And their responses showed them taking on more technical tasks and more responsibilities for supervising nonnursing personnel, for documenting, for discharge planning, and for teaching and referrals.

"Nurses judge whether a unit is safe by the intensity of care required," said Shindul-Rothschild.

"Granted, hospitals don't need nurses to take care of empty beds. But the patients are so acutely ill, and are discharged so fast, that the demands on nurses keep intensifying."

BIBLIOGRAPHY

Abdellah, FG: Nursing's Role in the Future: A Case for Health Policy Decision Making. A Case For Monograph Series. Sigma Theta Tau International Center Nursing Press, Indianapolis, 1991.

Aburdene, P and Naisbitt, J: Megatrends for Women: From Liberation to Leadership. Fawcett Columbine, New York, 1993.

American Nurses Association: Nursing Facts. American Nurses Publishing, Washington, DC, 1994.

Bagwell, MM: The politics of nursing. In Schoolcraft, V (ed): Nursing in the Community. John Wiley & Sons, New York, 1984.

Chalich, T and Smith, L: Nursing at the grassroots. Nurs Hlth Care, 13:242–244, 1992.

Curtis, B and Lumpkin, B: Political action committees. In Mason, D, Talbott, S, and Leavitt, J (eds): Policy and Politics for Nurses. WB Saunders, Philadelphia, pp 562–576.

Goldwater, M and Lloyd Zusy, MJ: Prescription for Nurses: Effective Political Action. CV Mosby, St. Louis, 1990.

Hopey, D: Close-Up. The Pittsburgh Post-Gazette, July 17, 1994, pp 3 and 11.

Kelly, L: Dimensions of Professional Nursing. Pergamon Press, New York, 1991.

Majewski, J: Local government. In Mason, D, Talbott, S and Leavitt, J (eds): Policy and Politics for Nurses. WB Saunders, Philadelphia, 1993, pp 421–432.

Mason, D, Talbott, S, and Leavitt, J (eds.): Policy and Politics for Nurses: Action and Change in the Workplace, Government, Organizations, and Community. WB Saunders, Philadelphia, 1993.

N-STAT (Nurses Strategic Action Team): Program Report: Victory in Key Committee. American Nurses Association, Washington, DC, 1994.

Pennsylvania Nurses Association: Action Plan to Immobilize PNA Nurses. Legislative Bulletin, PNA Publishing, Philadelphia, 1991.

Sharp, N: All politics is local: And other rules. Nurs Management 25:22–25, 1994.

Uhlman, M: Medical market in transition. Philadelphia Inquirer 24 July, 1994, pp A1 and A6.

Winter, K: Educating nurses in political process: A growing need. Cont Educ Nurs 22:143–146, 1991.

HISTORICAL PERSPECTIVES

Health Care and Nursing During and After World War I (1914–1918)

Although earlier wars had produced marked changes in health care, the effects of World War I (WWI) are still being felt today.

There were only about 400 nurses in the Army Nurse Corps at the beginning of the war. Through the increased number of Army hospital nursing schools, and programs* such as the Vassar Training Camp, by 1917 that number had swelled to 21,000. The American Red Cross also contributed a large number of nurses to the effort, and as many as 10,000 nurses from the United States were involved in providing nursing care to military personnel overseas.

Despite the best efforts of the nursing leaders of the time to provide high-quality nursing education for the many nurses who were being trained, many hospitals recruited untrained women to provide basic care. In response to this trend, a committee on nursing was established to set up standards, and eventually the Red Cross began a training program for nurse's aides.

This program, which taught women from all classes and education levels

---

*These were "pre-nursing" programs that taught the students basic courses such as anatomy and physiology, microbiology, epidemiology, and so on. When the students finished these programs, they could go directly into nursing schools.

how to provide basic care for the sick at home, was universally opposed by nursing leaders and nursing organizations of the time. The practice seemed to imply that, with only a minimal amount of training, anyone could be a nurse and that nursing was really a woman's job, much as housekeeping and having children were also women's work. The nurse's aide program was strongly supported by physicians.

Despite several major advancements in medical technology, particularly in the areas of anesthesia and surgery, WW I had an overall negative effect on health care in general, and on professional nursing in particular. The best efforts of the nursing leaders of the time to improve the quality of education for nurses were negated to a great degree by its dilution through the large number of nurse's aides programs that developed.

This tendency for nursing to "quick-fix" a nursing shortage situation by developing short programs with fewer educational requirements was repeated throughout the years following WW I. The nurse's aide program, initially developed to provide care in the home, was viewed by hospital administrators as a quick source of cheap labor. Nurse's aides soon began replacing trained nurses in the hospital setting.

In the years that followed WW I, nursing underwent many changes, and not all were positive. Many of the issues facing the profession today can be traced back to the years after WW I.

On the positive side, nurses began to recognize that due to their large numbers, they could, if organized, exert a significant impact on social and health care reforms. Private home care and public health nursing represented about 90% of the nursing care being provided at this time. Only about 10% of nurses worked in hospitals, which still had a reputation for being places of last resort to obtain health care. Public health nursing grew during this period, with the development of the U.S. Public Health Service, The Veterans Bureau, and the Indian Health Service. Rural areas were targeted because of the lack of quality health care available.

There was also a concurrent growth in university-based schools of nursing, but at a much reduced pace than seen during WW I. Nurses began expanding their practice to industry and other branches of the federal government besides the military.

On the negative side, many of the nurses who were trained and worked in the military services left nursing after WW I because of the poor image nursing was developing because of the widespread use of under-trained aides. This created a nursing shortage that was largely met by training more nurse's aides. Although women had gained the right to vote in 1920, nurses as a group, except for a few dedicated leaders, seemed uninterested in organizing and expanding their power base. Overall, the standards of nursing education were low and external quality controls such as licensure and accreditation were almost nonexistent. Anyone could work as a nurse so long as there was no use of the title Registered Nurse (RN).

The stock market crash of 1929 and the ensuing Great Depression sent economic ripples across the nation that had a profound effect on both health care and nursing. Many nurses who had been employed as private duty nurses by wealthy individuals lost their jobs as the funds available to pay them decreased. These private duty nurses migrated to the hospitals but found there that jobs were also scarce because the hospitals tended to use their own students as free labor, and nurse's aides as cheap labor. Many nurses ended up working for room and board just to have a place to sleep and eat. Nursing was viewed as a female occupation, and men were not admitted to nursing schools. The money for college-based nursing programs had also dried up, and many schools of nursing closed. What few remained open had difficulty finding qualified educators to train nurses.

Out of the general chaos of this period developed several important trends that would affect nursing. The federal government became one of the largest employers of nurses. Under Franklin Delano Roosevelt's Federal Emergency Relief Administration (FERA), some 10,000 nurses were put to work in hospitals, clinics, and public health facilities. The Joint Committee on the Distribution of Nursing Services was organized to deal with nursing and health care problems. This commission recommended that the smaller, substandard nursing schools be closed to reduce the number of unemployed nurses. They advocated that graduate and registered nurses, not nursing students, staff hospitals. In an attempt to increase the number of nurses employed, the Joint Committee suggested reducing the work day from 12 hours to 8 hours. Their recommendations were not widely implemented, and the underlying problems remained until World War II.

The real trend toward using hospitals as the central point of health care also began during this period. The combination of a lack of private home care with an aging population who were developing chronic diseases led to a focus on hospital care. Hospital insurance programs also furthered the idea that the hospital was the place to receive health care, and more and more nursing jobs became available in hospitals as the size of there institutions increased.

12

COLLECTIVE BARGAINING AND GOVERNANCE

Learning Objectives

After completing this chapter, the reader will be able to:

1 Define collective bargaining.
2 Analyze the key issues that concern nurses in collective bargaining.
3 Correlate the steps in the contract-negotiation process.
4 Distinguish between a mediator and an arbitrator.
5 Delineate the important elements in a contract.
6 Name alternate forms of governance.
7 Analyze the effect governance has on collective bargaining.

As nursing moves toward achieving its full status as a profession, the issue of collective bargaining becomes more important. Throughout its history of developing into a profession, nursing and its practices have often been defined by other groups, such as physicians and hospital administrators (Schutt, 1973). As nurses begin to accept the authority and responsibility of the profession, they need to consider whether or not joining a union will help them reach their goal of full professionalism. Without a doubt, this is one of the most highly charged issues that a nurse will face in professional practice.

The image of nursing has always been one of dedication, service to clients, and selflessness. In the past, nurses' pay and working conditions were often secondary considerations, and many felt that too much emphasis on money demeaned the profession. In today's society, nurses are beginning to realize that professionals with a career should have a say in matters that affect their practice including working conditions, staffing patterns, benefits, and income (Scott, 1993). They need to be able to express these concerns without loss of status or reputation with the general public and other health care professionals.

COLLECTIVE BARGAINING

Collective bargaining is the uniting of employees for the purpose of increasing their ability to influence their employer and to improve working conditions (Tappen, 1995). Collective bargaining is a conflict-based power strategy working on the principle that there is greater strength in large numbers. Its primary goal is to equalize the power between labor and management. The primary collective bargaining unit is the union.

Unions were initially formed to protect workers from exploitation by greedy and insensitive employers. Although confronted with much opposition, they did accomplish their goals and became very powerful entities themselves. Recently, unions have received a more negative image because of the use of destructive and sometimes illegal practices in the quest for additional power. The end result is that the union movement itself is now in a fight for survival because of decreasing membership (Strickland, 1994). For some, unions and collective bargaining arouse images of picket lines, rowdy strikes, and violence. Many professionals, including nurses, do not regard this as an activity that professionals should be involved in and tend to reject the idea of union membership outright.

Legislative Development of Collective Bargaining

Although the informal roots of collective bargaining can be traced back to the middle 1800s, formal collective bargaining in this country was first legally recognized in 1935 with passage of the National Labor Relations Act (NLRA). This act granted employees the right to self-organization and to form, and help in the organization of, labor unions that could then bargain collectively through representatives. The representatives would be appointed by the union and bargain with management for the purpose of collective bargaining, mutual aid, and protection (Raelin, 1989). Under NLRA, the National Labor Relations Board (NLRB) was established to supervise the implementation of the act (Bazerman, 1992).

Originally, the NLRA included nonprofit hospitals and other health care providers under its authority. In 1947, however, the Taft-Hartley Act excluded nurses in nonprofit hospitals from coverage under the NLRA. This legally prevented nurses from organizing collective bargaining units and going on strike. It was not until 1974 that the Taft-Hartley Act was amended to cover nurses in nonprofit hospitals, thus allowing nurses to form collective bargaining units.

In April of 1991, the U.S. Supreme Court ruled that the NLRB had the authority to define bargaining units for health care providers in all settings, including acute care hospitals. Under this ruling, the NLRB defined eight separate bargaining units that were appropriate for use in hospitals. These eight units were:

1 Nurses
2 Physicians
3 All professionals except nurses and physicians
4 All technical employees
5 All skilled maintenance employees
6 All business office clerical employees
7 All guards
8 All other nonprofessional employees (Supreme Court, 1991)

Ultimately, this ruling by the Supreme Court permitted all registered nurses' (RNs') bargaining units to be formed so that work issues important to professional nurses could be addressed. The current major representative for nurses is the Service Employees International Union, which represents almost 400,000 nurses and health care providers nationwide (Strickland, 1994). The ANA has been active in the support of collective bargaining throughout its history.

Although the ANA does not serve as a bargaining agent, it does support the State Nurses Associations (SNAs) to function as bargaining agents. As early as 1944, the ANA ruled that the SNAs could engage in collective bargaining. In response to the attempt to regulate nursing from the outside, the ANA presented a position paper in 1946 that stated the importance for nursing to assume responsibility for advancing the social and economic security of its practitioners rather than leaving it to organizations outside the profession (Tappen, 1995). Today the SNAs represent approximately 140,000 RNs in some 840 individual bargaining units across the United States. Since the ruling by the Supreme Court in 1991, there has been an increased interest in organizing additional bargaining units (Scott, 1993). The Workplace Advocacy Initiative was also initiated in 1991 to help RNs improve the work environment and gain more control over professional practice.

Goals of Collective Bargaining

Although the basic goal of collective bargaining is to equalize power between management and employees, the inequality of power between the two groups is not so great as it initially appears. Although the majority of employees in most organizations are located toward the bottom of the power structure hierarchy, the management relies on these employees to carry out the work of the organization. Employees are vital to the growth, development, and even the survival of the organization. Employees also far outnumber individuals in management (Nicotera, 1993). Collective bargaining takes advantage of these two factors when attempting to produce change in the organization. An individual employee is highly vulnerable when attempting to force the employer to change.

The main area of concern of collective bargaining is basic economic issues such as salaries and benefits. In some hospital settings, nurses are paid less than other individuals in the hospital who have less education and fewer responsibilities. Collective bargaining attempts to balance these inequities.

Other concerns of collective bargaining include shift differentials, overtime pay, holidays, personal days off, the number of hours required in a work week, sick leave, maternity and paternity leave, uniform reimbursements, lunch and coffee breaks, health insurance, pension plans, and severance pay (Tappen, 1995). These elements are all found in the employment contract and may vary greatly depending on the hospital and the power of the bargaining unit.

One of the most important goals of a bargaining unit is to protect the employee against arbitrary treatment and unfair labor practices. These can be anything from working five weekends in a row to being fired because a physician felt the nurse was acting in an insubordinate manner. Other issues that might be considered unfair labor practices include being passed over for promotion without an explanation, staffing and scheduling policies, excessive demands for overtime, rotating shifts, unfair on call time, transfers, layoffs, seniority rights, and failure to post job openings. The collective bargaining unit establishes a grievance procedure by means of which the employee can bring a complaint against management without fear of reprisals (Lippman, 1991). These grievance procedures also allow a mechanism for the employee to follow up on the complaint to a satisfactory conclusion.

An important goal of collective bargaining is to maintain and promote professional practice. Often overlooked by management, this goal is one way nurses can keep and increase control over their own professional practice. For example, some nurses' bargaining units have been able to include the entire ANA Code of Ethics into the contract with the hospital. Other units have been able to address issues such as staffing, standards of care, and quality of care in the contract negotiations.

Nurses' Concerns About Collective Bargaining

The profession of nursing is relatively new to the process of collective bargaining. Nurses' concerns about it include:

1   *Unprofessional*—Nurses have a great deal of difficulty in adjusting their image to that of a union member or a striker. It just does not seem to be professional. For many nurses it seems that there must be other ways to achieve the same goals without collective bargaining.

   Organizers of collective bargaining units stress that many other professionals are members of unions. The NLRB defines nurses as professionals because their work requires advanced and specialized education and skills.

They also make critical judgments that affect the health and well-being of others. Union organizers contend that it is even less professional to accept low pay and poor working conditions than it is to join a union to improve these elements. They also feel that collective bargaining will give nurses control over their practice, which is one of the keys to professionalism.

2 *Unethical*—One of the major beliefs of nurses is the priority of the client's health and well-being over the personal needs and gains of the health care provider. This concern conflicts with the methods commonly used by collective bargaining units, such as strikes or work slowdowns. There is a feeling among many health care providers that these types of actions constitute abandonment of their clients and therefore violate the code of ethics.

Those who support collective bargaining stress that poor or intolerable work conditions are as much a threat to that client's health and well-being as the work actions taken to correct these conditions. The ability of nurses simply to threaten to strike, even though it may never materialize, is often powerful enough to bring about change (Giovinco, 1993). Law requires that there must be a 10-day notice given before a strike takes place. This gives the hospital a chance to prepare for the strike and to make changes to ensure client safety, such as transferring critical-care clients to another hospital, eliminating elective surgeries, and refusing to admit new clients.

In the few instances when nurses have gone on strike, client safety and well-being have not been affected. There were always enough nurses who were willing to work to care for the few critical-care clients who could not be transferred. Strikes by nurses tend to more civilized than strikes by coal miners or truck drivers.

3 *Divisive*—The process of collective bargaining is adversarial by nature. It pits two groups, management and employees, against each other. Although this relationship is not always the most productive type, it allows the staff nurses to be heard and to initiate changes that affect the practice of nursing. Nurses have been attempting for years to improve working conditions in the health care setting. Administrators pay little attention to an individual nurse or to a small group of concerned nurses. When a collective bargaining unit speaks for all of the nurses, however, administration will listen (Anderson, 1993). Collective bargaining does not have to be adversarial, and in facilities where administration is open to change and the collective bargaining unit is realistic in its requests, the process can be very smooth and amicable.

4 *Threat to job security*—Although the main goals of collective bargaining are improvement of working conditions and protection from unfair labor practices, it can itself pose a threat to job security. In some cases employees who are active in the collective bargaining process become well known to management and may become the targets for reprisals, particularly if the col-

lective bargaining fails. Another threat to job security arises when the collective bargaining unit has been too successful in its attempts to improve wages and benefits. In some cases the salaries required by negotiation drain the organization so much that it has to cut back the number of employees. Occasionally this financial drain is so great that it impedes the growth of the organization and threatens its very survival.

Taking an action always carries risk. Nurses involved in collective bargaining have to weigh the risk-to-benefit ratio before they take action. Are the working conditions so poor and the pay so inadequate that they overshadow the risk of possible job loss? The first attempts at organizing a collective bargaining unit are usually the most dangerous in terms of job security. Initial attempts at organizing nurses are usually made outside the hospital between representatives of the SNA and the union. This type of activity prevents any individuals from becoming targets of management's anger and makes management's reprisals more difficult.

The Contract

After a collective bargaining unit has been selected, the next important step is to develop or negotiate a contract between the nurses and the hospital. The contract is a legal document by which both management and the union must abide after it is signed (Tappen, 1995). Contracts can be very specific and include just a few items or very broad and include many. Contracts often contain requirements for union membership by the employees and set the cost of dues for that membership.

In negotiating the contract, both management and employee groups form negotiating teams. One member of each of these teams is designated as the spokesperson who will be the main representative for the group. Before negotiations start, each team meets separately to decide what their positions are on various issues and on what they are willing to compromise. A list of demands is exchanged by the two sides; it ought include everything each might possibly want.

Generally, management is reluctant to give up any power or relinquish any money. The employees' group tries to gain some of management's power and gain benefits for its members. Often many meetings between the two groups are required before they discover the key issues and determine where compromise is possible. Posturing and showmanship play a big part in the initial negotiations. Later, when serious issues are discussed and dealt with, final agreements may be reached behind closed doors.

The law requires that each side bargain in good faith. Good faith bargaining requires that both parties must agree to meet at reasonable times, to send individuals to the negotiations who can make binding decisions, and to be willing to bargain with the other side (Tappen, 1995). A lack of willingness to negotiate is not bargaining in good faith.

When the sides are unable to reach a settlement, a stalemate occurs. Stalemates are sometimes resolved through mediation, in which a neutral third party provided by the Federal Mediation and Conciliation Service meets with each side. After determining the nature of the conflict, the mediator brings the two sides together to attempt to work out a settlement. Both sides must work with the mediator, but they are not required to accept the mediator's recommendations.

If mediation fails, the Federal Mediation and Conciliation Service may appoint a fact-finding panel to investigate the conflict and to make recommendations. The panel's report is made public and can exert pressure on both sides to accept the recommendations of the mediator.

In some situations an arbitrator with binding power may be appointed. This is a neutral third party who, like the mediator, investigates the conflict, meets with both sides, and makes a recommendation for settlement. Unlike that of the mediator, however, the arbitrator's recommendation *must* be accepted by both sides. Both labor and management try to avoid binding arbitration because it limits their negotiating powers and they may lose something gained during previous negotiations.

When all else fails, the final step in the contract negotiation process is work slowdowns or stoppages (strikes). Although strikes are usually the tool used by employees to gain power, management can use a form of enforced strike called a lock-out, whereby employees are not permitted to enter the work facility.

The prospect of a strike is usually accompanied by more intense negotiations that may lead to a last-minute settlement. Strikes are detrimental to both sides. Employees lose pay and benefits during a strike and management loses income. In addition, the overall public image of strikes is negative, and they have little support. Some collective bargaining units have developed alternate ways of achieving their goals without a strike. Methods such as disruption of services on a random basis or boycott of an organization can achieve the same effects as a full-blown strike without damaging the image of the union.

After a settlement has been reached, the contract must be ratified. The collective bargaining unit takes the contract back to the employees, who must approve it. Once it is approved by a majority of the employees, the contract becomes legally binding for both management and the employees.

A good contract should contain the following elements:

- A statement outlining the objectives of both management and the employees
- A description of the official collective bargaining group
- A description of the benefits included in the contract, such as wages and salary, overtime pay, holiday pay, shift differentials, differentials for advanced education or certifications
- A description of other benefits, such as health insurance, life insurance, retirement, legal benefits, among others

■ A description of acceptable in-house labor practices, such as transfers, promotions, seniority, lay-offs, and work schedules
■ A description of the procedure to be used when employees have disciplinary problems
■ A description of the grievance procedures and the due process to be followed
■ A description of what is expected of the professional, including standards of care and codes of ethics (Flanagan, 1992)

CONCERNS FOR PROFESSIONAL NURSES

Nurses have many concerns about collective bargaining. The simple truth of the matter is that if the employer of nurses has initiated a means for the nurses to practice with autonomy and professionalism on a long-term basis, they will probably not be interested in forming a collective bargaining unit. It is only when a large number of nurses are dissatisfied with several issues that affect the work environment that organization of a union is even considered.

Representation

One of the most difficult decisions that nurses have to make is who shall represent them as a collective bargaining unit. Many nurses believe that the profession is best represented by professional nursing organizations, such as an SNA. It is reasonable to conclude that only a professional organization that understands the complex and varied needs of the profession will be able to represent that profession in a collective bargaining situation.

The SNA may not have access to the skilled representatives that are required to negotiate contracts, however. Unions, by their nature, have years of experience with negotiations and large sums to spend on developing skilled negotiators (Scott, 1993). The union, however, will have to convince the nurse's group that it is able to represent the interests of the nurses more effectively than the SNA. Many SNAs have neither the commitment nor skills to carry out effective collective bargaining.

Union groups who attempt to represent nurses soon find that nurses have difficulties in forming a consensus concerning problems and issues. Individuals outside the nursing profession have difficulty understanding issues such as quality and standards of care, ethical dilemmas, or even the different levels of nursing education.

Nurses should also be concerned about the public image of the collective bargaining unit they select to represent them. Some nurses' groups have been represented by a machinists' union, a teamster's union, or even a meat cutters' union. In the eyes of the public, alignment with groups such as these seems to diminish the professional status of nursing. Although these unions are highly proficient at negotiating contracts to gain benefits for their members, the image of nursing may be tarnished in the process.

Nursing Supervisors—Employees or Management?

Everyone is familiar with the nursing supervisor. This is the older, more experienced nurse who is present in the hospital or nursing home to guide the less experienced nurses. Nursing supervisors make sure staffing is adequate for their assigned shifts, resolve problems that are beyond the skills of the staff nurse, act as mediators between physicians and nurses, and use their higher skill levels to assist the staff nurses with code blues or complicated procedures. The term **nursing supervisor** also includes nurse educators, directors of nursing, head nurses, unit supervisors, assistant head nurses, and sometimes even charge nurses on the 3 PM to 11 PM or 11 PM to 7 AM work shifts.

Under the amendments to the Taft-Hartley Act of 1974, a supervisor was defined as any individual with authority to hire, transfer, suspend, lay off, promote, assign, reward, or discipline another employee (Tappen, 1995). From this legal viewpoint, nursing supervisors were no longer employees but really members of the management. Management cannot be involved in collective bargaining activities and are therefore prevented from joining units. A careful reading of the definition of a supervisor as presented in the Taft-Hartley Act makes the category of supervisor open to interpretation. Anybody who assigns a task to another nurse could be considered a supervisor.

This provision in the Taft-Hartley Act has sometimes been used by management in the attempt to control the organization and function of collective bargaining units. Management, if so inclined, can use this distinction to induce tension between nursing staff and supervisors, thus reducing the cohesion of the group. Supervisors often serve on important hospital committees to develop standards of care, foster professional recognition, and support nurse advancement. When contracts are negotiated, the supervisors are on the opposite side of the table from the staff nurses. Often in the heat of negotiation, things are said that foster negative feelings. After the negotiations have ended, it is difficult to re-establish that sense of unity that contributes to high-quality client care.

Attempts have been made by some health care institutions to categorize all of their nurses as supervisors, thus preventing any of them from organizing into a collective bargaining unit.

1994 Supreme Court Decision

In a 5-to-4 vote, the Supreme Court of the United States supported the decision that licensed practical nurses (LPNs) at the Heartland Nursing Home in Urbana, Ohio, should be considered supervisors because they directed the work of nurses' aides "in the interest of the employer." Under this ruling, these LPNs were *not* protected under the NLRA. This ruling has been of great concern to all nurses, but particularly to the ANA's Department of Labor Relations and Workplace Advocacy committee.

The implications of this decision are far-reaching and pose a direct threat to the ability of registered nurses to pursue collective bargaining. Employers have already begun to use this ruling to fight nurses in collective bargaining units from Alaska to Washington, D.C. The ANA has been working toward developing language that would follow the description of a supervisor as found in the NLRA and the Taft-Hartley Act (see earlier discussion). Since the passage of the NLRA, nurses who provide client care have been considered to be acting within the professional nature of nursing and not in the interests of the employer (as a supervisor would primarily be).

Under the ANA's proposed revisions, the scope of the definition of supervisor would be narrowed to include only employees of health care institutions. This change would allow the NLRB to continue to determine, on a case-by-case basis, whether nurses were supervisors or professional or technical employees. This legislation should be introduced to Congress in 1996, and it is essential that every nurse support these revisions of the Supreme Court ruling.

GOVERNANCE

The term **governance** has a variety of meanings in different contexts. In general, the term describes the arrangement of the hierarchy of power within an organization and how that power flows through the organization. In relationship to nursing, governance has been defined as "the establishment and maintenance of social, political and economic arrangements by which nurses maintain control over their practice, their self-discipline, their working conditions, and their professional affairs" (Aydelotte, 1980). The traditional structure of authority in the health care industry has been based on the triad of the board of directors, the administrator, and the medical staff.

Authority is a type of power that has its origins in the position that an individual holds within an organization (Tappen, 1995). This individual has this power only because others are willing to accept the decisions made by the person in that position. This allows relatively few people in the organization's hierarchy to control large number of employees as well as the directions and functions of the rest of the organization.

At the top of the governance hierarchy is the **board of directors,** also called the trustees or governors. The board of directors is usually composed of influential and rich business people who are considered community leaders. Although they retain the ultimate legal and ethical responsibility for the operation of the organization, generally the day-to-day operation is delegated to the administrator. The board's main function is to set general policies and to plan for the long-range development of the organization. Most boards become directly involved in the facility's operations only when there is a crisis, such as a financial short fall or a major lawsuit.

The **administrator** is usually the highest-ranking member of the hierarchy who actually becomes involved in the daily operation of the facility. The administrator has the education and knowledge required to direct the highly complex and technologically advanced elements that are an essential part of today's health care system.

In most health care facilities, the medical staff also exerts a great deal of control over the governance structure. The medical staff itself usually has its own internal governance structure, however, with higher- and lower-level members. Although the physicians in a facility have a great deal of influence in the running of the facility, they are generally neither employed nor controlled by the facility and indeed may not even be loyal to it. In the business world, this arrangement would not be tolerated because of the abuse of power that could take place.

Nurses' Role in Governance

Traditionally, nurses have had little say in governance. They accepted the work hours assigned to them, withstood disrespect and abuse from physicians and administrators as part of the work environment, and were satisfied with the meager salaries paid to them because theirs was a profession of dedication (Maloney, 1986). This situation has, however, changed drastically over the past two decades.

As nursing responsibilities increased with advancing technology, nurses became aware of the fact that their responsibilities far exceeded their authority to influence their practice. They began to recognize that autonomy, authority, and accountability are essential for high-quality client care and the only way these attributes could be gained was through changes in the organizational structure of the health care facilities where the nurses were employed.

Nurses have challenged this traditional governance structure at a number of levels. Nursing service administrators are the leaders of the largest single group of health care professionals in most health care organizations—generally about 50% of all the employees (Tappen, 1995). Because of their education and experience, many nursing administrators have moved into positions of power in the health care system and are no longer willing to accept the traditional role to which nurses were relegated. As middle managers, nursing administrators are often caught in the middle of conflicting expectations. For example, the chief administrator may want to cut the budget by reducing staffing, while the nurses on the units are already complaining that they cannot provide high-quality nursing care because the staffing levels are too low.

Staff nurses often view themselves as located at the bottom of the hierarchy with very little power. This is rarely the case. Depending on the organization of the facility, nurses have positional authority over other nurses, LPNs, nursing assistants, and individuals from the laboratory and radiology department.

Nurses have begun to recognize that in order to gain greater control over their practice, specific changes in the organizational structures of health care facilities must take place. The changes include decentralization of authority, identification of professional nurses as peers, agreement on the philosophy and goals of nursing care, and more responsibility for all the care given to clients while they are in the facility (Maloney, 1986).

Alternate Models for Governance

In an attempt to redistribute power and authority within health care organizations, several alternate forms of governance have been developed. Some of these work better than others, depending on the facility and the willingness of the individuals involved to cooperate.

The Board of Nursing Model

In this model of governance, the nursing staff structure is similar to the medical staff structure. There is a general board of trustees at the top and, immediately below, at the same level, a medical board of directors, a nursing board of directors, a board of directors representing other professionals, and the hospital administration itself (Tappen, 1995). The nursing board of directors deals with such matters as credentials and standards of care and also promotes cooperation between nurses and the other professionals of the facility. Although this type of structure places nurses on an equal administrative footing with the physicians, administration, and other professionals in the facility, it does have the tendency to create a large number of administrative personnel. A tendency for conflicts to arise between the different board members does exist.

Contracting for Nursing Services Model

This model proposes that clients be billed for nursing care as a separate item, much the same way that they are billed for medical care by the physicians. Currently, when a client receives a hospital bill, the care provided by nurses is included in the overall room charge. In order to make this model work, nurses select individual clients for whom they wish to care and then accept responsibility for providing that care. Some type of scale would need to be developed so that the nurse could charge a higher rate for taking care of more seriously ill clients with more complex health care needs. Nurses would take responsibility for scheduling and for self-management. And as with physicians, there would have to be a peer review mechanism to monitor the quality of health care provided.

Although this model supports primary care and the expansion of the nurse's role and responsibility, it would be very difficult to implement. Some of the problems include establishing acceptable pay scales, ensuring adequate staffing, and paying ancillary help such as orderlies and nursing assistants. Probably the most significant single factor that affects the implementation of this model is the hospital administration's loss of control over the nursing staff. If the nurses' pay were to come directly from the client, rather than the hospital, nurses would tend to place the client's needs before the needs of the facility. This would be unacceptable to most facilities.

Shared Governance Model

In the shared governance model, power and authority are transferred to the nursing staff rather than being seated primarily in nursing administration. The key to shared governance is decentralization of the nursing administration structure. Its goal is to involve professional nurses in the decision-making process at all levels to ensure that their knowledge and expertise are used to deliver the highest-quality care possible (Maloney, 1986).

Shared governance allows the nurse autonomy in decisions about nursing practice, working conditions, staffing levels, standards of care, and other areas. It gives professional nurses the chance to be held accountable and responsible for their clinical judgment and the care they give to clients. It allows their peers a chance to recognize their knowledge and competence as true health care professionals.

In general, shared governance locates the source of power in the clinical areas rather than in the administrative areas. Several different types of shared governance exist.

In the **congressional shared governance** model, a group of professional nurses is organized into a congress. This congress develops by-laws, elects representatives, and forms committees to govern the activities of the nursing staff (Tappen, 1995). Composed entirely of professional nurses, the committees oversee professional practice, evaluate quality of care, provide continuing education, plan for staffing, conduct research, and discipline errant nurses. Although this is a highly effective method to provide nursing care and to increase the autonomy of nurses, it does require a tremendous initial expenditure of time, effort, and money. Many institutions are not willing to make that commitment.

In the **unit-based model,** the shared governance is on a smaller scale. Groups of nurses on each unit form councils for professional practice that perform many of the functions that the professional congresses perform. In order to make this model succeed, there must be a real transfer of decision-making power from the head nurse or unit supervisor to the staff nurses. Shared governance is a model that the staff is willing to undertake, rather than being forced into it by the administration. Unfortunately, many facilities that profess a shared governance structure really are using a traditional hierarchy structure with somewhat more open lines of communication. The test of a true shared governance model quickly becomes evident when difficult decisions have to be made. For example, if the staff nurses decide that more staffing is needed for their unit, but the administration refuses to make money available for new nurses, then it is not a true shared governance model.

Governance and Collective Bargaining

Forms of governance directly affect the issues in which professional nurses are likely to become involved when conducting collective bargaining. Although salary and benefits are important considerations in professional nursing, nurses feel much more strongly about issues of autonomy, accountability, and control of practice. In a health care facility with a form of governance that allows nurses to have a relatively large degree of control over their practice, the issues discussed at the bargaining table are more likely to revolve around a professional agenda. In facilities with a rigidly structured hierarchy of authority that gives nurses little autonomy, accountability, or control over their practice, collective bargaining is more likely to center on control and power issues.

Nurses are highly educated professionals. They recognize that they can practice autonomously and can make sound decisions about client care. They also recognize that an increased understanding of the governance process requires many of the same skills used in collective bargaining. Key elements in both processes require an understanding of negotiation, compromise, and consensus building to attain one's goals. Changes in methods of governance also will require major changes in the health care system. Professional nurses have the power to produce those changes and the ability to deal with the future of health care successfully.

CONCLUSION

Although few issues elicit such strong emotions among nurses as collective bargaining, it is a reality in today's health care system. Nurses are beginning to realize that they are not in a strictly altruistic profession, but rather one in which they use their knowledge and skills to provide high-quality services to clients. The knowledge and skills used in client care are gained at the cost of years of expensive education in schools of nursing and of dedication to an often underappreciated profession. Nurses no longer need to apologize or feel guilty about seeking payment for their work on a level commensurate with their knowledge and skills. Unfortunately, the money is often controlled by less than generous hospital managements.

Negotiation is the process of give and take between groups with the goal

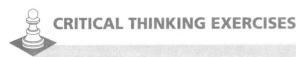

CRITICAL THINKING EXERCISES

1 Develop a position paper either supporting or opposing collective bargaining.
2 A nurse on your unit states one day: "Membership in the State Nurse's Association is a waste of time and money. They can't help you make a better living!" How would you respond to this nurse?
3 Develop an *ideal contract* for nurses. Which elements would receive the highest priority?
4 Develop a plan for shared governance in a facility you are familiar with. How would the organizational process take place? What are some of the major difficulties in developing this plan?
5 Develop a 5-year plan for your future after graduation, keeping in mind the proposed and likely changes in the health care system. Include the positions you would like to hold, any additional education that may be required, and any other life changes that are needed to achieve this plan.

of reaching an agreement acceptable to both sides. Although negotiations may be formal or informal, hostile or friendly, a cooperative atmosphere fostered by both sides that recognizes the similarity of each side's demands will be the most productive in reaching a satisfactory contract. Threats and antagonism usually have a negative effect on negotiations and may leave both sides feeling dissatisfied.

Collective bargaining is a rather new concept to professional nursing. Many nurses still feel that collective bargaining is unprofessional, unethical, divisive, and a fundamental threat to job security. Most of these same nurses, however, agree with the goals of collective bargaining, including improvement of economic benefits, better staffing and scheduling, fair treatment for all nurses, and improved quality of care for clients. Nurses must decide at some point in their careers if joining a collective bargaining unit will best help them to achieve these goals. This is not an easy decision to make, and each nurse should gather as much information as possible about the situation before making a decision.

Nurses need to recognize that the time has arrived to elevate the profession to a new level. Change in forms of governance is one method that nurses can use to change the health care system. Nursing as a profession at last has the opportunity to gain tremendous power and take its rightful place as an indispensable force in the health care system. All that is required is for nurses to become educated in the issues involved and to take an aggressive stance in the formation of the future.

COLLECTIVE BARGAINING AND GOVERNANCE: REDESIGNING HEALTH CARE

Nurses are quickly becoming familiar with a new buzzword in health care: **restructuring**. As the health care system responds to demands for improved efficiency in the delivery of client care, hospitals are undergoing a process of redesigning and re-engineering their internal structures. Often the major targets of this process are the traditional roles of caregivers and the departmental structure that provides that care. Sometimes it involves remodeling the facility to decentralize ancillary services so that they are located closer to the clients.

The goal of restructuring is to make the health care being provided more client centered and to provide a greater level of efficiency. The results of restructuring should be improved quality of care at a reduced cost.

Although a number of ways exist to achieve restructuring, several elements are common to most attempts to restructure. Usually ancillary staff are cross-trained so that they can complete several different types of client-care tasks. The RNs are often paired with multiskilled health care workers so that clients, rather than the functions of the individual department, are the focus of care.

Successful restructuring requires administrators with a high level of skill in establishing an environment where staff feel safe to take risks and challenge traditions. It also requires the staff to become involved early in the process so that there a common vision is shared by the entire institution. Staff members must be included in all planning stages and be allowed to make recommendations throughout the process. The most successful attempts at restructuring took place over an extended period to allow everyone to adjust to changes, new relationships, and new roles.

Institutions that have had the most difficulty with restructuring were those that did not include nursing administration in the process of change. Resistance from nurses at these facilities came from the feeling that the nurses were losing their leadership role on the client-care team. Nurses who were not involved in the long-term planning for restructuring viewed it as merely a short-term economic move to reduce costs by having nurses give up their professional roles.

The most successful attempts at redesigning health care programs occurred in institutions where changes were customized to adapt to the culture of the organization. It is important to recognize that each institution has its own goals and philosophical orientation and that only when the

COLLECTIVE BARGAINING AND GOVERNANCE: REDESIGNING HEALTH CARE (Continued)

changes made are in line with these unique elements will the health care teams function successfully. Many hospitals have managed to define their visions and have restructured in such a way as to enhance the quality of client care, increase the satisfaction of staff, and reduce the overall cost.

Modified from Clark, K.: Restructuring. The Oklahoma Nurse, 39:14–15, June 1995.

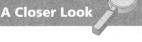

A Closer Look

COLLECTIVE BARGAINING AND GOVERNANCE: A NEW MODEL FOR COLLECTIVE BARGAINING

Traditionally, collective bargaining has been viewed as a struggle between two groups, one (usually employees) attempting to gain more power and another (usually management) attempting to retain power. This type of struggle often resulted in hurt feelings or impasses in negotiations. The Minnesota Nurses Association (MNA) recently ratified a contract with 12 Twin Cities–area hospitals using a new collective bargaining technique called **interest-based bargaining.**

Interest-based bargaining, also called mutual gains, win-win, and best-practice bargaining, is based on the idea that the way to achieve a mutually beneficial contract is to create an environment in which all parties can openly discuss all issues to the fullest extent. In interest-based bargaining, a highly structured six-step process is followed. These steps include: (1) selection of issues; (2) discussion of interests; (3) generation of options; (4) establishment of standards to measure the options; (5) measurement of the options; and (6) development of solutions. This step-by-step process prevents the parties involved in the bargaining from reverting to the traditional power struggle. All steps are done jointly, and even the 2-day training session that precedes negotiations requires participation by both management and labor.

Central to the contract negotiations by the MNA was ensuring that the role of the registered nurse as the primary assessor and planner of care be maintained. The contract included specific language stating that *only* RNs will assess, plan, and evaluate a client's nursing care needs. In order to guarantee this aspect of the contract in the future, the MNA negotiated greater participation by RNs in the hospital committees that establish

Continued on following page

COLLECTIVE BARGAINING AND GOVERNANCE: A NEW
MODEL FOR COLLECTIVE BARGAINING (Continued)

policies for labor-management relations, nurse staffing, client-care standards, and health and safety policies. This partnership between nurses and hospital administrators allowed for joint decision making when issues of nursing practice and delivery of care were involved.

Interest-based bargaining may be the trend for the future, particularly in the health care industry. Traditional collective bargaining methods are primarily adversarial and often leave the parties involved with deep-seated feelings of hostility toward each other. The old methods sometimes result in strikes or other types of work actions that harm the reputations of both nurses and the hospitals. Interest-based bargaining allows participants an opportunity to negotiate without hostility and to develop a more positive relationship after the contract has been agreed on.

Traditional Bargaining vs. Interest-Based Bargaining

Traditional Bargaining	Interest-Based Bargaining
Adversarial in nature	Collaborative
Victory-oriented goals	Multiple-gain goals
Negotiation process	Problem-solving process
Compromise on decisions	Consensus on decisions
Predetermined position	No prejudgment on issues
Controlled communication	Brainstorming
Limit information given	Open exchange of information

Modified from Himali, U.: MNA ratifies ground-breaking multi-employer contract. Am Nurse 271:10, 1995.

BIBLIOGRAPHY

American Nurses Association: Nursing's Agenda for Health Care Reform, American Nurses Association, Kansas City, 1992.
Anderson, K: Getting What You Want. Dutton, New York, 1993.
Aydelotte, MK: Governance, education are watchwords for the 80s. Am Nurse 12:4,1980.
Bazerman, MH: Negotiating Rationally. Free Press, New York, 1992.
Chenevert, M: Pro-Nurse Handbook. CV Mosby, Philadelphia, 1993.
Flanagan, L: How collective bargaining benefits nurses. Directions 22:8–22, 1992.
Giovinco, G: When nurses strike: Ethical issues. Nurs Management 24:86–90, 1993.
Johnston, W and Packer, A: Workforce 2000: Work and Workers for the Twenty-first Century. Hudson Institute, Indianapolis, 1987.
Lippman, H: Legally speaking: Expect to hear about unions. RN 54:68–72, 1991.
Maloney, MM: Professionalization of Nursing: JB Lippincott, Philadelphia, 1986.
Naisbitt, J and Aburdene, P: Megatrends 200: Ten New Directions for the 1990s. Morrow, New York, 1990.
Nicotera, AM: Beyond two dimensions: Handling conflict. Management Communication Quarterly 6:282–306, 1993.

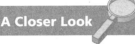

A Closer Look

DECIDING TO GO ON STRIKE

CASE STUDY

Sharon S., RN, was completing her charting on another busy 3 PM to 11 PM shift. While she was walking down the hall toward the time clock, she wondered who would be taking her place for the rest of the week. Like most of the other nurses at the Medical Center, she had decided to go on strike starting with the 7 AM to 3 PM shift the next day. The decision to strike had not been an easy one and had only been reached after much discussion (arguments?), many hours of meetings and conferences with the hospital negotiators, and animated discussion among the nurses' negotiating team.

Sharon could see both positive and negative sides to a strike. On the positive side, increased salaries, better fringe benefits, and improvements in working conditions and staffing would be a plus for all the nurses and clients at the Medical Center. Sharon herself had felt increasingly stressed during the past year because of the hospital's measures to reorganize. From what Sharon was able to see, reorganization meant saving money by cutting professional staff and partially replacing them with less trained, unlicensed individuals. This pattern of restaffing had led to longer hours, increased responsibilities for the RNs, and fewer support services. She also felt that the overall quality of care had decreased noticeably.

On the negative side, Sharon was experiencing a real ethical and emotional dilemma about going on strike. The quality of care was sure to deteriorate even further because of the reduced services caused by the strike. Was it really fair to decrease the services and care for clients who had nothing to do with the issues that brought on the strike? Of course, during the past 3 days, the clients who had been well enough were sent home early in anticipation of the strike. Some whose conditions were too complicated to be cared for at home were sent to other facilities for care. The hospital had severely restricted admissions, reducing the census to an all-time low.

Yet there were several clients who were too ill to transfer or send home. Mrs. Anderson, a 78-year-old client with renal failure, congestive heart failure, and a recent colostomy for a bowel obstruction, came to mind. Mrs. Anderson, and a number of other clients like her who had no family nearby and few resources, were highly dependent on the nursing staff to meet their needs for care. Mrs. Anderson was just beginning to be taught how to care for her colostomy. Even if she was discharged to a nursing home, there was no way to ensure that she could receive the teaching needed for her eventual self-care. Although there was to be a skeleton crew of nurses left in the

Continued on following page

DECIDING TO GO ON STRIKE (Continued)

hospital, they would be stretched very thin in trying to care for the remaining clients.

Sharon also thought about the ANA Code for Nurses she had been taught in nursing school, particularly the passage that stated "the nurse participates in the profession's effort to establish and maintain conditions of employment conducive to high-quality nursing care." The reason for the strike was to bring about improved working conditions that would benefit future clients in the hospital. But should these measures be carried out when nursing services were already operating at a reduced level of care and at a minimal level of safety? Didn't that somehow contradict the first statement in the Code, that "the nurse provides services with respect for human dignity?" When Mrs. Anderson was admitted to the hospital 4 days before, she came with the expectation of the best possible care under any circumstances. The Code seemed to have a split personality on strikes. While calling for service to the profession to maintain high standards and quality of care, the Code also insisted that the health, welfare, and safety of the client's should be the nurses' first consideration.

What should Sharon do? Does the overall welfare of the profession ever supersede the obligation to provide client care?

Raelin, JA: Unionization and deprofessionalization: Which comes first? J Organizational Behav 10(2):101–115, 1989.
Schutt, BG: Collective action for professional security. Am J Nurs 73:1946, 1973.
Scott, K: SNA representation means increased job satisfaction. Am Nurse 24:2, 1993.
Strickland, OL and Fishman, DJ: Nursing Issues in the 1990s. Delmar, Albany, 1994.
Supreme Court okays all-RN unit. Am Nurse 20:1, 1991.
Tappen, RM: Nursing Leadership and Management, FA Davis, Philadelphia, 1995.

 HISTORICAL PERSPECTIVES

Effects of War on Modern Nursing During and After World War II

The second world war (WW II) produced large numbers of sick and wounded, and there was another nursing shortage. Several measures were undertaken to meet the need. Congress passed the Bolton Nurse Training Act, establishing the Cadet Nurse Corps. Students who entered the program were sent to nursing schools near their homes, with all expenses paid. After graduation, they were obligated to work actively in nursing either in a hospital or in military service for 2 to 4 years. This program also established minimal educational standards that the nursing programs had to meet and forbade discrimination on the basis of race, creed, or sex. The Bolton Act also provided for shortening of the traditional hospital-based program from 36 months to 30 months. Although initially concerned about the quality of these shortened programs, many schools revised and improved their curriculums to meet the new standards.

Inactive nurses were strongly recruited back into active nursing during WW II. This practice opened the door for married nurses and encouraged hospitals to start the novel practice of hiring, on a part-time basis, nurses who had families. To encourage more nurses to enter the military, full commissioned status was granted, making nurses officers and raising their status. Unlike nurses in WW I, these nurses were also given the same pay as men with the same rank. Toward the end of WW II all discrimination was forbidden, and African-American and male nurses were also admitted to the services with full military rank.

WW II brought about many changes and advancements that continue to affect health care today. There was a rapid increase in medical knowledge during the war in such areas as the development of antibiotics, tranquilizers, new surgical techniques, dialysis, and the use of specialty units such as intensive care units, obstetrical units, operating rooms, and recovery rooms. Health care services were greatly expanded with the development of radiographs, laboratory tests, transfusions, and emergency department care. Hospitals became the focus of health care, and physicians became increasingly dependent on the services hospitals provided, particularly where expensive high-technology equipment was involved. The traditional belief that all nurses were interchangeable in the workplace began to be challenged. Nurses in the specialty units needed highly advanced and progressive education to meet the needs of the clients in those units. The philosophy long revered by hospital administrators and physicians that a nurse is a nurse is a nurse, although probably never true, was even less true during and after WW II.

The need for nurses increased even more dramatically after WW II, when many of the military nurses and most of the nurses trained under the Bolton Nurse Training Act opted to leave nursing to marry and to raise families. Nursing met this challenge by advocating the same quick-fix method it had used before. The origin of many licensed practical nurse (LPN) programs can be traced to this time. Designed to provide technical, bedside nurses in just 1 year, such programs were seen by the hospitals as a way of staffing their wards with inexpensive workers. The widespread acceptance of the team-nursing concept can also be traced to this time. The RN was the team leader who supervised the client care being provided by the LPNs and nurse's aides. Although this was a very efficient type of management style, it removed the most qualified of the nurses, the RN, from direct client care.

Other quick-fix measures to alleviate the postwar nursing shortage included hiring nurses from other countries and the development of the technical nursing programs, which granted associate degrees (ADs) in nursing at 2-year community colleges. These measures were supposed to be temporary, but as hospitals expanded, the baby-boom began, and the population increased, the need for nurses continued to grow. Under circumstances like these, quick-fix measures soon become permanent solutions. Although importation of foreign nurses leveled off and actually began to decline as practice standards were tightened, the AD nursing programs, originally designed to prepare nurses at an intermediate level between the professional BSN and the technical LPN, increased. By the middle 1960s, AD programs outnumbered both BSN and diploma programs. With their increasing numbers, AD nurses lobbied for and obtained the right to take the same licensing examination as the RN graduates from diploma and BSN programs.

Along with these changes, the period after WW II brought an interest in raising nursing to a professional level. With the health care system becoming increasing complicated, interest in baccalaureate nursing education began to grow and new nursing programs were established at 4-year colleges and universities. As the number of BSN graduates slowly increased, there was a corresponding slow but steady expansion of graduate-level nursing education to provide master's degrees, and even doctorates, in nursing.

13

NURSING LAW AND LIABILITY

Learning Objectives

After completing this chapter, the reader will be able to:

1 Distinguish between statutory law and common law.
2 Differentiate civil law from criminal law.
3 Explain the legal principles involved in:
   a unintentional torts.
   b intentional torts.
   c quasi-intentional torts.
4 Describe the trial process.
5 Provide methods to prevent litigation.

For many nurses, merely uttering the word **lawsuit** provokes high levels of anxiety. At first glance, the legal system often seems to be a large and confusing entity whose intricacies are designed to entrap the uninitiated. Many nurses feel that even a minor error in client care will lead to huge settlements against them and loss of their nursing license. In reality, even though the number of lawsuits against nurses has increased markedly during the past 10 years, the number of nurses who are actually sued remains relatively small.

It is important to remember that the legal system is just one element in the totality of the health care system. Laws are rules made by human beings to help protect other human beings and to keep society functioning. The ultimate goal of all laws is to promote peaceful and productive interactions between and among the people of that society.

An understanding of basic legal principles will augment the quality of care the nurse delivers. In our litigious society it is important to comprehend how the law affects the profession of nursing and the individual nurse's daily practice.

There are two major sources for laws in the United States, statutory laws and common law.

STATUTORY LAW

Statutory law consists of laws written and enacted by the Congress of the United States, the state legislatures, and other governmental entities such as cities, counties, or townships. Legislated laws enacted by the United States Congress are called **federal statutes**. State-drafted laws are termed **state statutes**. Individual cities and municipalities have legislative bodies that draft ordinances, codes, and regulations at their respective levels.

The laws that govern the profession of nursing are statutory laws. Most of these laws are written at the state level because licensure is a responsibility of the individual states. These laws include the Nurse Practice Act, State Board of Nursing, individual licensure procedures, and schedule of fees for the state.

COMMON LAW

Common law is different from statutory law in that it has evolved from the decisions of previous legal cases. These laws represent the accumulated results of the judgments and decrees that have been handed down by courts of the United States and Great Britain through the years. Common law often extends beyond the scope of statutory law. For example, no statutes require a person who is negligent and causes injury to another to compensate that person for the injury. Court decisions that have addressed the same legal issues over and over, such as negligence, however, have repeatedly ruled that the injured person should receive compensation. How each case is resolved creates a *precedent* or pattern for dealing with the same legal issue in the future. The common laws involving negligence or malpractice are most frequently encountered by the nurse.

Common law or case law is law that has developed over a long period. The principle of "stares decisis" requires a judge to make decisions similar to those that have been handed down in previous cases if the facts of the cases are identical. Common-law decisions are published in bound legal reports. Generally speaking, common law deals with matters outside the scope of laws enacted by the legislature.

In the U.S. legal system, there are many divisions in the law. A major example of such a division is the difference between criminal law and civil law.

CRIMINAL LAW

Criminal laws are concerned with providing protection for all members of society. When someone is accused of violating a criminal law, the government at the county, city, state, or federal level will impose punishments appropriate to the type of crime. Criminal law involves a wide range of violations ranging from minor traffic violations to murder.

Criminal law is regulated and created by the government through the enactment of statutes. Statutes are developed and enacted by the legislature (state or federal) and approved by the executive branch, such as a governor or the President. Criminal law is further classified into two types of offenses: (1) **misdemeanors**, which are minor criminal offenses, and (2) **felonies**, which are major criminal offenses.

In the criminal law system, an individual accused of a crime is called the **defendant**. The prosecuting attorney represents the people of the city, county, state, or federal jurisdiction who are accusing the individual of a crime. There are penalties imposed on the violators of criminal law. The penalties or sanctions that are imposed are based on the scope of the crime. They can involve a range of punishment from community service work and fines to imprisonment and death.

Nurses can become involved with the criminal system in their nursing practice in several ways. The most common violation by nurses of the criminal law is through failure to renew nursing licenses. In this situation, the nurse is, in effect practicing nursing without a license, which is a crime in all states. Nurses also become involved with the illegal diversion of drugs, particularly narcotics, from the hospital. This is a more serious crime that may lead to imprisonment for the nurse. Recent cases involving intentional or unintentional deaths of clients and assisted suicide cases have also led to criminal action against nurses.

CIVIL LAW

Nurses are much more likely to become involved in civil lawsuits than in criminal violations. Civil laws generally deal with the violation of one individual's rights by another individual. The court provides the forum that enables these individuals to have their disputes resolved by an independent third party, such as a judge or a jury of the defendants peers. The individual who brings the dispute to the court is called the **plaintiff**. The formal written document which spells out the dispute and the resolution sought is called the **complaint**. The individual against whom the complaint is filed is called the **defendant**. Civil law has many branches, including contract law, treaty law, tax law, and tort law. It is under the tort law that most nurses become involved with the legal system.

TORT LAW

A **tort** is generally defined as a wrongful act committed against a person or his property independent of a contract. A person who commits a tort is liable for damages to those who are affected by the person's actions. The word *tort*, derived from the Latin *tortus* (twisted), is a French word for injury or wrong. Torts can involve several different types of actions, including a direct violation of a person's legal rights or a violation of a standard of care that causes injury to a person. Torts are classified as unintentional, intentional, or quasi-intentional.

Unintentional Torts

Negligence is the primary form for unintentional torts. Negligence is generally defined as the omission of an act that a reasonable and prudent person would perform in a similar situation, or something a reasonable person would not do in that situation (Louisell, 1990).

There are four elements required for a person to make a claim of negligence. These are: "(1) duty was owed to the client; (2) the professional violated the duty and failed to conform to the standard of care; (3) the failure to act by the professional caused the resulting injuries; and (4) actual injuries resulted from the breach of duty" (Prosser, 1984).

Malpractice is often referred to as professional negligence. Because of their professional status, nurses are held to a higher standard of conduct than the ordinary layperson. The standard for nurses is what a reasonable and prudent nurse would do in the same situation: "A registered nurse is charged with utilizing the degree and skill and judgment commensurate with his or her education, experience and position" (Louisell, 1990).

Malpractice is more serious than mere negligence because it indicates professional misconduct or unreasonable lack of skill in performing professional duties. Malpractice suggests the existence of a professional standard of care and a deviation from that standard of care. An expert professional witness is often asked to testify in a malpractice case to help establish the standard of care to which the professional should be held accountable.

A 1988 case in South Dakota presents an example of nursing malpractice. The nurse failed to question the physician's order to discharge a client when she discovered that the client had a fever. In this case, a supervisory nurse provided expert testimony and reported to the judge that the general standard of care for nurses is to report a significant change in a client's condition, such as an elevated temperature. It is the nurse's responsibility to question the physician's order as to appropriateness of discharge. The records on this case indicated that the client's elevated temperature was charted after the physician had completed his rounds. The nurse did not notify the physician of the client's fever; and the client was subsequently discharged. The client was readmitted a short time after discharge and died in the hospital. The nurse was found negligent. The court held that negligence can be determined by failure to act as well as by the commission of an act.

Many other types of actions by nurses can produce malpractice law suits. Some of the more common actions include:

- Leaving foreign objects inside a client during surgery
- Failing to assess and observe a client as directed
- Failing to obtain a proper informed consent
- Failing to report a change in a client's condition, such as vital signs, circulatory status, and level of consciousness
- Failing to report another health care provider's incompetence or negligence
- Failing to take actions to provide for a client's safety, such as raising the siderails on the bed after giving the client narcotic medication
- Failing to provide a client with sufficient and appropriate education before discharge

If a nurse is found guilty of malpractice, several types of actions may be taken against the nurse. The nurse may be required to provide monetary compensation to the client for general damages that were a direct result of the injury including pain, suffering, disability, and disfigurement. In addition, the nurse is often required to pay for special damages that have resulted from the injury, such as all involved medical expenses and wages lost by the client while in the hospital. Optional damages, including emotional distress, mental suffering, and counseling expenses that were an outgrowth of the initial injury may be added to the total settlement. If the client is able to prove that the nurse acted with conscious disregard for the client's safety or acted in a malicious, willful, or wanton manner that produced injury, then an additional assessment of punitive or exemplary damages may be added to the award.

Intentional Torts

An **intentional tort** is generally defined as a willful act that violates another person's rights or property. Intentional torts can be distinguished from malpractice and acts of negligence by the following three requirements: (1) the nurse must intend to bring about the consequences of the act, (2) the nurse's act must be intended to interfere with the client or his property, and (3) the act must be a substantial factor in bringing about the injury or consequences.

The most frequently encountered intentional torts are assault, battery, false imprisonment, and intentional infliction of emotional distress. With intentional torts, the injured person does not have to prove that an injury has occurred, nor is the opinion of an expert witness required for adjudication. Punitive damages are more likely to be assessed against the nurse in intentional tort cases, and some intentional torts may fall under the criminal law if there is gross violation of the standards of care.

Assault

Assault is the unjustifiable attempt to touch another person or the threat of so doing. **Battery** is actual harmful or unwarranted contact with another person without his or her consent. Battery is the most common intentional tort seen in the practice of nursing.

For a nurse to commit assault and battery, there must be an absence of consent on the part of the client. Before any procedure can be performed on a competent, alert, and normally oriented client, the client must agree or consent to the procedure being done. Negligence does not have to be proven for a person to be successful in a claim for assault and battery.

A common example of an assault and battery occurs when a nurse physically restrains a client against the client's will and administers an injection against the client's wishes.

False Imprisonment

False imprisonment occurs when a client is confined or restrained with intent to prevent him or her from leaving the hospital. The use of restraints alone does not constitute false imprisonment when they are used to maintain the safety of a confused or disoriented client. In general, mentally impaired clients can be detained against their will only if they are a threat to injure themselves or others. The use of threats or medications that interfere with the client's ability to leave the facility can also be considered false imprisonment.

Intentional Infliction of Emotional Distress

Intentional infliction of emotional distress is another common intentional tort encountered by the nurse. To prove intentional tort, the following three elements are necessary: (1) conduct that exceeds what is usually accepted by society, (2) conduct that is calculated to cause mental distress, and (3) causation—the conduct must cause the mental distress. Any nurse who is charged with assault, battery, or false imprisonment is also at risk for being charged with infliction of emotional distress.

A 1975 a case is an example where there was infliction of emotional distress. In *Johnson v. Women's Hospital*, a mother wished to view the body of her baby who had died during birth. After she made the request, she was handed the baby's body floating in a gallon jar of formaldehyde (Guido, 1988). The Johnson case epitomizes the lack of respect and reasonableness that should have been extended to the mother. Handling a delicate situation with dignity and respect could have avoided this claim.

Quasi-Intentional Torts

A **quasi-intentional tort** is a mixture of unintentional and intentional torts. It is defined as a voluntary act that directly causes injury or distress without intent to injure or to cause distress. A quasi-intentional tort does have the elements of volition and causation without the element of intent. Quasi-intentional torts usually involve situations of communication and often violate a person's reputation, personal privacy, or civil rights.

Defamation of Character

Defamation of character, the most common of the quasi-intentional torts, is the harming of a person's reputation and good name. Defamation injures a person's reputation by diminishing the esteem, respect, goodwill, or confidence that others have for the person. It can be especially damaging when false statements are made about a criminal act, an immoral act, or false allegations about a client's having a contagious disease.

Defamation includes **slander**, which is spoken communication in which one person discusses another in terms that harm a third person's reputation, and **libel**, which is written communication in which a person makes statements or uses language that harms another person's reputation. To win a defamation lawsuit against the nurse, the client must prove that the nurse acted with malice, abused the principle of privileged communication, and wrote or spoke an untruth.

Medical record documentation is a primary source of defamation of character. Through the years, the client's chart has been the basis of many defamation lawsuits. Discussing client matters in the elevators, cafeteria, and other public areas can also lead to lawsuits for defamation if negative comments are overheard.

Invasion of Privacy

Invasion of privacy is a violation of a person's right to protection against unreasonable and unwarranted interference with one's personal life. To prove that invasion of privacy has occurred, the client must show: (1) the nurse intruded on the client's seclusion and privacy, (2) the intrusion is objectionable to a reasonable and prudent person, (3) the act committed intrudes on private or published facts or pictures of a private nature, and (4) public disclosure of private information was made (Fiesta, 1988). Examples of invasion of privacy include using the client's name or picture for the sole advantage of the health care provider, intruding into the client's private affairs without permission, giving out private client information over the telephone, and publishing information that misrepresents the client's condition.

Breach of Confidentiality

Confidentiality of information concerning the client must be honored. **Breach of confidentiality** results when a client's trust and confidence are violated by public revelation of confidential or privileged communications without the client's consent. Most breach of confidentiality cases involve a physician's revelation of privileged communications shared by a client. Nurses who overhear privileged communication or information, however, are held to the same standards as a physician with regard to that information.

Privileged client information can be disclosed only upon authorization by the client. Most health care facilities have specific guidelines dealing with client information disclosure. Disclosure of information to family members is also not acceptable unless authority is given by the client. For instance, a client may not wish to disclose to a family member a specific diagnosis, such as cancer, and if that is the case, the nurse should honor this request. Otherwise, it could be considered a violation of that client's privacy.

THE FIVE ELEMENTS OF INFORMED CONSENT

Informed consent is consent given by a client after the client receives sufficient information on:

1 Treatment proposed
2 Material risk involved
3 Acceptable alternatives
4 Outcome hoped for
5 Consequences of not having treatment

EXCEPTIONS TO INFORMED CONSENT

There are two exceptions to informed consent:

- In an emergency if the client is unconscious or incompetent.
- The health provider feels that it may be medically contraindicated to disclose the risk and hazards because it may result in illness, severe emotional distress, serious psychologic damage, or failure on the part of the client to receive life-saving treatment.

PATIENT SELF-DETERMINATION ACT

The Patient Self-Determination Act is a federal law that requires that all federally funded institutions inform clients of their right to prepare advance directives. The Patient Self-Determination Act of 1990 was sponsored by Senator John Danforth. The advance directives seek to encourage people to discuss and document their wishes concerning the type of treatment and care that they want (i.e., life-sustaining treatment) in advance, so that it will ease the burden on their families and providers when it comes time to make such a decision.

There are two types of advance directives: (1) the **living will**, which is a document stating what health care a client will accept or refuse after the client is no longer competent or able to make that decision and (2) the **medical durable power of attorney**, or **health care proxy**, which designates another person to make health care decisions for a person if the client becomes incompetent or unable to make such decisions. Each state outlines its own requirements for executing and revoking the medical durable power of attorney and living wills.

INCOMPETENT CLIENT'S RIGHT TO SELF-DETERMINATION

The courts are protective of incompetent clients and require high standards of proof before allowing a physician to terminate any life-sustaining treatment for that client. Nancy Cruzan was 30 years old and in a persistent vegetative state. She had a gastrostomy feeding and hydration tube inserted to assist with the feedings, which was consented to by her husband. Her parents, however, petitioned the court for removal of the tube. In the Cruzan case, the court held that the state had the right to err on the side of life. The U.S. Supreme Court recognized that a living will would have been sufficient evidence of Nancy Cruzan's wishes to sustain or to remove her feeding tube.

The issue before the U.S. Supreme Court was whether the state of Missouri could use its own standard of clear and convincing proof for removal of the tube or whether there was a 14th Amendment due process guarantee of a "right to die" that would override the state statute. It was decided that the constitutional right would not be extended and the state procedural requirement would be allowed, at which time the burden of proof was put on Nancy Cruzan's family to show that she would not have wanted to continue living in this manner.

THE NURSE'S ROLE

The nurse must know the laws of the state pertaining to advance directives and clients' rights. They must also know the policies and procedures of the institution. Nurses must inform clients of their right to formulate advance directives and to realize that not all clients can make such decisions. It is important to establish trust and rapport with your client and the client's family so that you can assist them to make decisions that are in the client's best interests. Nurses must also teach about advance directives (see Box 13–1 for common questions asked about advance directives) and document all critical decisions, discussions with the client and client's family about such decisions, and the basis for the decision-making process. Discrimination must be also prevented against clients and their families based on their decisions regarding their advance directives. If nurses *can* become involved in ethics committees at hospitals or nursing specialty groups at either local, state, or national levels, it is important that they participate. It is also important that the nurse determine

---

Box 13–1.　COMMON QUESTIONS ASKED ABOUT ADVANCE DIRECTIVES

Q. Which is better—a living will or a medical durable power of attorney for health care or health care proxy?

A. The documents are separate and allow the nurse to do two different things. The **living will** states what health care a client will accept or refuse after the client is no longer competent or able to make that decision. The **medical durable power of attorney** or **health care proxy** allows you as client to designate another person to make health care choices for you.

Q. If I change my mind and have a living will, can I cancel the living will or durable medical power of attorney?

A. Yes, each state has ways that your advance directives can be cancelled or negated. Most states require an oral or written statement, destruction of the document itself, or notification to certain individuals, such as the physician. Again, each state's statute should be checked for the specific details required.

Q. If I have a living will in one state, is it good in all states?

A. It may or may not be depending on the requirements for the living will. It is important that you have your living will checked by an attorney in order to determine whether or not it may be effective in the states in which you are traveling or working.

Q. If I have a living will and have medical durable power of attorney who should get copies?

A. Copies should be given to your next of kin, your physician and your attorney so that more than one person has a copy and knows what your intentions are. Some states will allow you to register your living will with certain state agencies such as the Secretary of State. Also there are national groups that will allow you to register your living will with them so that there is access to it.

---

whether or not the client has been coerced into making such decisions against his or her will.

DO-NOT-RESUSCITATE ORDERS

Do-not-resuscitate orders are separate and apart from advanced directives. In order to be legally protected there should be a *written* order for a "no code" or do-not-resuscitate order on the client's chart. Each hospital should have a policy and procedure that outlines what is required with regard to a client's condition for a do-not-resuscitate order. The do-not-resuscitate order should be reviewed, evaluated, and reordered. Different facilities have established different time periods. The nurse must also know if there is any law that regulates who should authorize a do-not-resuscitate order for an incompetent client or a client who is no longer able to make such a decision. Many times hospitals will have policies and procedures detailing what must be done and which clients fit the requirements for a do-not-resuscitate order. The American Nurses Association has published a position statement on nursing care and do-not-resuscitate decisions (Fig. 13–1).

Many ethical dilemmas face nurses when dealing with confusing or conflicting do-not-resuscitate orders. For example, it may be difficult to interpret a do-not-resuscitate order when it has been qualified, for instance, "do not resuscitate except for medications and defibrillation" or "no CPR or intubation." Many times lack of proper documentation in the medical records indicating how the do-not-resuscitate decision was reached can be an important and crucial issue if a medical malpractice case is involved and it is disputed whether or not the client or family actually gave consent for a do-not-resuscitate order.

Many facilities have developed do-not-resuscitate decision sheets for recording information about do-not-resuscitate discussions; or the sheets are dated and signed by the client and those family members who took part in the discussion. It then becomes a permanent part of the medical record. It is very important that nurses not stigmatize clients by the use of indicators for do-not-resuscitate orders, such as dots on the wristband or dots over the bed. Many times health care providers' attitudes change because they feel the client is "going to die anyway." It is very important that there is no abandonment of needed care with the client designated as a do-not-resuscitate client. It is also important for the nurse to know what the policies and procedures are with regard to transfer clients and do-not-resuscitate orders that accompany the incoming client. If there has not been a periodic review, is the order still in effect? If a client is transferred from one facility to another but has a do-not-resuscitate order that is time-limited and has not been reordered, what should a nurse do?

STANDARDS OF CARE

Standards of care are the *yardstick* that the legal system uses to measure the actions of a nurse involved in a malpractice suit. The underlying principle used to establish standards of care is based on the actions that would likely be taken by a reasonable person (nurse) who was placed in the same or similar circumstances. The standard usually includes both objective factors, such as the actions to be performed, and subjective factors, including the nurse's emotional and mental state. Specifically, a nurse is judged against the standards that are established within the nurse's profession and specialty area of practice. The American Nurses Association (ANA), as well as specialty groups within the nursing pro-

AMERICAN NURSES ASSOCIATION
Position Statement
on
Nursing Care and Do-Not-Resuscitate Decisions

ANA
AMERICAN NURSES
ASSOCIATION

Summary: Nurses bear a large responsibility at the time a patient experiences cardiac arrest for either initiating resuscitation or ensuring that unwanted attempts to resuscitate do not occur. Nurses face ethical dilemmas concerning confusing or conflicting DNR orders and this statement includes specific recommendations for the resolution of some of these dilemmas.

Background: Although cardiopulmonary resuscitation has been used effectively since the 1960s (Kouwenhoven et. al., 1960), the widespread use and possible overuse of this technique and the presumption that it should be used on all patients has been a subject of recent debate (U.S. Congress, 1987). The ways in which do-not-resuscitate (DNR) decisions are made and implemented continues to be a source of confusion and contention in the delivery of nursing care (Stenberg, 1988; MacIntosh, 1989). Practices regarding DNR decision-making and record-keeping vary from one health care institution to the next (Lo, 1991). There is a range of thinking about the nurse's participation in DNR decision-making. At some hospitals, the DNR policies actually indicate that the nurse is not to inquire about or initiate any discussion regarding extraordinary procedures with the patient; as this is perceived as the sole responsibility of the physician. Others have argued that nurses have a central role in DNR decision-making and have the competence and relevant authority to write DNR orders (Yarling, McElmurray 1983).

Nurses are actively involved in the decision-making about resuscitation and bear a large responsibility at the time a patient experiences cardiac arrest for either initiating resuscitation or ensuring that unwanted attempts to resuscitate do not occur (Stenberg, 1988). Nurses commonly face the following types of dilemmas concerning confusing or conflicting DNR orders:

1. Interpreting DNR orders especially in circumstances in which a "no code" order has been qualified as in "chemical code only," "or resuscitate but do not intubate" etc.;

2. Interpreting DNR orders in which there is some attempt to demonstrate or mimic a response, perhaps for the benefit of family members, that stops short of a full resuscitation effort as in "slow code" or "show code;"

3. DNR orders that are not accompanied by progress notes in the medical record indicating how the decision was made;

4. DNR orders that accompany patients from one facility to another with no periodic review or conversely DNR orders that are time-limited and therefore not in effect when a patient transfers from one facility to another;

5. Concerns about stigmatizing patients with DNR orders through the use of special symbols on armbands, etc.; and

6. Concerns about abandonment of other types of needed care for patients who are designated as DNR.

In view of the confusion and complexity that continue to surround DNR decisions and their implementation, ANA makes the following recommendations:

1. The choices and values of the competent patient should always be given highest priority, even when these wishes conflict with those of health care providers and families;

2. In the case of the incompetent or never competent patient, any existing advance directives or the decisions of surrogate decision-makers acting in the patient's best interest should be determinative;

Figure 13–1. ANA position on do-not-resuscitate decisions. (Reprinted with permission of the American Nurses Association, Washington, DC).

3. The DNR decision should always be a subject of explicit discussion among the patient, the family (one or more significant others as identified by the patient), any designated surrogate decision maker acting in the patient's best interest and the health care team and include consideration of the efficacy and desirability of CPR, a balancing of benefits and burdens to patients and therapeutic goals;

4. Nurses need to be aware of and have an active role in developing DNR policies within the institutions where they work;

5. DNR orders must be clearly documented, reviewed and updated periodically to reflect changes in the patient's condition (JCAHO, 1992);

6. A DNR order is separate from other aspects of a patient's care and there should be no implied implied or actual abandonment of other types of care for patients with DNR orders, which should continue to be evaluated on a burdens versus benefits basis;

7. Nurses have a duty to educate patients and their families about all types of termination of treatment decisions and should encourage patients and their families to think about these decisions before admission to health care facilities;

8. Nurses have a responsibility to educate patients and their families about various forms of advance directives such as living wills, durable power of attorney etc. (Omnibus, 1990);

9. Their should be clear mechanisms in place within each health care facility (preferably, the use of an interdisciplinary ethics committee with nurse members) for the resolution of disputes among health care professionals or among patients, families and health care professionals concerning DNR orders, and

10. If it is the nurse's personal belief that her moral integrity is compromised by her professional responsibility to carry out a particular DNR order, she should transfer the responsibility for the patient's care to another nurse.

The appropriate use of DNR orders can prevent suffering for many patients who choose not to extend their lives after experiencing cardiac arrest. As the primary continuous health care provider in health care facilities, the nurse must be involved in the planning as well as the implementation of resuscitation decisions. Clear DNR policies at the institutional level which include the basic features that ANA recommends, will enable nurses to effectively participate in this crucial aspect of patient care.

Figure 13–1. Continued.

fession like the American Association of Critical-Care Nurses (AACN), publish standards of care that are continually updated.

Both external and internal standards govern the conduct of nurses. **External standards** include nursing standards developed by the ANA, the State Nurse Practice Act of each jurisdiction, criteria from accrediting agencies such as the Joint Commission on Accreditation of Healthcare Organizations, guidelines developed by various nursing specialty practice groups, and federal agency regulations.

Internal standards include nursing standards defined in specific hospital policy and procedure manuals that relate to the nurse in the particular institution. The nurse's job description and employment contract are examples of internal nursing standards that define the duty of the nurse.

The rationale for advancing standards of care for the nurse is to ensure proper, consistent, and high-quality nursing care to all members of society. When nurses violate their duty of care to the client as established by the profession's standards of care, they leave themselves open to charges of negligence and malpractice. Until recently, nurses were held to the standards of the local community. National criteria have now replaced the *locality rule* standard. Individual nurses are held accountable not only to acceptable standards within the local community but to national standards as well.

Although standards of care may appear to be very specific, they are merely guidelines for nursing practice. Because every client's situation is different, the appropriate standard of care may be difficult to identify in a specific case. More than one course of nursing action may be considered appropriate under a proper standard of care. The final decision made must be guided by the nurse's judgment and understanding of the client's needs.

NURSE PRACTICE ACT

The **nurse practice** act defines nursing practice and establishes standards for nurses in each state. It is the most definitive legal statute or legislative act regulating nursing practice. Although nurse practice acts vary in scope from state to state, they tend to have similar wording based loosely upon the American Nurses Association model published in 1988. The nurse practice act provides a framework for the court on which to base decisions when determining whether a nurse has breached a standard of care.

Most state nurse practice acts define scope of practice, establish requirements for licensure and entry into practice, and create and empower a board of nursing to oversee the practice of nurses. In addition, nurse practice acts identify grounds for disciplinary actions such as suspension and revocation of a nursing license (Aiken, 1994).

The judicial interpretation of the Nurse Practice Act and its relationship to a specific case provides guidance for decisions about future cases. Many state legislatures have responded to the expanded role of the nurse by broadening the scope of their nurse practice acts. For example, adding the term **nursing diagnosis** to many states' acts reflects the legislature's recognition of the expansion of the nurse's role. In addition, occupational roles such a nurse practitioner and clinical nurse specialist are beginning to be included in nurse practice acts. It is important to remember that as the nurse's role expands, so does the legal accountability of the role itself.

WHEN THE NURSE IS SUED

Because of the rapid proliferation of lawsuits over the past decade, there is now a higher probability that a nurse, at some time in the nurse's career, will be involved either as a witness or a party to a nursing malpractice action. Knowledge of the litigation process increases the nurse's understanding of the way in which the nurse's conduct is evaluated before the courts.

Statute of Limitations

A malpractice suit against a nurse for negligence must be filed within a specified time. This period, called the **statute of limitations**, generally begins at the time of the injury, or when the injury is discovered and lasts until some specified future time. In most states, the limitation period lasts from 1 to 6 years, with the most common duration being 2 years. If the client fails to file the suit within the prescribed time, the lawsuit will be barred.

The Complaint

Filing the suit, also called the **complaint**, with the court begins the litigation process. The written complaint describes the incident that initiated the claim of negligence against the nurse. Specific allegations, including the amount of money sought for damages, are also stated in the complaint. The plaintiff, usually a client or a family member of a client, is the alleged injured party and the defendant (i.e., nurse, physician or hospital), is the person or entity being sued. The first notice of a lawsuit occurs when the defendant (nurse) is officially notified or served with the complaint.

The Answer

The defendant must respond to the allegations stated in the complaint within a specific time frame. This written response by the defendant is called the answer. If the nurse had liability insurance in force at the time of the negligent act, the insurer will assign a lawyer to represent the defendant nurse. In the answer, the nurse can outline specific defenses to the claims against him or her; failure to file within the prescribed time (statute of limitations) will result in the case being barred from trial.

The Discovery

After the complaint and answer are filed with the court, the discovery phase of the litigation begins. The purpose of discovery is to uncover all information relevant to the malpractice suit. The nurse may be required to answer a series of questions that relate to the nurse's educational background, emotional state, the incident that led to the lawsuit, and any other information the plaintiff's lawyer deems important. These written questions are called **interrogatories**.

In addition, the plaintiff's layer may seek **requests for production of documents**. These are actual documents related to the lawsuit including the plaintiff's medical records, the institution's policy and procedure manual concerning the specific situation, and the nurse's job description. The plaintiff is also required to disclose information as part of the discovery process that includes the plaintiff's past medical history.

The Deposition

The next step in the process is the taking of a deposition from each party to the lawsuit, as well as any potential witnesses, to assist the lawyers in the trial preparation. A **deposition** is a formal legal process that involves the taking of testimony under oath which is recorded by a court reporter. In some cases, videotaped depositions may be used. Nurses can prepare for a deposition by keeping some key points in mind (Box 13–2).

The deposition testimony is reduced to a written document for use at trial. If a witness during the actual trial changes testimony from that given at the deposition, the deposition can be used to contradict the testimony, a process called

---

**Box 13–2   PREPARING FOR A DEPOSITION
(AIKEN, 1994)**

1   Do not volunteer information.
2   Be familiar with the client's medical record and nurse's notes.
3   Remain calm throughout the process and do not be intimidated by the lawyers.
4   Clarify all questions before answering—ask the lawyer to explain the question if not understood.
5   Do not make assumptions about the questions.
6   Do not exaggerate answers.
7   Allow at least 5 seconds after a question is asked before answering it to allow objections from other lawyers.
8   Tell the truth.
9   Do not speculate about answers.
10   Speak slowly and clearly, using professional language as much as possible.
11   Look the questioning lawyer in the eye as much as possible.
12   If unable to remember an answer, simply state "I don't remember" or "I don't know."
13   Think before answering any question.
14   Bring a resume or curriculum vitae to the deposition in case it is requested.
15   Request a break if tired or confused.
16   Avoid becoming angry with the lawyers or using sarcastic language.
17   Avoid using absolutes in the answers.
18   If a question is asked more than once, ask the court recorder to read the answer given previously.
19   Be sure to read over the deposition just before the trial.

impeaching the witness. Impeaching a witness on a specific issue can create doubt about that witness's credibility and thus weaken other areas in the witness's testimony.

The Trial

The actual trial often takes place years after the complaint was filed. The first phase of the trial is the **voire dire process**, more commonly called **jury selection.** After jury selection, each attorney presents opening statements. The plaintiff's side is presented first. Each witness or party is subject to direct examination, cross-examination, and redirect examination. Direct examination involves open-ended questions by the attorney. Cross-examination is performed by the opposing lawyer, and questions are asked in such a way as to elicit short, specific responses. The redirect examination is composed of follow-up questions to address issues that were previously raised during the cross-examination. After both parties have presented their case, the lawyers deliver their closing arguments. The case then goes to the jury or the judge for deliberation. The decision or ruling made about the case can be appealed if either party is not satisfied.

Possible Defenses to a Malpractice Suit

Contributory Negligence Versus Comparative Negligence

Damages awarded vary from state to state and also with types of injuries sustained. In a state with **contributory negligence laws,** clients are not allowed to receive money for injuries if they contributed to that injury in any manner. For example, the nurse forgot to raise the bedrail after administering an injection of a narcotic pain medication to a client who had had an operation, but instructed the client to turn on the call light if he wanted to get out of bed. The client fell while attempting to go to the bathroom but because he did not use the call light, he had contributed to his own injuries and so could not receive compensation for them.

In a state with **comparative negligence laws,** the awards are based on the determination of the percentage of fault by both parties. For example, in the above case, if $100,000 was awarded by the jury, it may be determined that the nurse was 75% at fault and the client was 25% at fault. In that case, the client would receive $75,000. In general, if the client is 50% or more at fault, no award will be made. As can be seen, determination of these types of awards is highly subjective and is often appealed to a higher court.

Assumption of Risk

When the client signs the informed consent form for a particular treatment, procedure, or surgery, it is implied that he or she is aware of the possible complications of that treatment, procedure, or surgery. Under the **assumption-of-risk defense**, if one of those listed or named complications occurs, the client has no grounds to sue the health care provider. For example, a common complication from hip replacement surgery is some loss of mobility and range of motion of the affected leg. Even if a client, after having a hip replaced, is only able to walk using a walker, he still does not have any grounds for a lawsuit.

Good Samaritan Statutes

Health care providers are sometimes hesitant to provide care at accidents, in emergency situations, or disasters because they fear lawsuits. **Good samaritan laws** were written specifically to protect health care providers in these situations. A health care professional who provides care in an emergency situation cannot be sued for injuries that may sustained by the client if that care was given according to established guidelines and was within the scope of the professional's education. For example, a nurse who finds a person in cardiac arrest administers cardiopulmonary resuscitation (CPR) to revive the person. In the process, she fractures several of the client's ribs. The client would not be able to sue the nurse for the fractured ribs if the CPR was administered according to established standards.

Good samaritan laws do, however, have some limitations. They do not cover nurses for grossly negligent acts in the provision of care, nor for acts outside the nurse's level of education. For example, a person is choking on a piece of meat. The nurse initially attempts the Heimlich maneuver without success. As the person loses consciousness, the nurse decides to perform a tracheostomy. The client survives but can sue the nurse for injuries from the tracheostomy because this is not a normal part of a nurse's education.

Unavoidable Accident

Sometimes accidents happen without any contributing causes from the nurse, hospital, or physician. For example, a client is walking in the hall and trips over her own bathrobe, breaking an ankle. There were no puddles on the floor, no obstacles in the hall, and the client was alert and oriented. Because no one is at fault, there are no grounds for a law suit.

Defense of the Fact

This defense is based on the claim that the actions of the nurse followed the standards of care, or that even if the actions *were* in violation of the standard of care, the action itself was not the direct cause of the injury. For example, a nurse wraps a dressing too tightly on a client's foot after surgery. Later, the client loses his sight and blames the loss of vision on the nurse's improper dressing of his foot (Aiken, 1994).

Going through the litigation process can produce high levels of anxiety. Placing every aspect of the nurse's conduct under scrutiny in a trial is very stressful. All aspects of the alleged negligent act will be examined and re-examined. Every word of the nurse's notes and the medical record will be analyzed and questioned. Nurses can survive the litigation process by being honest and demonstrating that they were acting in the best interest of the client.

ALTERNATIVE DISPUTE FORUMS

Although most lawsuits against nurses are settled through the court system, there are other means for settling them. Due to the large number of cases and the resulting overload of the judicial system, other methods of resolving disputes have become increasingly popular. These alternative forums of dispute resolution (ADR) are being used for many types of conflicts and are seen more frequently in the area of torts, contracts, employment, and family law matters. Mediation and arbitration are the most commonly used alternatives to trial.

Mediation is a process that allows each party to present their case to a mediator, who is an independent third party trained in dispute resolution. The mediator listens to each side individually. This one-sided session is termed a **caucus**. The mediator's role is to find common ground between the parties and encourage resolution of the disputed matters by compromise and negotiation. The mediator aids the parties in arriving at a mutually acceptable outcome. The mediator does not act as a decision maker but rather encourages the parties to come to a "meeting of the minds."

Arbitration, on the other hand, allows a neutral third party to hear both parties' positions and then make a decision or ruling based on the facts and evidence presented. Arbitration, by agreement or by statutory definition, can be binding or nonbinding. Arbitrators or mediators can be, and frequently are, retired judges who work on an hourly basis. Often they are attorneys. In the family law areas, they are frequently social workers or specially trained mediators.

Negligence and malpractice issues are frequently resolved through arbitration and mediation.

PREVENTION OF LAWSUITS

What can the nurse do to avoid having to go through the very stressful, sometimes financially and professionally devastating process of litigation? The following guidelines provide some ways to avoid a lawsuit.

1   The medical record is the single most frequently used piece of objective evidence in a malpractice suit. Maintaining an accurate and complete medical record is an absolute requirement. The old adage "if it isn't written, it didn't

happen" remains true. Trying to recall specific events from 2 years previously without the benefit of written notes is almost impossible. In general, the client record should not contain personal opinion, should be legible, should be in chronological order, and should be written and signed by the nurse. An entry should never be obliterated or destroyed. If a nurse questions a physician's order, record must be made that the physician was contacted and the order clarified.

2   Establishing a rapport with the client through honest, open communication goes a long way in avoiding law suits. Treating clients and their families with respect and letting them know the nurse really cares about them may well prevent a lawsuit. Many people are willing to forgive a nurse's error if they have good rapport and a trusting relationship with a nurse they believe is interested in their well-being.

3   Keeping one's nursing knowledge and skills current is vital to prevent errors that may lead to lawsuits. It is better to refuse to perform an unfamiliar procedure than to attempt it without the necessary knowledge and skills. Taking advantage of in-services, workshops, and continuing nursing education classes is an important part of maintaining the nurse's skill level. Nurses must practice within their level of competence and scope of practice.

4   Recognizing the client who is lawsuit-prone can help reduce the risk of litigation. Some common characteristics of this type of client include constant dissatisfaction with the care given, constant complaints about all aspects of care, and negative comments about other nurses. This client often complains about the poor care given by nurses on the previous shift. This client may also have a history of lawsuits against nurses.

Being direct, solving problems with the client, and helping the client become involved in his or her care is helpful to diffuse this negative behavior. Also, even more careful documentation of the care provided and the client's responses to the care can be helpful if a lawsuit is later filed.

5   Maintaining proper liability insurance is a necessity. Nurses who do not carry liability insurance place themselves at high risk. The nurse's personal assets as well as the nurse's wages may be subject to a judgment awarded in a malpractice action. Even if the client does not win at the trial, the litigation process including hiring a lawyer and paying the costs of experts can be financially devastating.

Liability Insurance

A **professional liability insurance policy** is a contract with an insurer who promises to assume the costs paid to the injured party in exchange for payment of a premium. There are two types of malpractice policies: claims-made and occurrence. **Claims-made policies** protect only against claims made during the time the policy is in effect. **Occurrence policies** protect against all claims that occurred during the policy period, regardless of when the claim is made. Generally, the occurrence type of liability insurance offers more protection. Claims-made policy coverage can be broadened by also purchasing a *tail* which is a separate policy that extends the time of coverage.

Some hospitals have liability insurance policies for the nurse as a part of the nurse's employment package with the institution. This hospital policy may be limited to claims arising from nurse's employment and might not apply in a situation where a nurse renders care outside the institution, for instance, at an automobile accident site. It is preferable to have liability insurance coverage that includes all situations in which the nurse may be involved. Individual liability insurance coverage independent of the hospital is recommended (Box 13–3).

REGULATORY AND ADMINISTRATIVE LAW

Revocation of License

One of the most drastic punishments that a nurse can experience is revocation of the license to practice nursing. The nursing profession is responsible for monitoring and enforcing its own standards through the state licensing board. These actions may or may not be related to tort law, contract law, or criminal charges. Each state's licensing board is charged with the responsibility to oversee the professional nurse's competence.

The state's nursing board receives its authority to grant and revoke licenses from specific statutory laws. The underlying rationale for establishment of a licensing board is to protect the public from uneducated, unsafe, or unethical practitioners. If a nurse fails to adhere to the standards of safe practice and exhibits unprofessional behavior, he or she can be disciplined by the state nursing licensing board. One of the remedies that these boards can use is suspension or revocation of the nurse's license.

A disciplinary hearing is held to review the charges of the nurse's unprofessional conduct. This hearing is less formal than the trial process and the nurse is allowed to present evidence and be represented by legal counsel at the hearing. Due process requires that the nurse be notified in advance of the specific charges being made. The question of what constitutes *unprofessional conduct* is an issue frequently dealt with at the disciplinary hearing. Each respective state's nurse practice act provide guidance as to the specifies of unprofessional conduct.

Unprofessional conduct can be reported by a nursing peer, supervisor, client, or a client's family. Many cases are dismissed before the hearing takes place if the board finds there is no support for the allegation being made against the nurse. If a hearing is necessary, it is in the best interest of the nurse to seek legal counsel due to potential risk of license revocation.

Box 13–3 WHAT TO LOOK FOR IN AN INSURANCE POLICY

The following factors should be reviewed in order to determine what is the best policy for your type of nursing practice:

1 Type of insurance policy (claims-made or occurrence basis)
2 Insuring agreement.
The insurance company's promise to pay in exchange for premiums is called the **insuring agreement**. The insurance company agrees to pay a money award to a plaintiff who is injured by an act of omission or commission by a health care provider who is insured by the company.
3 Types of injuries covered.
The language must be scrutinized to determine whether it is broad or limiting. Some companies will agree to pay only if the insured nurse is sued for damages, which means the nurse must be sued for a money amount or award. If the nurse is sued for a specific performance lawsuit or an injunctive relief action, which means that the nurse will either have to perform something or discontinue doing something, that particular insurance policy may not be adequate. Also most insurance policies will not cover the nurse for disciplinary actions.
4 Exclusions.
Items that are not covered by policy are called **exclusions**. It is important to review the exclusions. Some of the more common exclusions include: sexual abuse of a client, injury caused while under the influence of drugs or alcohol, criminal activity, and punitive damages. These are damages that are used to punish the defendant for egregious acts or omissions.

WHO IS COVERED UNDER THE POLICY

The purchaser is the named insured who can either be an individual, institution or a group. Others who may be covered by the policy are nurses, employees, agents, and volunteers, among others.

LIMITATIONS AND DEDUCTIONS

In exchange for payment of the premium, the insurance company agrees to pay up to a certain amount on behalf of the insured. This amount is called the **limit of liability**. It is usually expressed in two ways. The amount that can be paid per incident (**per occurrence**), and the amount that will be paid for the entire policy year. For example, if you have a policy that states $1,000,000/$3,000,000, it means that the company will pay up to $1 million per incident and a total of $3 million per policy year.

Box 13-3 **WHAT TO LOOK FOR IN AN INSURANCE POLICY** (Continued)

FINANCIAL STRENGTH OF THE INSURANCE COMPANY

The insurance industry relies on the A. M. Best Company to evaluate both the financial size and relative strengths of insurance companies. An A. M. Best rating of A- or better should be a prerequisite for purchase of any policy.

THE RIGHT TO SELECT COUNSEL

Some insurance companies will allow nurses to select their own attorneys to represent them in a medical negligence claim. Others will retain attorneys or law firms and the nurse will not have the opportunity to make that selection.

THE RIGHT TO CONSENT TO SETTLEMENT

Some policies will allow the nurse to decide whether or not a case should be settled or go to trial, whereas others will not.

License revocation is a serious consequence for the nurse because it removes the nurse's right to practice. Drug abuse, administering medication without a prescription, practicing without a valid license, and any singular act of unprofessional or unethical conduct can constitute grounds for loosing a nursing license.

CONCLUSION

The legal system and its effects on the practice of nursing are ever-present realities in today's health care system. Nurses need to be aware of the implications of their actions but should not be so overwhelmed by fear that it reduces their ability to care for the client. The more advanced and specialized the nurse's practice becomes, the higher the standards to which the nurse is held. Nurses will be challenged throughout their career to apply legal principles in the day-to-day practice of nursing. An awareness of what constitutes malpractice and negligence will aid in the prevention of litigation.

BIBLIOGRAPHY

Aiken, TD: Legal, Ethical, and Political Issues in Nursing. FA Davis, Philadelphia, 1994.
Creighton, H: Law Every Nurse Should Know, ed 5. WB Saunders, Philadelphia, 1986.
Cushing, M: Nursing Jurisprudence. Appleton-Lange, Norwalk, CT, 1988.
Feutz-Harter, S: Nursing and the Law, ed 5. Professional Education Systems, Inc., New York, 1993.

CHARTING: WHAT YOU NEED TO KNOW

It would be difficult to find nurses who enjoy charting. In general, nurses view charting and most other kinds of paper work, as a necessary evil that should be if not avoided completely, at least put off for as long as possible. From a legal standpoint, however, it is one of the most important activities that nurses undertake. The following is a list of considerations that improve charting and help to make it a valuable element of patient care.

1 Be accurate because a client's condition changes throughout the shift. The time at which you performed a nursing action, as well as the time and nature of the client's response, can be very important when you are defending yourself from a lawsuit. When 2 or 3 years have elapsed after the action, the chart is the only hard evidence of what happened. Using a legal viewpoint, if it was not charted, it was not done.

2 Demonstrate the priority of nursing actions. It is important that the chart reflect not only *that* an action was taken, but also *why* it was taken. Showing that you treated a client's most serious, life-threatening problems first is essential to demonstrate that the actions you took are based on sound nursing judgment.

3 Incorporate standards of care. In any lawsuit, nurses are held to the applicable standards of care. If these standards are violated in the provision of care, it becomes difficult to defend yourself against a lawsuit. Charting should demonstrate that the overall nursing care was planned according to an acceptable standard of care. Charting should reflect any deviations from this plan, with rationales determined by the client's changing condition.

4 Chart all communications with physicians. A major element in many lawsuits is the failure of the physician to communicate with the nurse. Any telephone conversations, orders from the physician, and verbal exchanges while the physician is on the unit should be documented. If these exchanges involve information that has the potential to provoke a lawsuit, they should be charted in more detail.

5 Be careful with a physician's orders. Always check charts for new orders after physicians have handled them. When taking orders off, make sure that a line is drawn after the last order in such a way that the physician cannot add any orders on that sheet. Prewritten order sheets should be timed and dated for when they were received by the nurse. Always read back verbal or phone orders to the physician to doublecheck what was

CHARTING: WHAT YOU NEED TO KNOW (Continued)

said. Misinterpretation of a physician's orders is a frequent source of lawsuits against nurses.

6 Never change, recopy, or white out any part of a record: Obvious changes in medical records are a red flag to lawyers, indicating that someone is trying to hide something. If a part of a chart needs to be re-copied because it has become soiled or illegible, the original should remain with it.

7 Keep advanced directives on the chart. Living wills, durable powers of attorney, or other documents that describe the client's wishes, if clients are no longer are able to make decisions about their care, should be readily available in the chart. In situations where a client goes into cardiac or respiratory arrest, it is much easier for the health care providers to make decisions about what actions to take if this information is at hand. In addition, family members will be more comfortable with the actions taken if they can see the advance directives.

8 Record interactions with the family and client. Because of the stress on both client and family during a serious illness, misinterpretations of information often occur. Charting what was said to the client and family and their responses to the information is a good method to protect yourself from legal actions that may occur years later. Note any hostility or anger expressed by the family, but chart it in a nonjudgmental manner using direct quotes as much as possible. It is better to chart: client's husband states: "You nurses are really stupid in this hospital—nobody seems to know what is going on" rather than "client's husband seems hostile and angry." Angry families are more likely to sue than satisfied ones.

9 Be as descriptive as possible. Even if you do not know the exact medical term for what you are observing, try to describe it as clearly as possible. You may have forgotten that anasarca is the term that describes generalized body edema, but stating "+2 to +3 pitting edema of arms, hands, legs, feet, and torso" accomplishes the same goal. Avoid charting judgments and use of the words "seems" or "appears."

Despite universal distaste for it, charting is an important part of client care. It allows you to take credit for the care you have given and demonstrates your knowledge of the important patient responses to be evaluated. If you are ever sued for malpractice, the chart, if done well, will become your most important ally.

Modified from Calfee, BE: Tips for better charting. Nursing '94:32–33, December 1994.

A Closer Look

THE NATIONAL PRACTITIONER DATA BANK

The National Practitioner Data Bank was created by the Healthcare Quality Improvement Act of 1986. It became operational on September 1, 1990. The U.S. Congress enacted the law based on a belief that the need to improve the quality of care and slow the increasing rate of malpractice litigation could no longer rest solely with the licensing bodies and the states. The intent was to provide positive incentives, participation, and peer review in the form of good faith immunity for those providing information to the data bank. The data bank information is available upon request to hospitals and health care providers engaged in credentialing. The information should restrict the ability of incompetent practitioners to move from state to state.

The data bank supplies three different types of information:

1   Information relating to medical malpractice payments made on behalf of health care practitioners

2   Information relating to adverse actions taken against clinical privileges of the physician, osteopath, or dentist

3   Information concerning actions by professional societies that adversely affect membership

The types of information reported:

1   *Required*: adverse professional review actions against physicians, osteopaths, and dentists

2   *Required*: medical malpractice payments made on behalf of all health care providers

3   *Optional*: adverse professional review actions against other health care providers including nurses

Failure to report to the data bank carries fines and penalties for those identified as mandatory reporters.

Fiesta, J: The Law and Liability. A Guide for Nurses, ed 2. John Wiley and Sons, New York, 1988.
Guido, G: Legal Issues in Nursing. A Source Book for Practice. Appleton and Lange, Norwalk, CT, 1988.
Louisell, D, Hazard, G, and Colen, T: Pleading and Procedure, ed 5. The Foundation Press, New York, 1983.
Louisell, D and Williams, H: Medical Malpractice. Matthew Bender, New York, 1990.
Lynn, R: Jury Trial Law and Practice. John Wiley and Sons, New York, 1986.
Murchison, I, Nichols, T and Hansen, R: Legal Accountability in the Nursing Process, ed 2. CV Mosby, St Louis, 1982.

Prosser, W and Keeton, D: The Law of Torts, ed 5. St Paul, West Pub. 1984.
Rhodes, A and Miller, R: Nursing and the Law. Aspen Systems, Rockville, MD, 1984.

HISTORICAL PERSPECTIVES

The Effect of the Korean and Vietnam Conflicts on Nursing Today

Many of the medical practices that were initiated during the police action in Korea were further developed during the war in Vietnam. In Korea, the Mobile Army Surgical Hospital (MASH) and the use of the helicopter played important roles in saving lives. In Vietnam, the Medical Unit, Self-contained, Transportable (MUST) hospitals replaced MASH units because of the lack of distinct battle lines and a secure road system. The MUST units consisted of inflatable rubber shelters that were completely self-contained and generally located some distance from the combat areas. These hospitals were staffed with Army physicians, nurses, and ancillary help.

The first of some 5000 nurses to serve in the war in Vietnam started arriving in 1962. To encourage nurses to serve in the armed forces, the Warrant Officer Nurse Program was developed so that nurses who were graduates of 2-year associate's degree (AD) programs could be commissioned as Warrant Officers during the war. Up to this time, only nurses with bachelor's of science (BS) degrees could be commissioned in the armed services.

The nurses who served and cared for the wounded during the Vietnam war showed a high degree of professionalism, independence of practice, and great courage. They were an essential part of the health care team, an important morale booster for the troops, and participated in the development of new techniques for the care of the severely wounded. Four Navy nurses were awarded the Purple Heart for injuries they received during a Viet Cong assault on Saigon in 1964. One Army nurse, First Lt. Sharon Lane, was killed on June 8, 1969, during an attack on the hospital at Chu Lai.

Only recently have the efforts of these nurses and other women who served in the military during the Vietnam war been recognized in the Vietnam Womens' War Memorial. Gen. Colin L. Powell, former Chairman of the Joint Chiefs of Staff, said at the ground-breaking ceremony:

"I didn't realize, although I should have, what a burden you carried. I didn't realize how much your sacrifice equaled and even exceeded that of the men. . . . for male soldiers, the war came in intermittent flashes of terror, occasional death, moments of pain; but for the women who were there, for the women who helped before the battle and for the nurses in particular, the terror, the death and the pain were unrelenting, a constant terrible weight that had to be stoically carried."

14

ISSUES IN PROVIDING CARE

Learning Objectives

After completing this chapter, the reader will be able to:
1 Analyze the effect that computerized nursing systems have on management and ethical issues.
2 Compare quantitative and qualitative nursing research.
3 List the signs and symptoms of the chemically impaired nurse.
4 Name the steps in dealing with a chemically impaired nurse.
5 Discuss the need for maintaining competency in nursing.
6 Analyze the key issues involved in the mandatory versus voluntary continuing education for nurses.

Nursing is a dynamic profession in a constantly changing system of health care. This chapter discusses issues that challenge the profession of nursing today and will continue to challenge it into the future.

CARE DELIVERY MODELS

Various models may be used in the delivery of nursing care. Many health care facilities are currently in a period of transition from one model to another and may even incorporate several different models at the same time. The nurse must recognize which model is being used, as well as its strengths and weaknesses. These models include functional nursing, team nursing, primary-care nursing, and modular nursing.

Functional Nursing

Functional nursing (Fig. 14–1) has as its foundation a task-oriented philosophy—each person performs a specific job that is narrowly defined according to the needs of the unit. The medication nurse, for example, focuses on the duties concerned with administering and documenting medications for the assigned group of clients. In this organizational unit the nurse manager is called the *charge nurse* whose main responsibility is to oversee the various workers. This model relies on ancillary health workers, such as nurse's aides and orderlies. Some feel this model fragments care too much. Because many people have specific tasks, coordination can be difficult and the holistic perspective may be lost.

Team Nursing

Team nursing (Fig. 14–2) has a more unified approach to client care, with team members functioning together to achieve client goals. The team leader functions as the person ultimately responsible for the clients' well-being. More cohesiveness is present among the members of the team than is found in the functional model. Rather than having a narrow task to accomplish, team members focus on team goals under the coordination of the team leader. The team conference provides for effective communication and follow-up between and among team members and is the key to successful team nursing.

Primary Care Nursing

The primary-care nursing (Fig. 14–3) model provides nurses with the opportunity to focus on the whole person. The primary-care nurse provides, and is re-

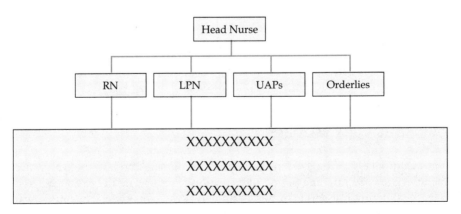

Clients

Figure 14–1. Organizational structure of functional nursing. (Adapted from Marquis, BL, and Huston, CJ: Management Decision Making for Nurses. JB Lippincott, Philadelphia, 1994.)

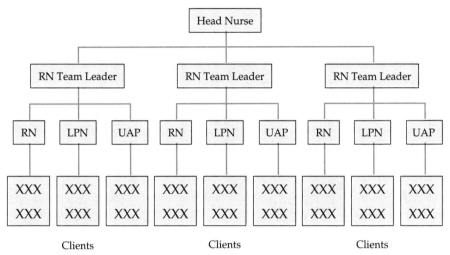

Figure 14–2. Organizational structure of team nursing. (Adapted from Marquis, BL, and Huston, CJ: Management Decision Making for Nurses. JB Lippincott, Philadelphia, 1994.)

sponsible for, all of the client's nursing needs. The nurse manager in this model becomes a facilitator for the primary-care nurses. Primary-care nurses are self-directed and concerned with consistency of care. The primary-care model is similar to the case management model which has one nurse caring for one client. Many home health care agencies use this method of assigning a registered nurse to work with an individual or family for the duration of the services rendered.

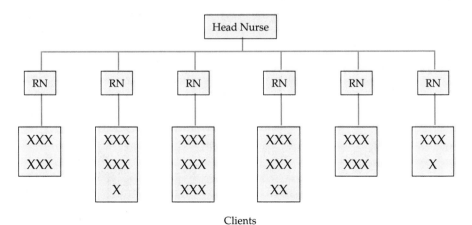

Figure 14–3. Organizational structure of primary-care nursing. (Adapted from Marquis, BL, and Huston, CJ: Management Decision Making for Nurses. JB Lippincott, Philadelphia, 1994.)

Modular Nursing

Modular nursing (Fig. 14–4), also called client-focused care, is a model which was developed in response to shortages of professional nursing personnel and to the downsizing of professional nursing staffs. This model is based on a decentralized organizational system that emphasizes close interdisciplinary collaboration. Redesigning the method of nursing care delivery takes much planning and input from the various departments involved, such as nursing, respiratory therapy, physical therapy, radiology, laboratory, and kitchen.

Important aspects of modular nursing include: relying on unlicensed assistive personnel (UAP, also called unit-service assistants) for the provision of direct care; grouping clients with similar needs; and emphasizing team concepts in small groups that remain constant. Cross-training of personnel is another important aspect of modular nursing; for example, using this system, respiratory therapists do not just provide respiratory treatments but also help clients to the bathroom and turn bedridden clients. Nurse managers in this system are responsible for providing explicit job descriptions, maintaining the work group's cohesiveness, carefully monitoring each staff person's abilities, assessing client conditions, delegating tasks as appropriate, and evaluating the effectiveness of care.

The role of UAPs is one area of the client-focused care model that needs more definition, particularly in relation to the registered nurse's accountability and responsibilities in supervising these workers. State boards of nursing across the country are in the process of considering possible changes in nurse practice acts necessitated by the use of unlicensed assistive personnel.

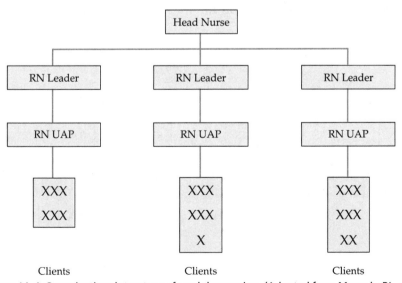

Figure 14–4. Organizational structure of modular nursing. (Adapted from Marquis, BL, and Huston, CJ: Management Decision Making for Nurses. JB Lippincott, Philadelphia, 1994.)

Benefits of this care-delivery model include decreased staffing cost and greater autonomy of cross-trained personnel. The nurse manager must be a strong leader for this model of care delivery to succeed (Clouten, 1994). Consistent collaboration between the nurse manager and physician is of utmost importance in planning client care.

Case Method

The **case method**, also called total-client care, is the assignment of one nurse to the total care of one or more clients. The nurse assumes total responsibility for meeting all the needs of clients the nurse is assigned to when on duty (Tappen, 1995).

This method of care was used widely when home care was the norm. It is still used by home health care nurses, community agencies, and private duty nurses. It was used in the hospital setting for some time, but was felt by administrators to be too expensive.

This form of care gives nurses a high degree of autonomy and responsibility. The lines of responsibility and accountability are clearly defined so the client receives consistent and unified care while the nurse is on duty. This mode of care is simple and direct and after the assignments are made, no further delineation of duties are required.

The greatest disadvantage of total-client care is when the nurse does not have adequate training to meet the care needs of the client. Due to nursing shortages, nurses with lower levels of education may be assigned to provide care for clients with problems they are not trained to meet. In this situation, a co-nurse may also be assigned, which destroys the total-client-care model.

Care Management

The goal of **care management**, also called **managed care**, is to provide the highest level of client care at the lowest cost. All the services that add up to the totality of care for a client are used so that the end costs are carefully controlled. In this model, the professional nurse coordinates care and provides direct care for his or her assigned clients. Health maintenance organizations and preferred provider organizations are the primary examples of managed-care systems. Because of their cost effectiveness, it is felt that managed-care systems will become the dominant mode of health care delivery in the future (Tappen, 1995).

Managed care uses a combination of primary-nursing and case-management models. The nurse assumes responsibility for both the clinical and economic outcomes associated with the client's care and is responsible for close monitoring of the client's progress toward recovery and discharge. In many institutions, a critical pathway is established for the client during admission. Critical pathways are blueprints for providing and monitoring care. The blueprint identifies the intermediate goals that the client should achieve while hospitalized. Through this process, the nurse is able to monitor the client's continued progress toward the ultimate goal of recovery and discharge within the time allowed by the diagnosis-related groups (DRGs) or other payment systems. Under the DRG method of reimbursement, the hospital is given a fixed sum of money for each client based on that client's medical diagnosis. (See Chapter 10.)

A critical pathway is a standardized plan of care that identifies predictable outcomes that must be achieved within a specific time frame. In a critical pathway, many activities depend on one another for completion. Wide numbers of variables affect the final outcome. Some of these factors are outside of the control of the planner but will need to be anticipated as much as possible (Table 14–1).

One of the most satisfying aspects of managed care is the holistic orientation it brings to the health care setting. In addition to following a client's progress from admission to discharge, the nurse plays an important role in all aspects of the client's care. Moreover, the client has one individual to whom to turn who understands all aspects of the client's care regimen. The improved coordination and better access to required services are also important advantages to this method.

Nursing-care management makes greater demands on individual nurses. The nurse needs to be more knowledgeable and flexible in the care provided. Managed care also requires a collegial relationship between physicians and nurses, a relationship with which some physicians feel uncomfortable. If the facility is not philosophically oriented toward this type of care and totally dedicated to it, it will probably not work.

COMPUTER APPLICATION

How do computers assist in the delivery of efficient, effective nursing care? Communication, research, client-care decisions, and documentation are examples of areas that are enhanced by use of computers. Most modern health care facilities use computers to link the various departments, thus enhancing communication. Rural facilities use computers as referral and consultation tools providing interaction with larger medical centers and specialty physicians. Computers help provide instant and continuous monitoring of the client's condition, for instance when they are used in monitoring vital signs and other physiologic properties.

At the nurse-management level, computers are used to determine personnel schedules and to improve communication among team members on the various shifts; they are also increasingly important tools in care documentation. One area in which computer systems have had a profound impact on nursing is medication administration. Computer-generated medication administration forms and rapid communication between nurse and pharmacist have improved care and decreased medication errors. The client's medications can be automatically cross-checked against the pharmacy's formulary for overdoses and interactions

TABLE 14–1. Critical Pathway of Care for the Client Experiencing a Manic Episode

Nursing Diagnoses and Categories of Care	Time Dimension	Goals and/or Actions	Time Dimension	Goals and/or Actions	Time Dimension	Discharge Outcome
Risk for Injury Related to Central Nervous System Agitation					Day 7	Client shows no evidence of injury incurred during ETOH withdrawal
					Day 7	Discharge with follow-up appointments as required
Referrals	Day 1	Psychiatrist Assess need for: Neurologist, Cardiologist, Internist				
Diagnostic studies	Day 1	Blood alcohol level Drug screen SMAC 27 Urinalysis Chest x-ray ECG	Day 4	Repeat selected diagnostic studies as necessary		
Additional assessments	Day 1	Vs q 4 hr	Day 2–3	Vs q 8 hr if stable	Day 4–7	VS bid; remain stable
	Day 1–5 Ongoing	I & O Restraints PRN	Day 6	DC I & O		

TABLE 14–1. Critical Pathway of Care for the Client Experiencing a Manic Episode (*Continued*)

Nursing Diagnoses and Categories of Care	Time Dimension	Goals and/or Actions	Time Dimension	Goals and/or Actions	Time Dimension	Discharge Outcome
	Ongoing	Assess withdrawal symptoms: tremors, nausea/ vomiting, tachycardia, sweating, high blood pressure, seizures, insomnia, hallucinations	Day 4	Marked decrease in objective symptoms	Day 7	Discharge: absence of objective withdrawal symptoms
Medications	Day 1 Day 2 Day 1–6 Day 1–7	Librium 200 mg Librium 160 mg Librium prn Maalox ac and hs	Day 3 Day 4	Librium 120 mg Librium 80 mg	Day 5 Day 6 Day 7	Librium 40 mg DC Librium Discharge; no withdrawal symptoms

Nursing Diagnoses and Categories of Care	Time Dimension	Goals and/or Actions	Time Dimension	Goals and/or Actions	Time Dimension	Discharge Outcome
Patient education			Day 5	Discuss goals of Alcoholics Anonymous (AA) and need for ongoing therapy	Day 7	Discharge with information regarding AA attendance or outpatient treatment or transfer to Behavioral Unit
Altered Nutrition: Less Than Body Requirements						
Referrals	Day 1	Consult dietitian	Day 1–7	Fulfill nutritional needs	Day 7	Nutritional condition has stabilized
Diet	Day 1	Bland as tolerated; fluids as tolerated	Day 2–3	Frequent, small, meals; easily digested foods; advanced as tolerated	Day 4–7	High-protein, high-carbohydrate diet

TABLE 14–1. Critical Pathway of Care for the Client Experiencing a Manic Episode *(Continued)*

Nursing Diagnoses and Categories of Care	Time Dimension	Goals and/or Actions	Time Dimension	Goals and/or Actions	Time Dimension	Discharge Outcome
Additional assessments	Day 1–7	Weight I & O Skin turgor Color of mucous membrane				
Medications	Day 1–4	Thiamine 100-mg injections	Day 2–7	Multiple vitamin tablet		
Patient education			Day 5	Principles of nutrition; foods for maintenance of wellness	Day 6–7	Client demonstrates ability to select appropriate foods for healthy diet

*From Doenges, ME, Moorhouse, MF, and Burley, JT: Application of Nursing Process and Nursing Diagnosis: An Interactive Text for Diagnostic Reasoning, ed. 2. FA Davis, 1995, with permission.

(Williams, 1994). Even with advanced computerized systems, the nurse is still ultimately responsible for the medications given; following the five rights of medication administration remains an imperative.

Computers also improve documentation of care. Bedside terminals, which are networked into a central system, provide multiple access points to client information. The nurse can enter client data into the system as well as access other important data, such as diagnostic reports and laboratory results, at the bedside. Information contained on the computerized client record is instantaneously available to health care providers. Although nurses must ensure correctness of data entered, the time previously spent on transcribing orders from the chart is decreased. One chief benefit of computer use is increased time for direct client care.

Issues of privacy and confidentiality apply to computer documents just as they apply to paper documents. Guarding access to terminals and ensuring privacy when reading computer screens are two areas that require the nurse's vigilance.

DEVELOPING RESEARCH-BASED NURSING PRACTICE

Research is the basis for making decisions and modifying care with the goal of improved client outcomes. Research helps build up the body of unique knowledge about nursing that acts as its scientific basis for practice. Examples of subjects for nursing research include questions about how specific nursing interventions influence client care, the effectiveness and side effects of medications, and how staffing patterns affect client safety.

Nature of Research

Frequently nurses in clinical settings have questions about nursing interventions, such as why one intervention is more effective than another. Research is the scientific process used to obtain knowledge about identified problems, to test theories, and to add to the profession's scientific basis. Four broad types of research questions have been identified: "What is this? What's happening here? What will happen if . . .?" and "How can I make . . . happen?" (Diers 1979). The two types of research aimed at answering these questions are qualitative research and quantitative research.

Qualitative Research

The term **qualitative research** is primarily used to describe phenomena rather than to identify or explain relationships between phenomena. Descriptive studies lay the groundwork for further research aimed at explaining, predicting, and controlling phenomena. Qualitative researchers strive to identify the meaning of a phenomenon as presented in the subject's natural setting. For example, if a researcher is investigating the current health practices of recent Chinese immigrants, the researcher would interview Chinese immigrants and observe events in their daily lives. This example illustrates a descriptive study aimed at exploring health practices within a particular culture. The researcher is concerned with the *concept* of health rather than *mere data* about health, such as blood-pressure measurements.

Quantitative Research

Quantitative research may also describe or classify a given phenomenon. For example, the nurse may want to list the health-promotion activities of single parents between 16 and 25 years of age. Questionnaires and interviews would be developed to collect the data. The researcher may then want to explore the relationship between the single parents' health-promotion activities and the health-promotion activities of their children.

Investigating the relationship among variables is the primary purpose of correlational research. It is important to note that correlational research does not establish cause and effect between the variables, but only shows a relationship.

Next, the researcher could try to manipulate the variables, such as a specific health-promotion activity, with the goal of answering the broad question, "What will happen if . . .?" The nurse researcher formulates hypotheses and tests them. This type of research attempts to predict the outcome of a situation. For example, the researcher might want to research the probability that the frequency of children performing daily exercise is based on the single parent's role modeling of that behavior. Thus, the researcher can predict the outcome: children who see their parents exercise will also exercise.

The next level of research seeks to reproduce an expected outcome. The researcher is interested in making an outcome happen, not in simply predicting its occurrence. For example, a nurse researching single parents might next formulate the question: What can be done to promote single parents' role modeling of exercise behaviors so that children will exercise more? In this type of research, the nurse wants not only to predict, but to intervene and affect outcomes.

Regardless of the type of research, the nurse can incorporate knowledge gained from current research studies into client-care practices. The nurse can also participate in research in a variety of ways, thus adding to the profession's body of knowledge.

Using Research in Client Care

Knowledge and its acquisition are parts of a dynamic process. Research is one method of augmenting nursing's body of knowledge. Nurses have an obligation to remain current with the latest research developments that may affect client care. Research is an important tool for improving client outcomes, thus it is fundamental for nurses to read and evaluate research findings. Participating in research and incorporating research findings into practice are also crucial to nursing's growth as a scientific profession.

How can beginning nurses become involved in research that may improve client care? One way is to read research journals and evaluate their articles. All nurses have several areas of the profession of greater interest to them than others. To discover the latest research on those topics begin by going to the library and using one or several indexes available there. The Cumulative Index to Nursing and Allied Health Literature (CINAHL), Index Medicus, and Nursing Abstracts are a few examples. These indexes are now in computerized databases and can be searched rapidly.

In addition there are nursing journals devoted specifically to research, such as Nursing Research and Research in Nursing and Health. Of course, other professional nursing journals, such as Heart and Lung, American Journal of Nursing, and Oncology Nursing Forum also include research articles.

A good way to evaluate selected articles is by discussing them with colleagues, both nurses and other health care providers. This provides a forum for putting the findings into practice. Not all research is good research, however, and not all findings are usable. A close and thoughtful reading of appropriate research is essential to good nursing care.

Through research nurses can identify a client at risk for a particular disease and then tailor the teaching accordingly. Recent studies have correlated diet, exercise, and smoking behaviors to the risk of heart disease. The nurse can use this information when teaching health-promotion behaviors to individuals or groups.

Throughout the country there are exciting developments in research. At the University of Iowa Hospitals and Clinics (UIHC), research is emphasized as an essential tool to ensure and promote quality care. In their 1994 article, Infusing Research into Practice to Promote Quality Care, Titler and co-workers discussed the process used at the Iowa clinics to critique research in a way that can be used to guide practice. Specific criteria are used, including actually trying the proposed changes in a pilot unit of the facility before research is incorporated. The quality assurance unit, known as Quality Assessment or Quality Improvement, can assist in identifying specific clinical problems that require attention and participate in monitoring the outcomes.

Besides reading research articles and incorporating their findings into practice, the nurse may be involved with development and implementation of specific research projects. The opportunity to collect data for a project, or to serve as a participant gives the nurse a unique perspective on the research process. These activities are another way for nurses to make a difference in clients' lives.

THE CHEMICALLY IMPAIRED NURSE

There are a large number of individuals who abuse alcohol and drugs. The national average for drug and alcohol abuse is 1 in 10 people (Williams, 1994). For the health care professions, including nursing, the average has been reported as 1 in 6 (Sullivan, 1991). It is likely that most nurses at some point in their careers will have to work with a colleague with an alcohol or drug problem. Most of the factors inherent in the work situation that produce burnout can also cause chemically dependent behavior. Easy access to a variety of addictive drugs adds to the problem.

Recognizing the Signs

Although different categories of drugs produce different types of behaviors, there are some characteristics that are common to all individuals who abuse drugs in the work place. These tell-tale signs can be divided into major categories: those affecting *personal* behavior and those affecting *work* behavior.

Characteristics Affecting Personal Behavior

It may be difficult for co-workers to detect alcohol or drug abuse unless they socialize with the nurse outside of work. Indications of abuse include social withdrawal, poor personal hygiene and unkempt appearance, slurred speech, unsteady gait, flushed or pale skin, blood-shot eyes, constantly dilated or constricted pupils, erratic mood swings, and memory loss (Fulton, 1981).

Characteristics Affecting Work Behavior

Observant co-workers can detect these signs: inability to complete assignments without help, frequent bathroom breaks, frequent absences from work, chronic tardiness to work, increased numbers of errors in client care, inability to concentrate or remember procedures, increased errors in narcotic counts when the person is working, frequent volunteering to give clients' pain medications, increased frequency of reported client requests for pain medications, increased client complaints that medications administered by this nurse do not relieve pain, preference for working the night shift (where there is less supervision) alcohol or other drug odors on the breath, refusal to accept complicated assignments, incoherent and sloppy charting, and falling asleep during the shift.

Legal and Ethical Obligations

A nurse who is working under the influence of alcohol or drugs is not competent to provide safe care. The ANA's ethical *Code for Nurses* requires the nurse to protect the client from the incompetent, unethical, or illegal practice of *any* person. The initial step, if any of the characteristics of drug abuse is observed, is to document the time, date, and circumstances, including the names of any witnesses to the behavior (Caroselli-Karinja, 1986). Because it is likely that other co-workers have observed the same behavior, it would be appropriate to have them verify the observations. These observations should then be reported to the supervisor of the suspected drug abuser. Direct confrontation with the nurse should be avoided by co-workers (Lowinson, 1992).

At this point, the supervising nurse must verify the observations and make personal judgments about the nurse's behavior. If the supervisor agrees that the behavior indicates drug or alcohol abuse, the nurse must be confronted with these suspicions. This is the most difficult step in the process. The confrontation must take place in as nonthreatening a manner as possible, providing the accused nurse with an opportunity to respond (Fulton, 1981). All of the nurse's options then need to be listed. These options usually include entering a drug rehabilitation program, immediate termination of employment, or, if narcotics have been taken from the hospital, reporting the incident to the legal authorities.

Often, if nurses are able to recognize that they have a drug problem and are willing to enter a rehabilitation program, no disciplinary action will be pursued by the hospital. In situations where the nurse denies the problem and accusations, due process is required before the nurses can be terminated. Due process often involves a hearing or trial and may likely be presented to the legal authorities for final disposition. The legal system has much less understanding and sympathy for nurses who abuse drugs than the institution attempting to help the nurse overcome the problem.

In general, nurses who have successfully completed rehabilitation programs can return to work (Sullivan, 1991). Often they are required to sign a special contract with the hospital that specifies conditions that must be met in order to remain employed. These may include regular attendance at AA meetings or group therapy sessions, submitting to random blood and urine tests for drugs, remaining drug-free both at home and work, and attending classes to improve self-esteem, manage stress, and learn to cope with tension. Such nurses may also be limited in their client-care activities. Recovering nurses may be forbidden to work the night-shift or to pass medications. If they are allowed to pass medications, it may only be under the close supervision of another nurse who must cosign all medication sheets.

Coworkers can play an important part in the recovering nurse's rehabilitation. Offering support and understanding during the important initial transition period from rehabilitation to work can ease the process of reassimilation into the unit. Helping the recovering nurse to develop strong support systems with both co-workers and others can provide an outlet for stress other than drugs. Inviting the recovering nurse to participate in group activities both inside and outside the workplace will reinforce acceptance and help the individual come to terms with a drug problem.

MAINTAINING COMPETENCY IN NURSING

Maintaining a level of knowledge and skill adequate for the competent practice of the professional nurse would seem to be a requirement in today's rapidly advancing health care system. Indeed, the fifth statement of the ANA *Code of Ethics for Nursing* states that the nurse "maintains competence in nursing." Even Florence Nightingale recognized the need for continuous updating of the nurse's knowledge and skills when she wrote in 1882: ". . . nurses have to learn new and improved methods in medicine, surgery and hygiene." All professional nurses agree on the need for continual self-development. There is disagreement, however, about how to achieve the goal of continuing education.

MANDATORY VERSUS INDEPENDENT CONTINUING EDUCATION

Many student nurses, when they graduate, realize that they are really just beginning their professional education, rather than completing it. Passing the NCLEX only establishes a minimum level of competency, not a high level of expert knowledge. Membership in the nursing profession demands a lifelong commitment to continuous self-development based on periodic self-evaluation and on-going education (Meservy, 1986). One method used to maintain currency in skills and knowledge is through continuing education programs.

Continuing education programs take a variety of forms, ranging from simple on-the-unit demonstrations of the use of new equipment to formal programs of education located on university campuses lasting several days or even weeks. In-hospital continuing education programs are usually administered by the hospital's Director of Education, or an individual with a similar title. Out-of-hospital programs may be organized by colleges, universities, or even organizations whose sole purpose is to offer continuing education classes.

One distinguishing feature of continuing education is that no academic credit is awarded for attendance at the classes. To recognize the importance of continuing education, the continuing education unit (CEU) was developed to establish a uniform way to quantify and recognize the efforts of individuals to maintain competency. Standards for educational programs were established, as well as guidelines and procedures for obtaining the units. In general, one CEU (1.0 CEU) represents 10 contact hours of class in a recognized program of continuing education.

CEUs are awarded by various agencies. In nursing, the American Nurses Association oversees all such activities. During the past 20 years, the ANA has recognized and approved some 60 individual entities for the awarding of CEUs. Today, CEUs are usually awarded by the specialty organization overseeing a particular area of practice. For example, a continuing education program on hemodynamic monitoring would be awarded CEUs by the American Association of Critical-Care Nurses (AACN), whereas a program presenting the latest techniques in breast feeding might be awarded CEUs by the Obstetrical Nurse's Association.

An issue that arises repeatedly in professional nursing is the requirement for mandatory CEUs for renewal of licensure. The twelve states that have mandatory requirements for CEUs have established a set number of CEUs that must be accumulated before nurses in these states may renew their licenses. The idea behind mandating CEUs for license renewal was that the practice would force nurses to maintain competency in nursing. The required CEU's range from a low of 2 hours to as high as 30 hours of classes.

The underlying question that opponents of mandatory CEUs ask concerns the notion that requiring nurses to attend a prescribed numbers of classes will automatically increase knowledge and competency. Even though evaluation methods are incorporated into approved courses for CEUs, little evidence proves that acquiring mandatory CEUs actually improves nursing practice.

Another important issue for opponents of mandatory CEUs is the arbitrary number of required hours. Why would a nurse in one state only need 2 hours to remain competent, whereas a nurse in another state will require 30 hours over the same period to remain competent?

Fundamental to the debate about mandatory CEUs is **accountability**. Nurses, as professionals, are accountable for the decisions they make and the actions they take in the provision of client care (Mead, 1985). It is the professional nurse's responsibility to maintain competence in his or her nursing practice as part of the professional role. Mandating that nurses take a certain number of course hours to remain competent implies that these nurses are not professional enough to attend these classes without outside supervision. Many nurses resent this implication and see it as an attack on their professionalism.

This debate is far from over. As a new health care system is developed in the United States, there will be even higher demand for professional accountability. A key element in meeting these higher standards, especially for nursing, will be enhancement of the nurse's knowledge and skills through life-long learning. Although mandating CEUs for licensure renewal may seem effective to achieve continued competency in nursing, forcing nurses to attend classes does *not* guarantee that they are actually learning anything there. Ultimately, the individual nurse has to make the decision and accept the responsibility for personal learning.

THE IMAGE OF NURSING

Sources

The image of nursing is important to the profession for several reasons. Those who belong to a profession need a strong and positive image on which to model themselves. As nursing students progress through their programs, their image of nursing changes from an abstract ideal to a more concrete and realistic one. Their image of what they are and what they should be is, however, influenced to some degree by the image of nurses from the past, as well through images presented in the current media, some of which are less than positive. Students who are not well grounded in the realities of nursing are in danger of subconsciously accepting such negative and stereotypical images. There is an unconscious tendency to reinforce and perpetuate these negative images if the students are not well grounded in the realities of nursing and the effects that image has on the profession and the professional (Young, 1992).

As previously discussed, nurses, as an identifiable group, developed rather recently. Because for most of history health care was provided in the home setting, a strong demand for nursing services did not exist. In the few cultures where health care was provided in a more hospital-like setting, the *nurses*, or those who attended the sick, were often men. Women, except in a few enlightened cultures, were considered second class, and usually were not permitted to engage in activities outside of the home.

Historically, images of nursing range from the ideal to the dissolute. Probably the earliest, and most enduring, image of the nurse is that of the nurturing, mother-like individual. Indeed, the word **nurse** comes from a Latin word that means nurturing, or one who nourishes. Even today, the word nursing is used for breast feeding a baby when used professionally in the context of the obstetrical unit. In most early cultures and civilizations, care of the sick at home was provided by the female members of the family. Although elements of this caring, gentle, nurturing image of nursing are still an essential part of the current image of nursing, it has been greatly modified throughout history by changes in society.

As the mores of the Roman Empire were modified by the influence of Christianity, the image of the nurse was also modified. Christianity added the elements of respect for all life and love of neighbor as key aspects of living a good life. From this point of view, care of the sick was not only a service to sick members of one's own family, but also an activity that should be provided for all people as a demonstration of belief in Christ's teachings. Large monasteries and convents were established throughout Europe with a primary goal of providing care for the sick. Under this influence, nursing took on a strong religious image. Indeed, in a time and age when medical care was primitive, saving the sick person's immortal soul became as important an element in health care as trying to cure the person's body.

One of the important elements in the lives of the individuals who joined these religious nursing orders was the vow of obedience. Members of these religious communities were obligated to subjugate themselves to those in authority. This idea of deferring to a higher authority persisted in nursing for many years.

Early Christians strongly believed in the equality of women with men and created many opportunities for women outside of the traditional home setting. In the early centuries, nearly equal numbers of religious men and women dedicated their lives to care of the sick. After the Reformation, and the subsequent breaking apart of the Holy Roman Empire, many of the male-dominated monasteries were disbanded by the new local political leaders because of their potential threat to the local ruler's power. Because they were less threatening, the convent hospitals run by women were often allowed to remain, although they were now to be under the joint authority of the Vatican and the local ruler. At this time, nursing obtained its predominantly female image.

Despite the great advances made in other areas of learning and science during the Renaissance, medical and nursing knowledge remained rooted in the traditions and methods of the past. In countries where the care for the sick was still being provided by religious orders, the Roman Catholic Church blocked introduction of new medical knowledge it considered unnatural. In predominantly Protestant countries, the social status of women eroded to an even more subservient level, and health care provided at home became the norm. The few institutions of the Protestant countries where care was provided outside the home were staffed by females from the lowest classes of the society.

As nursing entered the modern age, it was encumbered with these images from its history. Nurses were seen as primarily nurturing and caring females who were obedient to those in authority, especially to physicians. It was believed that nurses neither had nor were required to have anything more than a rudimentary education. This image of nursing, despite the best efforts of leaders in nursing like Florence Nightingale, persisted to modern times (Young, 1992).

In modern times, nurses fare better in the written news media, particularly in popular news magazines. Many insightful and realistic articles have been written about nurses who provide care for clients in a highly technical and very demanding environment. These articles may even include information about nursing education, salaries, working conditions, and relationships with other health-care workers. Newspapers, because of the demand for fast-paced current information, often ignore the less dramatic aspects of the everyday care provided by nurses. Newspapers do tend to report the more sensational events, such as nursing strikes, nurses who are accused of client euthanasia, convicted of crimes (especially when drug-related), or sued for malpractice (Alspach, 1989). In reality, these cases represent only a small proportion of nurses, yet the disproportionate reporting in the newspapers has an overall negative effect on the image of nursing.

Improving the Image of Nursing

The public image of nursing has a wide-ranging, profound effect on how nurses are viewed by those who control the money that funds the health care system. In these days of health care reform, the nurse's negative image may reduce public confidence in the profession and persuade legislators to decrease funding for nurses and nursing care. In the current climate of budget cutting, nurses must be viewed as well-educated and independent co-partners in the health care system (Bream, 1992). A loss of confidence in nurses, as well as the generally negative image portrayed by the media, can undermine respect for the profession at all levels. The results may be felt well into the next century.

Nurses can influence how they are depicted in the media. Most attempts to date have been under the auspices of the nursing organizations. For example, through letter writing and telephone campaigns organized by the ANA and directed at a TV-network, a program that presented a negative image of nursing students was quickly pulled from the prime-time lineup. In addition, several professional organizations have begun to produce their own videos for television to depict nurses in a more positive light. These can also be used for public education and nursing recruitment.

Individual nurses can help improve the image of nursing. One of the more important things a nurse can do is join a professional organization and support its activities. Individual nurses can also become involved in politics, particularly where health care issues are concerned. This action may be as simple as writing letters to the editor or as complicated as making presentations to public civic groups about important health care issues. Similarly, nurses can write and submit for publication realistic accounts of what is involved in providing competent, independent, and high-quality nursing care to clients in the contemporary health care system.

Probably the most important action that individual nurses can take to improve the image of nursing is to practice nursing themselves with a high level of professionalism (Young, 1992). Besides media coverage, personal contact with nurses in the health care system is the factor that most influences the image of nursing. If the public encounters nurses who act like the nurses on their favorite soap operas, the negative images are sure to be reinforced. On the other hand, if their experience is with nurses who practice with the highest professional, ethical, and personal standards, and deliver sensitive and high-quality care to their clients, the image of the professional nurse will be improved.

Each nurse is responsible for the image presented. It is to the advantage of that nurse, as well as the nursing profession as a whole, that the image presented is of the highest quality.

PREPARING FOR THE FUTURE

The future can be filled with excitement and anticipation or it can be fraught with danger and fear. Nurses should continually reevaluate and reaffirm their attitudes about the future and about the need for change. They should look as far as possible into the future so that they can help to shape it, to be part of it, and to anticipate changes they may need to make in their education to be prepared for it. It is not an easy task, particularly in a profession that is so strongly rooted in tradition.

That is not to say all change is progress or that the traditions and values of the past will have no place in the future. On the contrary, some of the changes taking place in health care today can be considered regressive. The change toward functional team nursing and the use of unlicensed assistive personnel is a throwback to an earlier time in health care when there were not enough qualified licensed nurses to provide care for clients. Although they may cost less than the primary care or total patient care models that were popular up until the early 1990s, the functional and team nursing models lower the overall quality of care (Johnston, 1987).

Likewise, there will always be a place for certain traditions and values that nursing has maintained from its earliest days. Even in a society saturated by advanced technology, the traditional values of caring, helping, and empathizing are still pillars of the nursing profession. The strong personal relationship between the nurse and the client is the bedrock upon which good nursing practice is built. The challenge for nurses is clear in this regard. Nurses must develop the skills necessary to use all the complex technology necessary for the care of clients in today's health care system. But they must also combine it with the caring, sensitivity, and humanism that have made nursing an essential part of the health care system for centuries. It is difficult to be technologically proficient and sensitive at the same time, yet this is exactly what nurses are being called upon to do on a daily basis.

KEEPING NURSING A HIGH-TOUCH PROFESSION IN A HIGH-TECH WORLD

Although technologic competence is vital, nurses must never forget what makes nursing unique in the health care system. As noted in many states' nurse practice acts, **nursing** is defined as the "diagnosis and treatment of human responses to actual or potential health care problems." This is a very powerful statement about the nature of the work nurses perform. No matter how technically proficient nurses may be, if they are unable to identify the human responses of a client, they have lost the heart of what it means to be a nurse. The ability to recognize human responses to health care problems is a significant undertaking deserving of professional status. This element is what makes nursing a high-touch profession in a high-tech world (Naisbitt, Aburdene, 1990).

To be able to be proficient in technologic skills while retaining the ability to deal with clients humanely will require greater skill and knowledge than nurses have possessed in the past or present. Nursing education must be

CRITICAL THINKING EXERCISES

1 Discuss with a classmate some area of nursing practice that interests you as a possible research topic. What type of research question is your imaginary research trying to answer?
2 How would you, as the nurse in charge of a unit in the hospital, react to the client's father trying to access the bedside computer's data? How would you intervene?
3 Discuss the legal and ethical implications of allowing a chemically impaired nurse to continue practicing.

THE NURSE'S ROLE IN CLIENT-FOCUSED CARE

The federal government's desire to reduce the cost of acute care hospitalizations has already slowed the increases in Medicare reimbursements. Even without enactment of official legislative reform, health care in the United States is changing. Out-patient services are rapidly increasing, whereas in-patient services are decreasing. Although hospital beds remain empty, the number of home health care agencies is increasing.

Are all nurses going to have to work in home health care in order to find a job? The answer is no, but to survive in the acute-care setting, nursing care will need to be radically redesigned.

One of the models of care that is receiving a great deal of attention is the "patient-focused care" model. Central to this model is a recognition that client care in the acute setting should be organized to maximize efficiency and to meet clients' needs. This model recognizes that client care is the responsibility of the entire range of client-care services, including medicine, nursing, respiratory therapy to food services and housekeeping. In this model, nurses retain the core responsibilities of assessment and client teaching and coordinate the care provided by other services.

The client-focused care model advocates that single-service providers, such as respiratory therapists, laboratory personnel, pharmacists, and unlicensed workers become involved in direct client care in units rather than in centralized departments. In addition, this model would require that these providers, along with nurses, be cross-trained to perform tasks that had not previously been considered part of their job. For example, respiratory therapists would be able to run electrocardiographic (ECG) equipment and draw blood as well as give therapy. Nurses would be able to draw laboratory work samples, run ECGs, give respiratory treatments, and provide education to patients.

This model requires that nurses surrender some duties and assume new ones. The goal is for nurses to gain greater job satisfaction as they are freed from clerical and housekeeping tasks, and thus to be able to devote more time to client care. It is recognized that the number of RN positions will be reduced as future reforms take place.

The nurses who remain at work in the acute-care setting need to become actively involved in shaping reforms. One of the best ways to influence reform is to serve on hospital-wide committees and task forces that are set up to plan and design reform. Nurses on these committees must voice their concerns about proposed changes on such issues as nurse-to-patient ratios, licensed and unlicensed care giver ratios, systems for classifying acuity,

THE NURSE'S ROLE IN CLIENT-FOCUSED CARE (CONTINUED)

procedures for ordering supplies, and job descriptions for unlicensed personnel that might compromise client care.

With or without reform, the role and nature of the work done by RNs is going to change. If nurses participate in the changes, there is a much better chance that the reforms will be done well, and that RNs will retain their central position in the health care system.

Modified from Porter-O'Grady, T: Working with consultants on a redesign. Am J Nurs 94:33–37, 1994.

able to meet the demands of preparing nurses to deal with the widened scope and increasingly complex responsibilities of a rapidly changing health care system.

Society demands and deserves nurse practitioners who are prepared to function at a high level of quality in a changing health care system. Only with society's support and recognition of nursing as an independent profession will nursing be able to emerge from the cloud of subservience to other professions in which it has been hidden for so long.

SUMMARY

Today's health care system is in a state of rapid change. Many factors affect nursing both as a profession and in its day-to-day practice. By understanding the issues and their effect on nursing, nurses can become involved in activities to further the profession. Every change made in the health care system offers an opportunity to advance the profession of nursing.

Nurses must also strive for excellence in nursing care and attempt to make a positive difference in each client's life. They should appreciate the advantages a broad base of knowledge and a wide range of skills gives them and should avoid becoming too specialized or narrowly focused in their practice. They should be enthusiastic about the work they do and the services they provide; then translate that enthusiasm into a life-long commitment to the profession.

Nurses need to recognize that the time has arrived to take the profession to a new level. Nursing as a profession now has the opportunity to gain tremendous power and take its rightful place as an indispensable force in the health care system. All that is required is for nurses to become educated in the issues and to taken an aggressive stance in the formation of the future.

A Closer Look

GOVERNMENT MANDATES AFFECT NURSING CARE

An example of how a government mandate can affect nursing care is seen in the Patient-Self Determination Act of 1990. This Act mandated that all nursing homes, hospitals, home health care agencies, hospices, and health maintenance organizations be required to ask clients about their desires for health care if they are to be unable to make decisions in the future. Basically, they were to be asked if they had a living will, and if not, whether they would like to make one.

The intent of the Act was based on the principle that adults have the right to make decisions about their medical care. It was hoped by increasing the number of clients with living wills, there would be less difficulty in health care decision making for clients when they became incompetent, and less confusion among the providers of care. Although the Act mandated that some type of advance directive be provided to clients, and that the results be documented in the client's record, no specific guidelines were developed to do so. Each state was required to develop its own guidelines and to submit them for approval to the federal government.

All states have currently implemented some procedure to meet the mandates of the Act. These procedures generally require that the nurse who is admitting the client ask, as part of the admission assessment, whether the client has a living will, and if not, whether the client would like to make one. Many of the admission assessment forms have been revised with a section added that deals with advanced directives.

Nursing care is influenced by many different factors. The government, through its mandates, has a wide-ranging effect on what nurses do. It is important that nurses recognize this fact and, through their professional organizations, work to make sure that the changes implemented are reasonable and in the best interests their clients.

Modified from Barnett, CW and Pierson, DA: Advanced directives: Implementing a program that works. Nurs Management 10:58–65, 1994.

BIBLIOGRAPHY

Alspach, JG: Making an impact, Crit Care Nurse 9:2, 1989.
American Nurses Association: Registered Professional Nurses and Unlicensed Assistive Personnel. American Nurses Publishing, Washington, D.C., 1994.
Anderson, H: Hospitals seek new ways to integrate health care. Hospitals 66:26–36, 1992.
Bream, TL, Bower, FL, Stanton, M, et al: Beyond the ordinary nursing image. Nurs Management 23:44, 1992.
Caroselli-Karinja, M and Zbory, SD. The impaired nurse. Journal of Psychosoc Nurs Ment Health Serv 24:14–19, 1986.

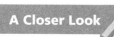
A Closer Look

ACUTE-CARE NURSE PRACTITIONER—SUPPORTED BY AMERICAN ASSOCIATION OF CRITICAL-CARE NURSES

A new category of nurse practitioners—acute-care nurse practitioners—has developed recently. They practice advanced nursing in the hospital setting, often in the critical-care unit. As might be imagined, difficulties about their scope of practice, role, and functions have arisen.

The American Association of Critical-Care Nurses (AACN) supports this role of advanced nursing practice. The AACN views this new role for nurses as an element in the development of a health care system driven by the needs of patients and their families rather than the needs of hospitals and physicians.

Among other efforts, the AACN is collaborating with the National Organization of Nurse Practitioner Faculty, the Oncology Nursing Society, and other organizations, on advanced practice issues, such as building a state and national database on advanced practice nurses, promoting the development of educational guidelines, and planning continuing education for advanced practice nurses. One of the most important undertakings of the AACN is to support legislation that eliminates restrictions and regulations imposed on advanced practice nurses. Some of the long-term goals include gaining prescriptive authority, allowing hospital privileges, and supporting reimbursement mechanisms for all advanced practice nurses.

Although the current number of acute-care nurse practitioners remains small, efforts to define and widen their scope of practice promotes the role. Nurses who are interested in practicing acute or critical care at an advanced level should seek the appropriate educational programs.

Modified from Caterinicchio, MJ: Advanced practice. AACN News, February 1995, page 3.

Clouten, K and Weber R: Patient-focused care . . . playing to win. Nurs Management 25:34–36, 1994.

Diers, D: Research in Nursing Practice. JB Lippincott, Philadelphia, 1979.

Fulton, K: Drug abuse among nurses: What nursing management can do. Supervisor Nurse 12:18–20, 1981.

Hegner, BR and Caldwell, E: Nursing Assistants: A Nursing Process Approach. Delmar Publications, Albany, 1995.

Hull, M: Your nursing image: Tending the flame. Nursing '93 23:116, 1993.

Johnston, W and Packer, A: Workforce 2000: Work and Workers for the Twenty-First Century. Hudson Institute, Indianapolis, 1987.

Kirkwood, C: Your Services Are No Longer Required: The Complete Job Loss Recovery Book. Plume Books, New York, 1993.

Lowinson, V, Ruiz, J, Millman, H: Substance Abuse: A Comprehensive Textbook. Williams & Wilkins, Baltimore, 1992.

Mattson, MT: Atlas of the 1990 Census. Macmillian, New York, 1992.

Mead, MD, Berger, S and Nicksic, E: Contracts for continuing education. J Cont Educ Nurses 16:121–126, 1985.

Meservy, D and Monsond, MA: Impact of continuing education on nursing practice and quality of patient care. J Cont Educ Nurses 18:214, 1986.

Naisbitt, J and Aburdene, P: Megatrends 2000: Ten New Directions for the 1990s. Morrow, New York, 1990.

Sabatino, F: Foundations' Funding Priorities Shift from Acute to Primary Care. Hospitals 65:34–37, 1991.

Shugars, DA, O'Neill, EH and Bader, JD: Health America: Practitioners for 2005, An Agenda for Action. Pew Health Professions Commission, Durham, N.C. 1991.

Simpson, RL: Ensuring patient data, privacy, confidentiality and security. Nurs Management 25:18–20, 1994.

Sullivan, E, Bissell, L and Williams, E. Chemical Dependency in Nursing—The Deadly Diversion. Addison, Menlo Park, 1991.

Titler, MG, Kleiber, C, and Steelman, V: Infusing research into practice to promote quality care. Nurs Res 43, 307–313, 1994.

Williams, D and Brown, DL: Automation at the point of care. Nurs Management, 25:32–35, 1994.

Young, J: Changing nursing's image through professionalism. Imprint 34:50, 1992.

APPENDIX A

NUMBERS AND DEMOGRAPHICS

Registered nurses are the largest segment of the health care work force. 2,239,816 people living in the U.S. are educated and licensed to practice as registered nurses (RNs), and 1,853,024 are employed RNs. RNs come from every socio-economic class, every state, every neighborhood in America. What follows is a statistical portrait of today's RN, compiled from *The Registered Nurse Population, Findings from the National Sample Survey of Registered Nurses, March 1992*, U.S. Department of Health & Human Services, Public Health Service, Health Resources and Services Administration.

WHO CHOOSES NURSING

Gender

Historically, more women than men have chosen nursing. But the trend may be changing. In 1992, only 4.3 percent of RNs employed in nursing were men. However, that number reflects a 97 percent increase from 1980 to 1992, in the number of men entering the profession. In the same period, the number of RNs grew by 35%.

Ethnic/Racial Background

Roughly 10 percent of the employed RN population come from racial/ethnic backgrounds. Black RNs make up 4 percent of the population. Asian/Pacific Islander account for 3.4 percent. Hispanics are 1.4 percent, and American Indian/Alaskan Native are 0.4 percent of the RN population.

Age

As the typical American citizen ages, so does the typical RN. In 1992, only 11 percent of all RNs were under 30. More than 60 percent of RNs were 30–49 years old, with the average age being 43 years. For RNs who graduated in 1987 or later, the average age at graduation was 30 years. Now, RNs enter the work force later, with more life experience to bring to the profession.

The Second-Career RN

The older RN also brings specialized training to the workplace. Almost 30 percent of RNs had worked in a health care occupation just before they entered nursing school. About two-thirds had worked as nursing aides, and another 29 percent were licensed practical nurses or licensed vocational nurses. Another 8 percent had post-high school academic degrees—more than half had baccalaureates, and almost 27 percent of these had majored in liberal arts, followed by health-related majors (24 percent).

Family Status

A majority—72 percent—of registered nurses are married. Less than 17 percent are widowed, divorced or separated. The remainder have never married. More than half—55 percent—have children living at home, and 21 percent of all RNs have children under the age of 6. Almost a third of the RNs who are employed full-time in nursing have children.

Basic Nursing Education

Over the past 20 years, RNs have changed dramatically in the mode they have chosen for their basic nursing education.

In 1977, three-quarters of RNs graduated from diploma programs. Diploma programs were the first form of organized education for nurses. Usually associated with a hospital, the Diploma in Nursing combines classroom and clinical instruction. As nursing education has shifted from hospitals to academic institutions, fewer nurses are choosing this route. By 1992, the percentage of nurses who received their basic nursing preparation in a diploma program dropped to 34 percent. Associate degree nurses accounted for 28%; nurses with bachelor's degrees made up 27% of the group. There was an obvious trend toward associate degree graduation—with 59 percent of all RNs who had graduated within the past five years getting an associate's degree. During that same period, 31 percent were baccalaureate graduates. Overall, 3 percent of the RNs in 1992 received their basic nursing education in a foreign country.

About 21 percent of the RNs completed additional education. Aside from those who sought graduate and post-graduate degrees, associate degree RNs and diploma nurses also returned for baccalaureate degrees. More than 60 percent of the RNs returning to school were enrolled in baccalaureate programs. Typically, the returning RNs attend class part-time while working full-time as nurses (65%).

Advanced Nursing Education

In 1992, 7.5 percent of the RNs had a Master's degree in nursing or a related field. The percentage of doctorally-prepared nurses was 0.5 percent. Of those with a Master's degree, 43 percent focused their graduate work on clinical practice. The doctorally-prepared RNs concentrated more often on education (36.8 percent) or on research (33.5 percent).

Financing Nursing Education

To pay for their education, 72 percent of RNs use personal resources. Employer reimbursement plans were used by 56 percent of RNs in 1992. Scholarships, grants, loans, and fellowships were listed by less than 15 percent of the nurses as the means they employed to finance their basic or graduate nursing education.

WHERE NURSES WORK

Hospitals

In 1992, about two-thirds of employed RNs worked in hospitals, with almost 70 percent employed full-time. In the hospital, full-time RNs worked an average 41.6 hours during a survey week as opposed to the scheduled 39.4 hours. 84 percent of all employed RNs under 30 worked in hospitals. Only half of those 50 and over did so.

Within the hospital, 40 percent of RNs worked on general medical or surgical units. More than 18 percent worked in intensive care units. Just over 8 percent worked in operating rooms, and almost 7 percent staffed emergency rooms.

The types of patients that these RNs cared for at least 50 percent of the time included: coronary care, 16.7 percent; newborn infants and psychiatric patients, 7.5 percent each; pediatrics, 7 percent; obstetrics/gynecology, 5 percent; multiple units, 4 percent; chronic care, 3.3 percent; rehabilitation, 2.8 percent; and neurology, 2.4 percent. Just over 34 percent of RNs in hospitals had associate's degrees as their highest nursing education.

Community/Public Health

Almost 10 percent of RNs worked in community or public health settings in 1992, including health departments, visiting nurse services, non-hospital home health agencies, and substance abuse outpatient facilities, among others. More than 35 percent of those RNs held baccalaureate degrees.

Ambulatory Care

Almost 8 percent of RNs worked in ambulatory care settings, most of them physicians' offices. Other settings include nurse-based practices, freestanding clinics, health maintenance organizations and mixed professional practice groups. Just over 40 percent of these RNs had diplomas as their highest nursing educational preparation.

Nursing Home/Extended Care

Seven percent of RNs worked in nursing homes in 1992, which included those based in and out of hospitals, facilities for the mentally retarded and retired home residences. More than 45 percent of these RNs held diplomas as their highest nursing educational preparation.

Other Areas

The remainder of nurses worked in: nursing education, 2 percent; student health, 2.7 percent; occupational health, 1 percent; and in miscellaneous areas, such as for state boards of nursing, health planning agencies and correctional facilities, 3 percent.

JOB TITLES

In general, RNs with diplomas and associate degrees spent more time (67 percent of their work time) in direct patient care. RNs with Master's degrees spent less than a third of their time in patient care. RNs with doctorates spent less than 7 percent of their time in hands-on patient care.

Of the registered nurses surveyed in 1992, 66 percent listed their position title as staff nurse. Smaller proportions listed their position titles as follows: administrators—6.2 percent, instructors—3.5 percent, and supervisors—5 percent.

Advanced Practice Nurses

Almost 140,000 RNs in 1992 reported having the education and credentials to work as advanced practice nurses. There are four categories of advanced practice nurses: clinical nurse specialists, nurse practitioners, nurse anesthetists and nurse-midwives.

Clinical Nurse Specialist

To be a clinical nurse specialist, an RN must have earned a Master's degree in nursing that confers specialized knowledge, skills and training. Usually, the clinical nurse specialist works in a hospital, teaching patients and staff as well as consulting on complex cases. The RNs who fit this description numbered 58,185.

Nurse Practitioner

The 48,237 nurse practitioners received advanced education that culminated in a certificate or Master's degree. The practice area is an evolving one in which many states are allowing nurse practitioners to write prescriptions and provide primary care.

Nurse Anesthetists

The oldest advanced nursing specialty is that of nurse anesthetist. Approximately 25,238 nurses in 1992 were nurse anesthetists. These RNs complete formal preparation beyond their basic nursing education, usually a two-year program. They administer anesthesia in a variety of settings from operating rooms to dentists' offices.

Nurse-Midwives

The smallest group of advanced practice nurses is that of nurse-midwife. Slightly more than 7,400 RNs were nurse-midwives in 1992. They had completed formal education of at least 9 months in length after their basic nursing preparation. Nurse-midwives attend to or assist in childbirth in various settings, including hospitals, birthing centers and homes. They are also involved in well-woman care.

CERTIFICATIONS

The 1992 survey found that certification made a difference in the employment status of advanced practice nurses. No information was given for RNs other than those in advanced practice positions.

- For clinical nurse specialists, 7,877 were certified by a national organization. The certified clinical nurse specialists were more likely to be employed than their noncertified peers, and also they were more likely to have a position title of clinical nurse specialist.
- About 58 percent of nurse practitioners were certified by national organizations. Of those who were certified, 95 percent were employed in nursing and were more likely to have the title of nurse practitioner.
- For nurse anesthetists, most had national certification. Of the certified registered nurse anesthetists (CRNAs), 93 percent were employed in nursing.
- Two-thirds of the nurse-midwives were certified by national organizations. At least half of these practiced nursing with the title of certified nurse-midwife.

GEOGRAPHIC DISTRIBUTION

The geographic distribution of RNs reflected the general population spread of the United States. Accordingly, more RNs practiced on the East Coast (approx. 42 percent) and in cities than anywhere else (approx. 69 percent). The concentration of nurses was densest in New England with 991 employed nurses per 100,000 population, and it was sparsest in the West South Central states with 537 employed nurses per 100,000 population.

New England: Connecticut, Maine, Massachusetts, New Hampshire, Rhode Island, Vermont

This region represented 7 percent of the employed RN population. Fewer RNs were employed in hospitals in this region (62 percent), and more RNs worked in nursing homes (11 percent). It had the largest percentage of nurses with a diploma as the highest nursing preparation (41.9 percent), and the largest percentage of its population had a Master's degree in nursing (6.4 percent). Almost 3 percent of this region's RN population was from a racial/ethnic background.

Middle Atlantic: New Jersey, New York, Pennsylvania

This region represented 18 percent of the employed RN population. A larger portion (4.5 percent) of this RN group worked in student health service than any other region. About 12.5 percent of this region's RN population was from a racial/ethnic background.

East North Central: Illinois, Indiana, Michigan, Ohio, Wisconsin

This region represented 18 percent of the employed RN population. Approximately 5.4 percent of this region's RN population was from a racial/ethnic background.

West North Central: Iowa, Kansas, Minnesota, Missouri, Nebraska, North Dakota, South Dakota

This region represented 8 percent of the employed RN population. Slightly more than 3 percent of this region's RN population was from a racial/ethnic background.

South Atlantic: Delaware, District Of Columbia, Florida, Georgia, Maryland, North Carolina, South Carolina, Virginia, West Virginia

This region represented 17 percent of the employed RN population. A tenth of this region's RN population was from a racial/ethnic background.

East South Central: Alabama, Kentucky, Mississippi, Tennessee

This region represented 5.5 percent of the employed RN population. A larger portion (11.8 percent) of the RN workforce practiced in community/public health than any other region, and the smallest percentage (1.6 percent) worked in student health. Almost 38 percent of the RN population had an associate's degree as the highest nursing preparation. It had the highest proportion of RNs who were 29 years and younger (14.9 percent). About 8% of this region's nurses was from a racial/ethnic background, including the largest proportion (6.7 percent) of RNs who were identified as black (non-Hispanic).

Salaries are the lowest of all the regions.

West South Central: Arkansas, Louisiana, Oklahoma, Texas

This region represented 8 percent of the employed RN population. It had the highest proportion of RNs in the age groups of 30–49 years old (65.6 percent) and the lowest proportion of RNs who were 50–64 years old (15.7 percent). About 11.2 percent of the RN population in this region was from a racial/ethnic background.

Mountain: Arizona, Colorado, Idaho, Montana, Nevada, New Mexico, Utah, Wyoming

This region represented the smallest proportion of RNs nationally—5 percent of the employed RN population. Almost 6 percent of this region's RN population was from a racial/ethnic background. It includes the largest portion (0.9 percent) of American Indian/Alaskan Native RNs.

Pacific: Alaska, California, Hawaii, Oregon, Washington

This region represented 13 percent of the employed RN population. Of all the regions, it had both the highest percentage of RNs in the 50–64 age group (24.1 percent) and the lowest percentage of RNs in the category of 29 years and younger (6.1 percent). This region had the largest portion (16 percent) of RNs from a racial/ethnic background, with the most represented group being Asian/Pacific Islander (9.5 percent). Also, the Pacific region included the largest portion (2.7 percent) of Hispanic RNs.

Salaries are the highest of all the regions.

Appendix A reprinted, in part, with permission from Today's registered nurse—numbers and demographics. American Nurses Association, pub. no. PR-17, ANA Publications, Washington, D.C., 1994.

APPENDIX B

GLOSSARY

Term	Definition
abandonment	Leaving a client without the client's permission; terminating the professional relationship without providing for appropriate continued or follow-up care by another equally qualified professional.
accountability	Concept that each individual is responsible for his or her own actions and the consequence of those actions; professional accountability implies a responsibility to perform the activities and duties of the profession according to established standards.
accreditation	Approval of a program or institution by a voluntary professional organization to provide specific education or service programs.
act	Legislation that has become law.
active euthanasia	Acts performed to help end a sick person's life.
actual health problem	A client's health problem that exists now.
acute–severe	Health problem of sudden onset; a serious illness or condition.
adaptation	Process of exchange between a person and the environment to maintain or regain personal integrity; the key principle in the *Roy Model of Nursing*.
administrative agency	A governmental agency that implements legislation.
administrative rule or regulation	An operating procedure that describes how a government agency implements the intent of a statute; state boards of nursing implement the nurse practice act.

Term	Definition
advanced nursing education	Master's or doctoral level education that provides knowledge and skills in areas such as research, education, administration, or clinical specialties.
advanced practice	Extended role; increased responsibilities and actions undertaken by an individual because of additional education and experience; nurse practitioners are advanced practice nurses.
advanced placement	A process by which a student is given credit for a required course through transfer or examination rather than by enrolling in and completing the course.
advocate	One who pleads for a cause or proposal; one who acts on behalf of another.
affidavit	Written sworn statement.
affiliation agreement	A formal agreement between an educational institution and another agency that agrees to provide clinical areas for student practice.
aggressiveness	Harsh behavior that may result in physical or emotional harm to others.
allied health	Group of health care providers that assists or complements the work of primary health care providers such as physicians and nurse practitioners; examples are physical therapists, laboratory staff, radiology technicians, dietary personnel, and social workers.
ambulatory care center	Type of primary care facility that provides treatment on an outpatient basis.
answer	Document filed in the court by the defendant in response to the complaint.
anxiety	Uneasiness or apprehension caused by an impending threat or fear of the unknown.
apathy	Lack of interest.
appeal	Request to a higher court to review a decision in the hopes of changing the ruling of a lower court.
appellant	Person who seeks an appeal.
arbitrator	Neutral third party who assesses facts independently of the judicial system.
articulation	Type of education program that allows easy entry from one level to another; for example, many BSN programs have articulation for nurses with an associate degree.
artificial insemination	Insertion of sperm into the uterus with a syringe.
assault	Touching another person without permission.

Term	Definition
assertiveness	Ability to express thoughts, feelings, and ideas openly and directly without fear.
assessment	Process of collecting information about a client, to help plan care.
associate degree nursing program	Type of nursing education program that leads to an associate degree with a major in nursing; usually located in a community or junior college, these programs nominally last 2 years.
audit	Close review of records or documents to detect the presence or absence of specific information.
auscultation	Assessment technique that requires listening with a stethoscope to various parts of the body to detect sounds produced by organs.
autonomy	State of being self-directed or independent; the ability to make decisions about one's future.
autopsy	Examination of a body after death to determine the cause of death.
baccalaureate degree nursing program	Type of nursing education program that leads to the bachelor's degree with a major in nursing; usually located in a college or university, the length of the program is 4 years.
bargaining agent	Organization certified by a governmental agency to represent a group of employees for the purpose of collective bargaining.
bargaining unit	Group of employees, recognized as representatives of the majority, with the right to bargain collectively with their employer and to reach an agreement on the terms of a contract.
baseline data	Initial information obtained about a client that establishesthe norms for comparison as the client's condition changes.
battery	Nonconsensual touching of another person that does not necessarily cause harm or injury.
behavioral objectives	Statements of specific observable client behavior that leads to achievement of a client goal; should be client centered, time oriented, and measurable.
behaviorism	Psychologic theory based on the belief that all behavior is learned over time through conditioning.
behavior modification	Method to change behavior through rewards for positive behavior.

Term	Definition
belief	Expectations or judgments based on attitude verified by experiences.
beneficence	Ethical principle based on the beliefs that the health care provider should do no harm, prevent harm, remove existing harm, and promote the good and well-being of the client.
bereavement	State of sadness brought on by the loss or death of a significant other.
bill	Proposed law that is moving through the legislative process.
bill of rights	List of statements that outline the claims and privileges of a particular group, such as the Client's Bill of Rights.
bioethical issues	Issues that deal with the health, safety, life, and death of human beings often arising from advances in medical science and technology.
biofeedback	Ability to control autonomic response in the body through conscious effort.
body substance isolation (BSI)	Universal precautions; guidelines established by the Centers for Disease Control (CDC) and the Occupational Safety and Health Administration (OSHA) to protect health care professionals and the client from diseases carried in the blood and body fluids, such as HIV and hepatitis B; involves the use of gloves whenever one is in contact with blood or body fluids and the use of masks, gowns, and eye covers if a chance of aerosol contact with fluids exists.
brain death	Cerebral death; irreversible destruction of the cerebral cortex and brain stem manifested by all absence of reflexes; absence of brain waves on an electroencephalogram.
breach of contract	Failure by one of the parties in a contract to fulfill all the terms of the agreement.
burden of proof	Requirement that the plaintiff submit sufficient evidence to prove a defendant's guilt.
cadaver donor	Clinically or brain-dead individual who previously agreed to allow organs to be taken for transplantation.
capricious	Unpredictable; arbitrary.
career ladder	Articulation of educational programs that permits advancement from a lower level to a higher level without loss of credit or repetition of coursework.

Term	Definition
career mobility	Opportunity for individuals in one occupational area to move to another without restrictions.
case management	Health care delivery in which a client advocate/health care coordinator helps the client through the hospitalization to obtain the most appropriate care.
certification	Official recognition of a degree of education and skills in a profession by a national specialty organization; recognition that an institution has met standards that allow it to deliver certain services.
challenge examination	Examination that assesses levels of knowledge or skill to grant credit for previous learning and experience; passing a challenge examination gives the individual credit for a course not actually taken.
chart	Legal document that contains all the pertinent information about a client who is in a hospital or clinic; usually includes medical and nursing history, medical and nursing diagnosis, laboratory test results, notes about the client's progress, physician's orders, and personal data.
charting	Process of recording (written or computer-generated, for example) specific information about the client in the chart or medical record.
civil law	Law concerned with the violation of the rights of one individual by another; it includes contract law, treaty law, tax law, and tort law.
client	More modern term for patient; an individual seeking or receiving health care.
client goal	Statement about a desired change, outcome, or activity that a client should achieve by a specific time.
clinical education	Hands-on part of a nursing program that allows the student to practice skills on actual clients under the supervision of a nursing instructor.
clinical ladder	Type of performance evaluation and career advancement in which nursing positions for direct client care have two or more progressive levels of required skill leading to advancement in salary and responsibility; it allows nurses to remain in direct client care while making career advancements rather than having to move into administration.
closed system	System that does not exchange energy, matter, or information with the environment or with other systems
code of ethics	Written values of a profession that act as guidelines for professional behavior.

Term	Definition
collaboration	Cooperation between two or more individuals or agents to achieve a goal.
collective bargaining	Negotiations for wages, hours, benefits, and working conditions for a group of employees.
committee	Group of legislators, in the House or Senate, assigned to analyze bills on a particular subject.
common law	Law based on past judicial judgments made in similar cases.
comparable worth	Method for determining employees' salaries within an organization so that the same salary is paid for all jobs that have equivalent educational requirements, responsibilities, and complexity regardless of external market factors.
competencies	Behaviors, skills, attitudes, and knowledge that an individual or professional has or is expected to have.
competency-based education	Courses or programs based on anticipated student outcomes.
complaint	Legal document filed by a plaintiff, to initiate a lawsuit, claiming that the plaintiff's legal rights have been violated.
compliance	Voluntary following of a prescribed plan of care or treatment regimen.
computer technology	Use of highly advanced technologic equipment to store, process, and access a vast amount of information.
concept	Abstract idea or image.
conceptual framework	Concept, theory, or basic idea around which an educational program is organized and developed.
conceptual model	Group of concepts, ideas, or theories that are interrelated but in which the relationship is not clearly defined.
confidentiality	Right of the client to expect the communication with a professional to remain unshared with any other person unless a medical reason exists or unless the safety of the public is threatened.
consensus	General agreement between two or more individuals or groups regarding beliefs or positions on an issue or finding.
consent	Voluntary permission given by a competent person.
consortium	Two or more agencies that share sponsorship of a program or an institution.
constitutional law	Law contained within a federal or state constitution.

Term	Definition
consultation	Discussion or deliberation between two or more individuals.
continuing care	Nursing care generally provided in geriatric day care centers or in the homes of elderly clients.
continuing education	Formal education programs and informal learning experiences that maintain and increase the nurse's knowledge and skills in specific areas.
continuing education unit (CEU)	Specific unit of credit earned by participating in an approved continuing education program.
contract	Legally binding agreement between two or more parties.
contractual obligation	Duty to perform a service identified by a contract.
coping	Process of managing a crisis successfully.
coping strategies	Learned methods of dealing with a crisis.
core curriculum	Curriculum design that enables a student to leave a career program at various levels, with a career attained and with the option to continue at another higher level or career; it is organized around a central or core body of knowledge common to the profession.
coroner	Elected public official, usually a physician, who investigates deaths from unnatural causes.
credentialing	Process whereby individuals, programs, or institutions are designated as having met minimal standards for the safety and welfare of the public.
crime	Violation of criminal law.
criminal action	Process by which a person charged with a crime is accused, tried, and punished.
criminal law	Law concerned with violation of criminal statutes or laws.
criterion-referenced examination	Test that compares an individual's knowledge to a predetermined standard rather than to the performance of others who take the same test.
curriculum	Group of courses that prepare an individual for a specific degree or profession.
damages	Money awarded to a plaintiff by a court in a lawsuit that covers the actual costs incurred by the plaintiff.
data	Information.
database	Information collected by a computer program on a specific topic in a specified format.
defamation of character	Communication of information that is false or detrimental to a person's reputation.

Term	Definition
defendant	Person accused of criminal or civil wrongdoing. A party to a lawsuit *against whom* the complaint is served.
delegation	Assignment of specific duties by one individual to another individual.
deontology	Teleology; an ethical system based on the principle that the right action is guided by a set of unchanging rules.
dependent nursing function	Nursing action that is a result of a physician's order.
dependent practitioner	Provider of care who delivers health care under the supervision of another health care practitioner; for example, a physician assistant is supervised by a physician, or an LPN is supervised by an RN.
deposition	Sworn statement by a witness that is made outside the court room; sworn depositions may be admitted as evidence in court when the individual is unable to be present.
diagnosis	Statement that describes or identifies a client problem and is based on a thorough assessment.
diagnosis-related groups (DRGs)	Prospective payment method used by the U.S. government and many insurance companies that pay a flat fee for treatment of a person with a particular diagnosis.
differentiated practice	Organizational process of defining nursing roles based on education, experience, and training.
dilemma	Predicament in which a choice must be made between two or more equally balanced alternatives; it often occurs when attempting to make ethical decisions.
directed services	Health care activities that require contact between a health care professional and a client.
discharge planning	Assessment of anticipated client needs following discharge from the hospital and development of a plan to meet those needs before the client is discharged.
disease	Illness; a functional disturbance resulting from an individual organism's inability to adapt to certain stressors; an abnormal physiologic state caused by micro-organisms, cancer, or other conditions.
distributive justice	Ethical principle based on the belief that the right action is determined by that which will provide an outcome equal for all persons and will also benefit the least fortunate.

Term	Definition
due process	Right to have specific procedures or processes followed before the deprivation of life, liberty, or property; the guarantee of privileges under the Fifth and Fourteenth Amendments to the U.S. Constitution.
duty	Obligation to act created by a statute, contract, or voluntary agreement.
emerging health occupations	Health care occupations that are not yet officially recognized by government or professional organizations.
employee	Individual hired for pay by another.
employer	Individual or organization that hires other individuals for pay to carry out specific duties during certain hours of employment.
empowerment	Process in which the individual assumes more autonomy and responsibility for his or her actions.
endorsement	Reciprocity; a state's acceptance of a license issued by another state.
end product	Output of a system not reusable as input.
energy	Capacity to do work.
entropy	Bound energy not capable of conversion into work; the tendency of a system toward disorder and disintegration.
entry into practice	Minimal educational requirements to obtain a license for a profession.
environment	Internal and external physical and social boundaries of humans; all those things that are outside a system.
equifinality	Principle that states that open systems may attain similar states independent of initial conditions and different interactions with the environment; internal stability of a system.
essentials for accreditation	The minimal standards that a program must meet to be accredited.
ethical system	System of moral judgments based on the beliefs and values of a profession.
ethics	Principles or standards of conduct that govern an individual or group.
ethnic group	Individuals who share similar physical characteristics, religion, language, or customs.
euthanasia	Mercy killing; the act or practice of killing, for reasons of mercy, individuals who have little or no chance of recovery by withholding or discontinuing life support or by administering a lethal agent.

Term	Definition
evaluation	Fifth step in the nursing process used to determine whether goals set for a client have been attained.
evaluation criteria	Outcome criteria; desired behaviors or standards.
expanded role	Extended role; increased responsibilities and actions undertaken by an individual because of additional education and experience.
expert witness	Individual with knowledge beyond the ordinary person because of special education or training who testifies during a trial.
external degree	Academic degree granted when all the requirements have been met by the student; a type of outcomes-based education in which credit is given when the individual demonstrates a certain level of knowledge and skill, regardless of how or when these skills are attained; challenge examinations are often used.
false imprisonment	Intentional tort committed by illegally confining or restricting a client against his or her will.
family	Two or more related individuals living together.
Federal Tort Claims Act	Statute that allows the government to be sued for negligence of its employees in the performance of their duties; many states have similar laws.
feedback	Reentry of output into a system as input that helps to maintain the internal balance of the system.
fellowship	Scholarship or grant that provides money to individuals who are highly qualified or highly intelligent.
felony	Serious crime that may be punished by a fine of more than $1000, more than 1 year in jail or prison, death, or a combination thereof.
foreign graduate nurse	Individual graduated from a school of nursing outside the United States. This individual is required to pass the US NCLEX-RN CAT to become a registered nurse in the United States.
fraud	Deliberate deception in provision of goods or services; lying.
functional nursing	Nursing care in which each nurse provides a different aspect of care; nurses are assigned a set of specific tasks to perform for all clients, such as passing medications.
general systems theory	Set of interrelated concepts, definitions, and propositions that describes a system.

Term	Definition
genetics	Scientific study of heredity and related variations.
gerontology	Study of the process of aging and of the effects of aging on individuals.
goal	Desired outcome.
Good Samaritan Act	Law that protects health care providers from being charged with contributory negligence when they provide emergency care to persons in need of immediate treatment.
grievance	Complaint or dispute about the terms or conditions of employment.
health	Complete physical mental and social well-being; a relative state along a continuum ranging from severe illness to ideal state of being; the ability to adapt to illness and to reach the highest level of functioning.
health care consumer	Client or patient; an individual who uses health care service or products.
health care team	Group of individuals of different levels of education who work together to provide help to clients.
health maintenance organization (HMO)	Prototype of the managed health care system; method of payment for a full range of primary, secondary, and tertiary health care services; members pay a fixed annual fee for services and a small deductible when care is actually given.
health policy	Goals and directions which guide activities to safeguard and promote the health of citizens.
health practitioner	Individual, usually licensed, who provides health care services to individuals with health care needs.
health promotion	Interventions and behaviors that increase and maintain the level of well-being of persons, families, groups, communities, and society.
health systems agency (HSA)	Local voluntary organization of providers and consumers that plans for the health care services of its geographic region.
hearsay	Evidence not based on personal knowledge of the witness and usually not allowed in courts.
holistic	Treatment of the total individual, including physical, psychologic, sociologic, and spiritual elements, with emphasis on the interrelatedness of parts and wholes.
home health care	Health care services provided in the client's home.
homeostasis	Equilibrium of a system in a steady state.

Term	Definition
hospice care	Alternative way of providing care to terminally ill clients in which palliative care is used; the major goals of hospice care are control of pain, provision of emotional support, promotion of social interaction, and preparation for death; family support measures and anticipatory grieving counseling are also used if appropriate.
hospital privileges	Authority granted by a hospital, usually through its medical board, for a health care practitioner to admit and supervise the treatment of clients within that hospital.
hypothesis	Prediction or proposition related to a problem, usually found in research.
illness	Disease; a functional disturbance resulting from an individual organism's inability to adapt to certain stressors; an abnormal physiologic state caused by micro-organisms, cancer, or other conditions.
implementation	Fourth step in the nursing process, in which the plan of care is carried out.
incidence	Number of occurrences of a specific condition or event.
incident report	Document that describes an accident or error involving a client or family member that may or may not have resulted in injury; the purpose of the incident report is to track incidents and to make changes in the situations that caused them; the incident report is not part of the chart.
incompetency	Inability of an individual to manage personal affairs because of mental or physical conditions; the inability of a professional to carry out professional activities at the expected level of functioning because of lack of knowledge or skill or because of drug or alcohol abuse.
indemnity insurance	Method of payment for health care services; policy holders pay fixed periodic payments for insurance and are compensated, in whole or in part, for their health care expenses, usually through payment to the provider.
independent nurse practitioner	Nurse who has a private practice in one of the expanded roles of nursing.
independent nursing function	Nursing actions within the scope of nursing practice that are carried out without a physician's order.
independent practitioner	Health care provider who delivers health care independently with or without supervision by another health care practitioner.

Term	Definition
indirect services	Health care actions that do not require direct client contact but that still facilitate care, such as the supply and distribution department of a hospital.
informed consent	Permission granted by a person based on full knowledge of the risks and benefits of participation in a procedure or surgery for which the consent has been given.
injunction	Court order specifying actions that must or must not be taken.
input	Matter, energy, or information entering a system from the environment.
inquest	Formal inquiry about the course or manner of death.
institutional licensure	Authority for an individual health care provider to practice that is granted by the individual's employing institution; the institution determines the educational preparation, training, and functions of each category of providers it employs; no longer legally permitted, UAPs act under a form of de facto institutional licensure.
interrogatories	Written questions directed to a party in a lawsuit by the opposing side as part of the discovery process.
intervention	Nursing actions taken to meet specific client goals.
invasion of privacy	Disturbance or revelation of those things an individual holds as confidential.
judgment	Decision of the court regarding a case.
jurisdiction	Authority of a court to hear and decide lawsuits.
justice	Fairness; giving people their due.
Kardex	Portable card file that contains important client information and a care plan.
law	Formal statement of a society's beliefs about interactions among and between its citizens; a formal rule enforced by society.
legal complaint	Document filed by a plaintiff against a defendant claiming infringement of the plaintiff's legal rights.
legislator	Elected member of either the House of Representatives or the Senate.
legislature	Body of elected individuals invested with constitutional power to make, alter, or repeal laws.
liable	Obligated or held accountable by law.
libel	Written defamation of character.

Term	Definition
license	Permission to practice granted to an individual by the state after he or she has met the requirements for that particular position; licensing protects the safety of the public.
licensed practical nurse (LPN)	Licensed vocational nurse; technical nurse licensed by any state, after completing a practical nursing program, to provide technical bedside care to clients.
licensing board	Government agency that implements the statutes of a particular profession in accordance with the Professions Practice Act.
licensure	Process by which an agency or government grants an individual permission to practice; it establishes a minimal level of competency for practice.
licensure by endorsement	Method of obtaining a license to practice by having a state acknowledge the individual's existing comparable license in another state.
licensure by examination	Method of obtaining a license to practice by successfully passing a state board examination.
living wills	Signed legal document in which individuals make known their wishes about the care they are to receive if they should become incompetent at a future date; usually specify what types of treatments are permitted and what types are to be withheld.
lobbyist	Person who attempts to influence political decisions as an official representative of an organization, group, or institution.
malfeasance	Performance of an illegal act.
malpractice	Negligent acts by a licensed professional based on either omission of an expected action or commission of an inappropriate action resulting in damages to another party; not doing what a reasonable and prudent professional of the same rank would have done in the same situation.
managed care	System of organized health care delivery systems linked by provider networks; health maintenance organizations are the primary example of managed care.
mandatory licensure	Law that requires all who practice a particular profession to have and to maintain a license in that profession.

Term	Definition
manslaughter	Killing of an individual without premeditated intent; different degrees of manslaughter exist, and most are felonies.
Medicaid	State health care insurance program, supported in part by federal funds, for health care services for certain groups unable to pay for their own health care; amount and type of coverage vary from state to state.
medical examiner	Coroner; a physician who investigates deaths that appear to be from other than natural causes.
midwife	Individual experienced in assisting women during labor and delivery; they may be lay midwives, who have no official education, or certified nurse midwives, who are RNs in an expanded role, having received additional education and passed a national certification examination.
misdemeanor	Less serious crime than felony punishable by a fine of less than $1000 or a jail term of less than 1 year.
morality	Concept of right and wrong.
mores	Values and customs of a society.
mortality	Property or capacity to die; death.
motivation	Internal drive that causes individuals to seek achievement of higher goals; desire.
multicompetency technician	Allied health care provider who has skills in two or more areas of practice.
multiskilled practitioner	Health care professional who has skills in more than one area of health care, such as an RN who has training in physical therapy.
national health insurance	Proposed system of payment for health care services whereby the government pays for the costs of the health care.
negative entropy	Tendency toward increased order in a system.
negligence	Failure to perform at an expected level of functioning or the performance of an inappropriate function resulting in damages to another party; not doing what a reasonable and prudent person would do in a similar situation.
no code order	Do not resuscitate (DNR) order; an order by a physician to withhold CPR and other resuscitative efforts to a client.
nonfeasance	Failure to perform a legally required duty.

Term	Definition
nonmaleficence	Ethical principle that requires the professional to do no harm to the client.
nontraditional education	Methods of education that do not follow the traditional lecture and clinical practice methods of learning; may include computer-simulated learning, self-education techniques, or other creative methods.
norm-referenced examination	Examination scored by comparison with standards established on the performance of all others who took the same examination during a specific time; the NLN achievement examinations are norm referenced.
nurse clinician	Registered nurse with advanced skills in a particular area of nursing practice; if certified by a professional organization, a nurse clinician may also be a nurse practitioner, but more often this designation refers to nurses in advanced practice roles such as nurse specialists.
nurse practice act	Part of state law that establishes the scope of practice for professional nurses, as well as educational levels and standards, professional conduct, and reasons for revocation of licensure.
nurse practitioner	Nurse specialist with advanced education in a primary-care specialty such as community health, pediatrics, or mental health who is prepared independently to manage health promotion and maintenance and illness prevention of a specific group of clients.
nurse specialist (clinical nurse specialist)	Nurse who is an expert in providing care focused on a specialized field drawn from the range of general practice, such as cardiac nurse specialist.
nurse theorist	Usually, a nurse who analyzes and attempts to describe what the profession of nursing is and what nurses do through nursing models or nursing theories.
nursing assessment	Systematic collection and recording of client data, both objective and subjective, from primary and secondary sources using the nursing history, physical examination, and laboratory data, for example.
nursing diagnosis	Statement of a client's actual or potential health care problems or deficits.
nursing order	Statement of a nursing action selected by a nurse to achieve a client's goal; may be stated as either the nurse's or the client's expected behavior.
nursing process	Systematic, comprehensive decision-making process used by nurses to identify and treat actual and potential health problems.

Term	Definition
nursing research	Formal study of problems of nursing practice, the role of the nurse in health care, and the value of nursing.
nursing standards	Desired nursing behaviors established by the profession and used to evaluate nurses' performance.
omission	Failure to fulfill a duty or carry out a procedure recognized as a standard of care; often forms the basis for claims of malpractice.
oncology	Area of health care that deals with the treatment of cancer.
open curriculum	Educational system that allows a student to enter and leave the system freely; often uses past education and experiences.
open system	System that can exchange energy, matter, and information with the environment and with other systems.
ordinance	Local or municipal law.
outcome criteria	Standards that measure changes or improvements in clients' conditions.
output	Matter, energy, or information released from a system into the environment or transmitted to another system.
palliative	Treatment directed toward minimizing the severity of a disease or illness rather than curing it; for example, for a client with terminal cancer, relief of pain is the main goal (palliative), rather than cure.
patient	Client; an individual seeking or receiving health care.
patient day	Client day; the 24-hour period during which hospital services are provided that forms the basis for charging the patient, usually from midnight to midnight.
pediatrics	Study and care of problems and diseases of children below the age of 18.
peer review	Evaluation against professional standards of the performance of individuals with the same basic education and qualifications; formal process of review or evaluation by co-workers of an equal rank.
percussion	Physical examination involving the tapping of various parts of the body to determine density by eliciting different sounds.
perjury	Crime committed by giving false testimony while under oath.

Term	Definition
permissive licensure	Law that allows individuals to practice a profession as long as they do not use the title of the profession; no states now have permissive licensure.
plaintiff	Individual who charges another individual in a court of law with a violation of the individual's rights; the party who files the complaint in a lawsuit.
planning	Second step in the nursing process that establishes the goals for the client while receiving health care.
political action	Activities on the part of individuals that influence the actions of government officials in establishing policy.
political involvement	Group of activities that, individually or collectively, increase the voice of nursing in the political or health care policy process.
politics	Process of influencing the decisions of others and exerting control over situations or events; includes influencing the allocation of scarce resources.
potential health problems	Clients at high risk for the development of certain health care problems based on past illness or surgeries; for example, a postoperative client is at high risk for infection due to the procedure.
practical nursing program	Vocational nursing program; a program of study leading to a certificate in practical nursing, usually 12 to 18 months in length; these programs are located in a vocational or technical school or in a community or junior college; after passing the NCLEX-LPN CAT examination, students become licensed practical nurses (LPNs).
precedent	Decision previously issued by a court that is used as the basis for a decision in another case with similar circumstances.
preceptor	Educated or skilled practitioner who agrees to work with a less educated or trained individual to increase the individual's knowledge and skills; often, staff nurses who work with student nurses during their senior year.
preferred provider organization (PPO)	Method of payment for employee health care benefits in which employers contract with a specific group of health care providers for a lower cost for their employees' health care services but require the employee to use the providers listed.
prescriptive authority	Legal right to write prescriptions for medications, granted to physicians, veterinarians, dentists, and advanced practice nurses.
preventive care	Well care; nursing care provided for the purpose of maintaining health and preventing disease or

Term	Definition
	injury, often through community health clinics, school nursing services, and storefront clinics.
primary care	Type of health care for individuals and families in which maintenance of health is emphasized; first-line health care in hospitals, physician's offices, or community health clinics that deal with acute conditions.
primary-care nurse	Hospital staff RN assigned to a primary-care unit to provide nursing care to a limited number of clients, who are followed by the same nurse from admission to discharge.
private-duty nurse	Nurse in private practice; nurse self-employed for providing direct client care services either in the home or the hospital setting.
privileged communication	Information imparted by a client to a physician, lawyer, or clergyman that is protected from disclosure in a court of law; communication between a client and a nurse is not legally protected, but nurses can participate in privileged communication when they overhear information imparted by the client to the physician.
profession	Nursing; an occupation that meets the criteria for a profession, including education, altruism, code of ethics, public service, and dedication.
professional review organization (PRO)	Multilevel program to oversee the quality and cost of federally funded medical care programs.
professionalism	Behaviors and attitudes exhibited by an individual that are recognized by others as the traits of a professional.
proprietary hospital	For-profit private hospital.
prospective payment system (PPS)	System of reimbursement for health care services that establishes the payment rates before hospitalization based on certain criteria, such as diagnostic related groups (DRGs).
protocol	Written plan of action based on previously identified situations; standing orders are a type of protocol often used in specialty units that have clients with similar problems.
provider	Person or organization who delivers health care including health promotion and maintenance and illness prevention and treatment.
proximate cause	Nearest cause; the element in a direct cause-and-effect relationship between what is done by the professional and what happens to the client, such as when a nurse fails to raise the side rails on the bed of a client who receives a narcotic medication and then falls out of bed and breaks a hip as a result.

Term	Definition
public policy	Decision made by a society or its elected representatives that has a material effect on citizens, other than on the decision makers.
quality	Level of excellence based on pre-established criteria.
quality assurance	Activity conducted in health care facilities that evaluates the quality of care provided to ensure that it meets pre-established quality standards.
recertification	Periodic renewal of certification by examination, continuing education, or other criteria established by the accrediting agency.
reciprocity	Endorsement; a state's acceptance of a license issued by another state.
registration	Listing of a license with a state for a fee.
registry	Published list of those who are registered; the agency that publishes the list of individuals who are registered.
regulations	Rules or orders issued by various regulatory agencies, such as a state board of nursing, which have the force of law.
rehabilitation	Restoration to the highest possible level of performance or health of an individual who has suffered an injury or illness.
relative intensity measures (RIMs)	Method for calculating nursing resources needed to provide nursing care for various types of clients; helps to determine the number and type of staff required based on client acuity and needs.
respondeat superior	Legal doctrine that holds the employer or supervisor responsible for the actions of the employees, or of those supervised; for example, under this doctrine, RNs are held responsible for the actions of unlicensed assistive personnel under their supervision.
responsibility	Accountability; the concept that all individuals are accountable for their own actions and for the consequences of those actions.
restorative care	Curative care; nursing care that has as its goal cure and recovery from disease.
resume	Curriculum vitae; a summary of an individual's education, work experience, and qualifications.
retrospective payment system	Payment system for health care in which reimbursement is based on the actual care rendered, rather than on preset rates.

Term	Definition
right	Just claim or expectation that may or may not be protected by law; legal rights are protected by law, whereas moral rights are not.
risk management	Evaluating the risk of clients and staff for injuries and for potential liabilities and implementing corrective and preventive measures.
sanatorium	Early Greek type of hospital that provided therapy, diet, exercise programs, and baths for the prevention of disease; individuals with diseases were not permitted to enter sanatoria.
secondary care	Nursing care usually provided in short-term and long-term care facilities to clients with commonly occurring conditions.
significant other	Individual who is not a family member but is emotionally or symbolically important to an individual.
slander	Oral defamation of character.
slow-code order	Physician's order that the efforts for resuscitation of a client who is terminally ill should be initiated and conducted at a leisurely pace; the goal of a slow-code order is to allow the client to die during an apparent resuscitation; slow-code orders are not acceptable practice and do not meet standards of care.
staff nurse	Nurse generalist who works as an employee of a hospital, nursing home, community health agency, or some other organization providing primary and direct nursing care to clients.
standards	Norms; criteria for expected behaviors or conduct.
standards of care	Written or established criteria for nursing care that all nurses are expected to meet.
standards of practice	Written or established criteria for nursing practice that all professional nurses are expected to meet.
standing order	Written order by physician for certain actions or medication administration to be initiated or given in certain expected circumstances; similar to protocols.
statute	Law passed by a government's legislature and signed by its chief executive.
statute of limitations	Specific time period in which a lawsuit must be filed or a crime must be prosecuted; most nursing or medical lawsuits have a 2-year statute of limitation from the time of discovery of the incident.
statutory law	Law passed by a legislature.

Term	Definition
stereotype	Fixed or predetermined image of or attitude toward an individual or group.
stress	Crisis situation that causes increased anxiety and initiation of the flight-or-fight mechanism.
stressor	Internal or external force to which a person responds.
structure criteria	Physical environmental framework for client care.
subpoena	Court document that requires an individual to appear in court and provide testimony; individuals who do not honor the subpoena can be held in contempt of court and jailed or fined.
subsystem	Smaller system within a large system.
summary judgment	Decision by a judge in cases in which no facts are in dispute.
Sunset Law	Law that automatically terminates a program after a pre-established period of time unless that program can justify its need for existence.
support system	Environmental factors and individuals who can help an individual in a crisis cope with the situation.
systems theory	Theory that stresses the interrelatedness of parts in any system in which a change in one part affects all other parts; often, the system is greater than the sum of its parts.
taxonomy	Classification system.
team nursing	Method of organizing nursing care in which each client is assigned a team consisting of RNs, LPNs, and nursing assistants to deliver nursing care.
technician	Individual who carries out technical tasks.
technology	Use of science and the application of scientific principles to any situation; often involves the use of complicated machines and computers.
teleology	Utilitarianism; an ethical system that identifies the right action by determining what will provide the greatest good for the greatest number of persons; this system has no set, unchanging rules; rather, it varies as the situation changes.
tertiary care	Nursing care usually provided in long-term care and rehabilitation facilities for chronic diseases or injuries requiring long recovery.
testimony	Oral statement of a witness under oath.
theory	Set of interrelated constructs (concepts, definitions, or propositions) that presents a systematic view of phenomena by specifying relations among variables with the purpose of explaining and predicting phenomena.

Term	Definition
therapist	Individual who has professional knowledge and skills to administer certain types of services to help clients recover; examples include respiratory therapist, physical therapist, speech therapist, and occupational therapist.
third-party payment	Payment for health care services by an insurance company or a government agency rather than directly by the client.
throughput	Matter, energy, or information as it passes through a system.
tort	Violation of the civil law that violates a person's rights and causes injury or harm to the individual. Civil wrong independent of an action in contract which results from a breach of a legal duty; a tort can be classified as unintentional, intentional, or quasi-intentional.
tort feasor	Person who commits a tort.
Tri-Council	Nursing group composed of the American Nurses Association (ANA), National League for Nursing (NLN), American Association of Colleges of Nursing (AACN), and American Organizatoin of Nurse Executives (AONE).
trial	Legal proceedings during which all relevant facts are presented to a jury or judge for legal decision.
two plus two (2 + 2) program	Nursing education program that starts with an associate (2-year) degree and then moves the individual to a baccalaureate degree with an additional 2 years of education.
Uniform Anatomical Gift Act	Legal document signed by an individual indicating the desire to donate specific body organs or the entire body after death.
universal precautions	Body substance isolation; guidelines established by the Centers for Disease Control (CDC) and the Occupational Safety and Health Administration (OSHA) to protect health care professionals and clients from diseases carried in the blood and body fluids, such as HIV and hepatitis B; involves the use of gloves whenever in contact with blood or body fluids and masks, gowns, and eye covers if a chance exists of contact with aerosol fluids.
upward mobility	Movement toward increased status and power in an organization through promotion.
utilitarianism	Teleology; an ethical system that identifies the right action by determining what will provide the greatest

Term	Definition
	good for the greatest number of persons. This system has no set, unchanging rules; rather it varies as the situation changes.
value	Judgment of worth, quality, or desirability based on attitude formed from need or experience; a strong belief held by individuals about something important to them.
values clarification	Process by which individuals list and prioritize the values they hold most important.
veto	Signed refusal by the President or a governor to enact a bill into law. If the President vetoes a bill, the veto may be overridden by a two-thirds vote of the memberships of both the House and Senate.
vicarious liability	Imputation of blame on a person for the actions of the other.
vocational nursing program	Licensed practical nursing program in Texas and California; a program of study leading to a certificate in vocational nursing, usually 12 to 18 months in length; these programs are located in a vocational or technical school or a community or junior college; after passing the NCLEX-LPN CAT examination, students become licensed vocational nurses (LVNs).
xenodochium	Early Hebrew hospital that provided shelter and nursing care for travelers.

APPENDIX C

NATIONAL COUNCIL OF STATE BOARDS OF NURSING, INC. BOARDS OF NURSING

Alabama

Alabama Board of Nursing
PO BOX 303900
Montgomery, Alabama 36130-3900
Phone: (334) 242-4060
Fax: (334) 242-4360
Judi Crume, Executive Officer

Street Address:
RSA Plaza, Suite 250
770 Washington Avenue
Montgomery, Alabama 36130-3900

Alaska

Alaska Board of Nursing
Department of Commerce and Economic
   Development
Division of Occupational Licensing
3601 C Street, Suite 722
Anchorage, Alaska 99503
Phone: (907) 561-2878
Fax: (907) 562-5781
NCNET: NCZ026
Dorothy Fulton, Executive Director

Alaska Board of Nursing
P.O. Box 110806
Juneau, Alaska 99811-086
Phone: (907) 465-2544
Fax: (907) 465-2974
Linda Gohl, Licensing Examiner

American Samoa

American Samoa Health Service
Regulatory Board
LBJ Tropical Medical Center
Pago Pago, American Samoa 96799
Phone: (684) 633-1222 Ext. 206
Fax: 011-684-633-1869
Telex No.: #782-573-LBJ TMC
Marie F. Ma'o, Director of Nursing Services

Arizona

Arizona State Board of Nursing
1651 E. Morten Avenue, Suite 150
Phoenix, Arizona 85020
Phone: (602) 255-5092
Fax: (602) 255-5130
Fran Roberts, Executive Director

Arkansas

Arkansas State Board of Nursing
University Tower Building, Suite 800
1123 South University
Little Rock, Arkansas 72204
Phone: (501) 686-2700
Fax: (501) 686-2714
Linda Murphy, Executive Director

California-RN

California Board of Registered Nursing
P.O. Box 944210
Sacramento, California 94244-2100
Phone: (916) 322-3350
Fax: (916) 327-4402
NCNET: C.Puri 132:NCZ030
Ruth Ann Terry, Executive Officer
Street Address:
400 R Street, Suite 4030
Sacramento, California 95814-6200

California-VN

California Board of Vocational Nurse and
    Psychiatric Technician Examiners
2535 Capitol Oaks Drive, Suite 205
Sacramento, California 95833
Phone: (916) 263-7800
Fax: (916) 263-7859
Theresa Bello-Jones, Executive Officer

Colorado

Colorado Board of Nursing
1560 Broadway, Suite 670
Denver, Colorado 80202
Phone: (303) 894-2430
Fax: (303) 894-2821
Karen Brumley, Program Administrator

Connecticut

Connecticut Board of Examiners for
    Nursing
150 Washington Street
Hartford, Connecticut 06106
Phone: (203) 566-1041
Fax: (203) 566-1464
Marie T. Hilliard, Executive Officer

For Examination Information:
Examinations and Licensure Division of
    Medical Quality Assurance
Connecticut Department of Health
    Services
150 Washington Street
Hartford, Connecticut 06106
Phone: (203) 566-1032
Joseph Gillen, Section Chief of Applications

Delaware

Delaware Board of Nursing
Margaret O'Neill Building
P.O. Box 1401
Dover, Delaware 19903
Phone: (302) 739-4522
Fax: (302) 739-2711
Iva Boardman, Executive Director

District of Columbia

District of Columbia Board of Nursing
614 H. Street, N.W.
Washington, District of Columbia 20001
Phone: (202) 727-7468
Fax: (202) 727-7662
Barbara Hagans, Contact Person
For Examination Information:
Phone: (202) 727-7454
Clifford Cooks, Program Administrator

Florida

Florida Board of Nursing
111 Coastline Drive, East, Suite 516
Jacksonville, Florida 32202
Phone: (904) 359-6331
Fax: (904) 359-6323
Marilyn Bloss, Acting Executive Director
For Examination Information:
Same as above
Roberta Long, Professional Specialist II

Georgia-PN

Georgia State Board of Licensed Practical
    Nurses
166 Pryor Street, S.W.
Atlanta, Georgia 30303
Phone: (404) 656-3921
Fax: (404) 651-9532

Patricia N. Swann, Executive Director
For Examination Information:
Exam Development & Testing Unit
Phone: (404) 656-3903
Lila Quero

Georgia-RN

Georgia Board of Nursing
166 Pryor Street, S.W.
Atlanta, Georgia 30303
Phone: (404) 656-3943
Fax: (404) 651-7489
Shirley Camp, Executive Director

Guam

Guam Board of Nurse Examiners
P.O. Box 2816
Agana, Guam 96910
Phone: 011-(671) 475-0251
Fax: 011-(671) 477-4733
*Teofila P. Cruz, Nurse Examiner
   Administrator*

Hawaii

Hawaii Board of Nursing
P.O. Box 3469
Honolulu, Hawaii 96801
Phone: (808) 586-2695
Fax: (808) 586-2689
Kathleen Yokouchi, Executive Officer

Idaho

Idaho Board of Nursing
P.O. Box 83720
Boise, Idaho 83720-0061
Phone: (208) 334-3110
Fax: (208) 334-3262
NCNET: ID NC2022
Leola Daniels, Executive Director

Illinois

Illinois Department of Professional
   Regulation
320 West Washington Street, 3rd Floor
Springfield, Illinois 62786
Phone: (217) 785-9465
            (217) 785-0800
Fax: (217) 782-7645

For Examination Information:
Mary Jo Southard, Chief Testing Officer
Illinois Department of Professional
   Regulation
100 West Randolph, Suite 9-300
Chicago, Illinois 60601
Phone: (312) 814-2715
Fax: (312) 814-3154
*Jackie Waggoner, Nursing/Acting
   Coordinator*
Application Requests
Licensure Information
Assisting Nursing/Acting Coordinator
Phone: (217) 782-0458
            (217) 782-8556
            (217) 785-9465

Indiana

Indiana State Board of Nursing
Health Professions Bureau
402 West Washington Street, Room 041
Indianapolis, Indiana 46204
Phone: (317) 232-2960
Fax: (317) 233-4236
Laura Langford, Executive Director

Iowa

Iowa Board of Nursing
State Capitol Complex
1223 East Court Avenue
Des Moines, Iowa 50319
Phone: (515) 281-3255
Fax: (515) 281-4825
Lorinda K. Inman, Executive Director

Kansas

Kansas State Board of Nursing
Landon State Office Building
900 S.W. Jackson, Suite 551-S
Topeka, Kansas 66612-1230
Phone: (913) 296-4929
Fax: (913) 296-3929
Patsy L. Johnson, Executive Administrator
Departments:
General Information
Continuing Education
Practice or Disciplinary
Phone: (913) 296-4929
            (913) 296-3782
            (913) 296-4325

Kentucky

Kentucky Board of Nursing
312 Wittington Parkway, Suite 300
Louisville, Kentucky 40222-5172
Phone: (502) 329-7000
Fax: (502) 329-7011
Sharon M. Weisenbeck, Executive Director

Louisiana-PN

Louisiana State Board of Practical Nurse
  Examiners
3421 N. Causeway Boulevard, Suite 203
Metairie, Louisiana 70002
Phone: (504) 838-5791
Fax: (504) 838-5279
Terry L. DeMarcay, Executive Director

Louisiana-RN

Louisiana State Board of Nursing
912 Pere Marquette Building
150 Baronne Street
New Orleans, Louisiana 70112
Phone: (504) 568-5464
Fax: (504) 568-5467
NCNET: NCZ018
Barbara Morvant, Executive Director

Maine

Maine State Board of Nursing
State House Station #158
Augusta, Maine 04333-0158
Phone: (207) 624-5275
Fax: (207) 624-5290
NCNET: NCZ010
Jean C. Caron, Executive Director

Maryland

Maryland Board of Nursing
4140 Patterson Avenue
Baltimore, Maryland 21215-2299
Phone: (410) 764-5124
Fax: (410) 358-3530
Donna Dorsey, Executive Director

Massachusetts

Massachusetts Board of Registration in
  Nursing
Leverett Saltonstall Building
100 Cambridge Street, Room 1519
Boston, Massachusetts 02202
Phone: (617) 727-9961
Fax: (617) 727-2197
Theresa M. Bonanno, Executive Director

Michigan

Bureau of Occupational and Professional
  Regulation
Michigan Department of Commerce
Ottawa Towers North
611 West Ottawa
Lansing, Michigan 48933
Phone: (517) 373-1600
Fax: (517) 373-2179
Doris Foley, Licensing Administrator
For Examination Information:
Office of Testing Services
Michigan Department of Commerce
P.O. Box 30018
Lansing, Michigan 48909
Phone: (517) 373-3877
Fax: (517) 335-6696
Kara L. Schmitt, Executive Director

Minnesota

Minnesota Board of Nursing
2700 University Avenue, West #108
St. Paul, Minnesota 55114
Phone: (612) 642-0567
Fax: (612) 642-0574
Joyce M. Schowalter, Executive Director

Mississippi

Mississippi Board of Nursing
239 N. Lamar Street, Suite 401
Jackson, Mississippi 39201
Phone: (601) 359-6170
Fax: (601) 359-6185
Marcia Rachel, Executive Director

Missouri

Missouri State Board of Nursing
P.O. Box 656
Jefferson City, Missouri 65102
Phone: (314) 751-0681
Fax: (314) 751-0075
Florence Stillman, Executive Director
Street Address:
3605 Missouri Blvd.
Jefferson City, Missouri 65109

Montana

Montana State Board of Nursing
111 North Jackson
P.O. Box 200513
Helena, Montana 59620-0513
Phone: (406) 444-2071
Fax: (406) 444-7759
NCNET: NCZ032
Dianne Wickham, Executive Director

Nebraska

Bureau of Examining Boards
Nebraska Department of Health
P.O. Box 95007
Lincoln, Nebraska 68509
Phone: (402) 471-2115
Fax: (402) 471-0383
Charlene Kelly, Associate Director
Street Address:
301 Centennial Mall South
Lincoln, Nebraska 68508

Nevada

Nevada State Board of Nursing
P.O. Box 46886
Las Vegas, Nevada 89114
Phone: (702) 739-1575
Fax: (702) 739-0298
Lonna Burress, Executive Director
Street Address:
4335 S. Industrial Road, Suite 430
Las Vegas, Nevada 89103
Nevada State Board of Nursing (2nd
Office)
1755 East Plumb Lane, Suite 260
Reno, Nevada 89502
Phone: (702) 786-2778
Fax: (702) 322-6993

New Hampshire

New Hampshire Board of Nursing
Health & Welfare Building
6 Hazen Drive
Concord, New Hampshire 03301-6527
Phone: (603) 271-2323
Fax: (603) 271-6605
Doris Nuttelman, Executive Director

New Jersey

New Jersey Board of Nursing
P.O. Box 45010
Newark, New Jersey 07101
Phone: (201) 504-6493
Fax: (201) 648-3481
Sr. Teresa Harris, Executive Director
Street Address:
124 Halsey Street, 6th Floor
Newark, New Jersey 07102

New Mexico

New Mexico Board of Nursing
4206 Louisiana Blvd., NE, Suite A
Albuquerque, New Mexico 87109
Phone: (505) 841-8340
Fax: (505) 841-8347
Nancy Twigg, Executive Director

New York

New York State Board of Nursing
State Education Department
Cultural Education Center, Room 3023
Albany, New York 12230
Phone: (518) 474-3843/3845
Fax: (518) 473-0578
Milene Sower, Executive Secretary
For Examination Information:
Division of Professional Licensing
  Services
State Education Department
Cultural Education Center
Albany, New York 12230
Phone: (518) 474-6591
Susan Mekus, Supervisor

North Carolina

North Carolina Board of Nursing
P.O. Box 2129
Raleigh, North Carolina 27602
Phone: (919) 782-3211
Fax: (919) 781-9461
NCNET: NCZ014
Carol Osman, Executive Director
Street Address:
3724 National Drive
Raleigh, North Carolina 27612

North Dakota

North Dakota Board of Nursing
919 South Seventh Street, Suite 504
Bismarck, North Dakota 58504-5881
Phone: (701) 328-2974
Fax: (701) 328-4614
Karen Macdonald, Executive Director

Northern Mariana Islands

Commonwealth Board of Nurse
　Examiners
Public Health Center
P.O. Box 1458
Saipan, MP 96950
Phone: 011-670-234-8950 thru 8954
Fax: 011-670-234-8930
Elizabeth Torres-Untalan, Chairperson
Telex Number is 783-744,
Answer back code is PNESPN744.
When calling, ask for Public Health
　Center (ext. 2018 or 2019)

Ohio

Ohio Board of Nursing
77 South High Street, 17th floor
Columbus, Ohio 43266-0316
Phone: (614) 466-3947
Fax: (614) 466-0388
Rosa Lee Weinert, Executive Director

Oklahoma

Oklahoma Board of Nursing
2915 North Classen Boulevard, Suite 524
Oklahoma City, Oklahoma 73106
Phone: (405) 525-2076
Fax: (405) 521-6089
Sulinda Moffett, Executive Director

Oregon

Oregon State Board of Nursing
800 NE Oregon Street, Box 25,
　Suite 465
Portland, Oregon 97232
Phone: (503) 731-4745
Fax: (503) 731-4755
Joan Bouchard, Executive Director

Pennsylvania

Pennsylvania State Board of Nursing
P.O. Box 2649
Harrisburg, Pennsylvania 17105-2649
Phone: (717) 783-7142
Fax: (717) 787-7769
Miriam H. Limo, Executive Secretary
Street Address:
124 Pine Street
Harrisburg, PA 17101
For Examination Program/Contract
　Requirements:
Use same address as Pennsylvania State
　Board of Nursing
Joanne E. Mercer, Administrator

Puerto Rico

Commonwealth of Puerto Rico
Board of Nurse Examiners
Call Box 10200
Santurce, Puerto Rico 00903
Phone: (809) 725-8161 or
　　　(809) 725-7904
Fax: (809) 725-7903
Jose A. Perez Otero, Executive Director

Rhode Island

Rhode Island Board of Nurse Registration
　& Nursing Education
Cannon Health Building
Three Capitol Hill, Room 104
Providence, Rhode Island 02908-5097
Phone: (401) 277-2827
Fax: (401) 277-1272
Peter Petrone, Administrative Officer

South Carolina

South Carolina State Board of Nursing
220 Executive Center Drive, Suite 220
Columbia, South Carolina 29210
Phone: (803) 731-1648
Fax: (803) 731-1647
NCNET: NCZ023
Renatta Loquist, Executive Director
Departments:
Legal & Disciplinary Services
Education/Examination/Accounting/Computer Services
Phone: (803) 731-1667
Fax: (803) 731-1648

South Dakota

South Dakota Board of Nursing
3307 South Lincoln Avenue
Sioux Falls, South Dakota 57105-5224
Phone: (605) 367-5940
Fax: (605) 367-5945
Diana Vander Woude, Executive Secretary

Tennessee

Tennessee State Board of Nursing
283 Plus Park Boulevard
Nashville, Tennessee 37217-1010
Phone: (615) 367-6232
Fax: (615) 367-6397
Elizabeth Lund, Executive Director

Texas-RN

Texas Board of Nurse Examiners
P.O. Box 140466
Austin, Texas 78714
Phone: (512) 835-4880
Fax: (512) 835-8684
Louise Waddill, Executive Director
Street Address:
9101 Burnet Road
Austin, Texas 78758
Departments:
Practice & Compliance
Administration/Education/Examination
Phone: (512) 835-8686
        (512) 835-8650

Texas-VN

Texas Board of Vocational
    Nurse Examiners
9101 Burnet Road, Suite 105
Austin, Texas 78758
Phone: (512) 835-2071
Fax: (512) 835-1367
Marjorie A. Bronk, Executive Director

Utah

Utah State Board of Nursing
Division of Occupational and Professional
    Licensing
P.O. Box 45805
Salt Lake City, Utah 84145-0805
Phone: (801) 530-6628
Fax: (801) 530-6511
Laura Poe, Executive Administrator
Street Address:
Heber M. Wells Building, 4th Floor
160 East 300 South
Salt Lake City, Utah 84111

Vermont

Vermont State Board of Nursing
109 State Street
Montpelier, Vermont 05609-1106
Phone: (802) 828-2396
Fax: (802) 828-2853
Anita Ristau, Executive Director
For Mailing by UPS or FedEx:
81 River Street
Montpelier, Vermont 05602-1106

Virgin Islands

Virgin Islands Board of Nurse
    Licensure
P.O. Box 4247, Veterans Drive Station
St. Thomas, U.S. Virgin Islands 00803
Phone: (809) 776-7397
Fax: (809) 777-4003
Winifred L. Garfield, Executive Secretary
Street Address:
Plot #3, Kongens Gade
St. Thomas, U.S. Virgin Islands 00803

Virginia

Virginia Board of Nursing
6606 West Broad Street, Fourth Floor
Richmond, Virginia 23230-1717
Phone: (804) 662-9909
Fax: (804) 662-9943
Corinne F. Dorsey, Executive Director

Washington

Washington State Nursing Care Quality
   Assurance Commission
Department of Health
P.O. Box 47864
Olympia, Washington 98504-7864
Phone: (360) 753-2686
Fax: (360) 586-5935
Pat Brown, Executive Director

West Virginia-RN

West Virginia Board of Examiners for
   Registered Professional Nurses
101 Dee Drive
Charleston, West Virginia 25311-1620
Phone: (304) 558-3596
Fax: (304) 558-3666
Janet Fairchild, Executive Secretary

West Virginia-PN

West Virginia State Board of Examiners
   for Practical Nurses
101 Dee Drive
Charleston, West Virginia 25311-1688
Phone: (304) 558-3572
Fax: (304) 558-3666
(Please indicate for PN Board)
Nancy R. Wilson, Executive Secretary

Wisconsin

Wisconsin Department of Regulation &
   Licensing
1400 East Washington Avenue
P.O. Box 8935
Madison, Wisconsin 53708-3935
Phone: (608) 266-0257
Fax: (608) 267-0644.
Tom Neumann, Administrative Officer
For Application Information:
EXAMINATIONS:
Phone: (608) 266-0070
Jan Johnson, Administrative Assistant
ENDORSEMENT:
Phone: (608) 266-8957
Patsy Strasburg, Program Assistant

Wyoming

Wyoming State Board of Nursing
Barrett Building, Second Floor
2301 Central Avenue
Cheyenne, Wyoming 82002
Phone: (307) 777-7601
Fax: (307) 777-6005
Toma Nisbet, Executive Director

APPENDIX D

SPECIALTY NURSING ORGANIZATIONS

Academy of Medical-Surgical Nurses (AMSN)
North Woodbury Road, Box 56
Pitman, New Jersey 08071
Phone: (609) 589-6677
Fax: (609) 589-7463

American Academy of Ambulatory Care Nursing (AAACN)
North Woodbury Road, Box 56
Pitman, New Jersey 08071
Phone: (609) 582-9617
Fax: (609) 589-7463

American Association of Critical-Care Nurses (AACN)
101 Columbia
Aliso Viejo, California 92656-1491
Phone: (800) 899-2226/(714) 362-2000
Fax: (714) 362-2020

American Association of Diabetes Educators (AADE)
444 N. Michigan Avenue
Suite 1240
Chicago, Illinois 60611-3901
Phone: (312) 664-2233/(800) 644-2233
Fax: (312) 644-4411

American Association of Neuroscience Nurses (AANN)
224 N. Des Plaines #601
Chicago, Illinois 60661
Phone: (312) 993-0043

American Association of Nurse Anesthetists (AANA)
222 South Prospect Avenue
Park Ridge, Illinois 60068-4001
Phone: (708) 692-7050
Fax: (708) 692-6968

American Association of Occupational Health Nurses (AAOHN)
50 Lenox Pointe
Atlanta, Georgia 30324
Phone: (404) 262-1162
Fax: (404) 262-1165

American Association of Spinal Cord Injury Nurses (AASCIN)
75-20 Astoria Boulevard
Jackson Heights, New York 11370-1177
Phone: (718) 803-3782
Fax: (718) 803-0414

American College of Nurse-Midwives (ACNM)
1522 K Street, NW, Suite 1000
Washington, District of Columbia 20005
Phone: (202) 289-0171
Fax: (202) 289-4395

American Nephrology Nurses Association (ANNA)
North Woodbury Road, Box 56
Pitman, New Jersey 08071
Phone: (609) 589-2187
Fax: (609) 589-7463

American Psychiatric Nurses' Association (APNA)
6900 Grove Road
Thorofare, New Jersey 08086
Phone: (609) 848-7990
Fax: (609) 848-5274

American Society of Ophthalmic Registered Nurses, Inc. (ASORN)
655 Beach Street
PO Box 193030
San Francisco, California 94119
Phone: (415) 561-8513
Fax: (415) 561-8575

American Society of Plastic and Reconstructive Surgical Nurses, Inc. (ASPRSN)
North Woodbury Road, Box 56
Pitman, New Jersey 08071
Phone: (609) 589-6247
Fax: (609) 589-7463

American Society of Post Anesthesia Nurses (ASPAN)
11512 Allecingie Parkway
Richmond, Virginia 23235
Phone: (804) 379-5516
Fax: (804) 379-1386

American Urological Association Allied, Inc. (AUAA)
11512 Allecingie Parkway
Richmond, Virginia 23235
Phone: (804) 379-1306
Fax: (804) 379-1386

Association for Practitioners In Infection Control (APIC)
505 E. Hawley Street
Mundelein, Illinois 60060
Phone: (708) 949-6052
Fax: (708) 566-7282

Association of Operating Room Nurses, Inc. (AORN)
2170 S. Parker Road, #300
Denver, Colorado 80231-5711
Phone: (303) 755-6300
Fax: (303) 750-2927

Association of Pediatric Oncology Nurses (APON)
11512 Allecingle Parkway
Richmond, Virginia 23235
Phone: (804) 379-9150
Fax: (804) 379-1386

Association of Rehabilitation Nurses (ARN)
5700 Old Orchard Road, First Floor
Skokie, Illinois 60077-1057
Phone: (708) 966-3433
Fax: (708) 966-9418

Association of Women's Health, Obstetric, and Neonatal Nurses (AWHONN)
700 14th Street, NW, Suite 600
Washington, District of Columbia 20005-2019
Phone: (202) 662-1600
Fax: (202) 737-0575

Dermatology Nurses' Association (DNA)
North Woodbury Road, Box 56
Pitman, New Jersey 08071
Phone: (609) 582-1915
Fax: (609) 589-7463

Emergency Nurses' Association (ENA)
216 Higgins Road
Park Ridge, Illinois 60068-5736
Phone: (708) 698-9400
Fax: (708) 698-9406

International Society of Nurses in Genetics, Inc. (ISONG)
University of North Dakota
Department of Pediatrics/Genetics
501 Columbia Road
Grand Forks, North Dakota 58203
Phone: (701) 777-4243

Intravenous Nurses Society, Inc. (INS)
Two Brighton Street
Belmont, Massachusetts 02178
Phone: (617) 489-5205
Fax: (617) 484-6992

National Association of Nurse Practitioners in Reproductive Health (NANPRH)
2401 Pennsylvania Avenue, NW #350
Washington, District of Columbia 20037-1718
Phone: (202) 466-4825
Fax: (202) 466-3826

National Association of Nurse Massage Therapists (NANMT)
6851 Yumuri Street, #8
Coral Gables, Florida 33146
Phone: (305) 667-6821

National Association of Orthopaedic Nurses (NAON)
North Woodbury Road, Box 56
Pitman, New Jersey 08071
Phone: (609) 582-0111
Fax: (609) 589-7463

National Association of Pediatric Nurse Associates and Practitioners (NAPNAP)
1101 Kings Highway North, Suite 206
Cherry Hill, New Jersey 08034
Phone: (609) 667-1773
Fax: (609) 667-7187

National Association of School Nurses, Inc. (NASN)
PO Box 1300
Scarborough, Maine 04070-1300
Phone: (207) 883-2117
Fax: (207) 883-2683

National Flight Nurses Association (NFNA)
6900 Grove Road
Thorofare, New Jersey 08086-9447
Phone: (609) 384-6725
Fax: (609) 848-5274

National Nurses Society on Addictions (NNSA)
5700 Old Orchard Road, First Floor
Skokie, Illinois 60077-1057
Phone: (708) 966-5010
Fax: (708) 966-9418

Oncology Nursing Society (ONS)
501 Holiday Drive
Pittsburgh, Pennsylvania 15220-2749
Phone: (412) 921-7373
Fax: (412) 921-6565

Society of Gastroenterology Nurses & Associates, Inc. (SGNA)
1070 Sibley Tower
Rochester, New York 14604
Phone: (716) 546-7241
Fax: (716) 546-5141

Society of Otorhinolaryngology and Head-Neck Nurses, Inc. (SOHN)
116 Canal Street, Suite A
New Smyrna Beach, Florida 32168-7004
Phone: (904) 428-1695
Fax: (904) 423-7566

AFFILIATE MEMBERS

American Association of Nurse Attorneys (TAANA)
720 Light Street
Baltimore, Maryland 21230
Phone: (410) 752-3318
Fax: (410) 752-8295

American Holistic Nurses Association (AHNA)
4101 Lake Boone Trail, Suite 201
Raleigh, North Carolina 27607
Phone: (919) 787-5181
Fax: (919) 787-4916

National Association of GCRC Nurse Managers (NAGCRCNM)
Clinical Research Center
The Center for Health Sciences
27-066 CHS 169747
10833 Le Conte Avenue
Los Angeles, California 90024-169747
Phone: (310) 825-5225
Fax: (310) 206-9440

National Association for Health Care Recruitment (NAHCR)
PO Box 5769
Akron, Ohio 44372
Phone: (216) 867-3088
Fax: (216) 867-1630

National Student Nurses' Association, Inc. (NSNA)
555 West 57th Street
New York, New York 10019
Phone: (212) 581-2211
Fax: (212) 581-2368

Index

The letter "b" following a number indicates a box, the letter "t" indicates a table, and the letter "f" indicates a figure.